Atlas of Vulvovaginal Disease in Darker Skin Types

There is a significant increase in cross-migration of women from various ethnicities, cultures, and with varying skin color. With publications focused mainly on Fitz Skin types 1–4, accurate vulvar disease diagnosis in darker skin types may be compromised, resulting in suboptimal therapeutic outcomes. Diseases look quite different as the color disguises much of the erythema, which is prominently seen in the Caucasian population. This book is focused on female genital dermatoses and fills in those gaps for healthcare workers looking to accurately diagnose and manage such patients.

Key features

- Provides inclusive and consolidated contents on disorders of female genital skin and mucosa.
- Features more than 300 high-quality illustrations and impressive treatment algorithms, making it a ready reckoner for dermatologists, gynecologists, and general physicians.
- Facilitates diagnosis and further management of vulvar disease in the darker skin types, thus optimizing patient care.
- Features collective contributions from experts across the country.
- Simplifies the patient consult by providing ready answers to frequently asked questions.

Atlas of Vulvovaginal Disease in Darker Skin Types

Edited by
Dr Nina Madnani

Assisted by
Dr Kaleem Khan
Dr Nisha Chaturvedi

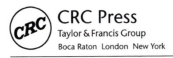

CRC Press
Taylor & Francis Group
Boca Raton London New York

CRC Press is an imprint of the
Taylor & Francis Group, an **informa** business

First edition published 2023
by CRC Press
6000 Broken Sound Parkway NW, Suite 300, Boca Raton, FL 33487-2742

and by CRC Press
4 Park Square, Milton Park, Abingdon, Oxon, OX14 4RN

CRC Press is an imprint of Taylor & Francis Group, LLC

© 2023 selection and editorial matter, Nina Madnani; individual chapters, the contributors

Library of Congress Cataloging-in-Publication Data

Names: Madnani, Nina, editor.
Title: Atlas of vulvovaginal disease in darker skin types / edited by Dr Nina Madnani.
Description: First edition. | Boca Raton : CRC Press, 2023. | Includes bibliographical references and index.
Identifiers: LCCN 2022053364 (print) | LCCN 2022053365 (ebook) | ISBN 9781032255897 (hardback) | ISBN 9781032255880 (paperback) | ISBN 9781003284116 (ebook)
Subjects: MESH: Vulvar Diseases--pathology | Vaginal Diseases--pathology | Skin Pigmentation | Atlas
Classification: LCC RG261 (print) | LCC RG261 (ebook) | NLM WP 17 | DDC 618.1/6--dc23/eng/20230119
LC record available at https://lccn.loc.gov/2022053364
LC ebook record available at https://lccn.loc.gov/2022053365

ISBN: 9781032255897 (hbk)
ISBN: 9781032255880 (pbk)
ISBN: 9781003284116 (ebk)

DOI: 10.1201/9781003284116

Typeset in Warnock Pro
by KnowledgeWorks Global Ltd.

This book is dedicated to individuals who changed my life:My teachers, Dr. V.R. Mehta and Dr. R. G. Valia, who nurtured my journey through Dermatology.

Dr Lynette Margesson who has encouraged and supported all the way

The Late Dr William Danby, who was a constant inspiration for me

My brilliant sister, the Late Emeritus Professor Vimla Nadkarni, who in her gentle way always encouraged me to follow my dreams. "Be Fearless and Forthright, and Rule the World" was her motto.

This book is the culmination of one of those dreams.

CONTENTS

PREFACE

As you pick up the *Atlas of Vulvovaginal Disease in Darker Skin Types*, you wonder about the need for one more book on the same subject. Yes, there are several great publications out there, but most of them showcase diseases in Fitzpatrick Types 1–3. Today, with globalization and the relocation of individuals across the world, there is a need to recognize the disease in patients with darker skin. India, a huge country, boasts of diversity in skin color and cultural habits. With all our collective experiences, there is enough clinical material to serve as a great reference for any healthcare individual interested in managing vulvar disease in darker skin types.

Dermatology is a very visual field, and the more one sees the easier it gets to arrive at a diagnosis. Hence, we have included more than 300 images in Fitzpatrick IV–VI skin types. Flowcharts of a few of the common presentations will make it easier for clinicians to manage their patients. A separate chapter on pediatric vulvar disease showcases various conditions in children. Although dermoscopy has not been standardized for vulvar skin conditions, we have included some images where relevant. Often, it gets tricky answering patients' queries about their conditions. To assist the caregivers, we have included a section on FAQs (frequently asked questions).

This atlas does not claim to be a comprehensive textbook on vulvar disease. But it is certainly more than an atlas to guide dermatologists, gynecologists, family physicians, and post-graduate students in the diagnosis and management of patients with the vulvar disease.

We wish you happy reading.

ACKNOWLEDGMENT

A big "Thank you" to all the contributors from India and across the world who have readily shared their expertise.

Dr Ashwini Gandhi Bhalerao, a contributor in this book, for her encouragement and active participation in jointly setting up the First Vulvar Clinic in India.

The P.D. Hinduja Memorial Hospital & MRC for giving us the platform to achieve this milestone.

Dr Kaleem Khan & Dr Nisha Chaturvedi, who, together with me, became the infamous trio, pouring over chapters, night after night propped up with several cups of coffee.

And a special hurrah for my husband Amar, son Mikhail, and my mother-in-law Mira for supporting me all the way.

CONTRIBUTORS

Dr Sowmya Aithal, MD, DVL
Senior Resident
Department of Dermatology
Mysore Medical College
Mysore, Karnataka, India

Dr Kavitha Athotha, MD
Consultant, Dermatology
Dr Paruchuri Rajaram Memorial Skin &
    Laser Centre
Guntur, Andhra Pradesh, India

**Dr Ashwini Bhalerao-Gandhi, MD, DGO,
FCPS**
Consultant, Gynecology
Hinduja Hospital - Mahim and Khar
Mumbai, Maharashtra, India

Dr Nisha Chaturvedi, MD, DNB, DDVL
Consultant, Dermatology
Surya Hospital, Dr Indu's Newborn and
    Childcare Centre
Mumbai, Maharashtra, India

Dr Rishi Goel, MD
Senior Resident
Department of Dermatology
Dr Baba Saheb Ambedkar Hospital and
    Medical College
Delhi, India

Dr Vrushali Kamale, MBBS, DGO
Consultant, Gynecology
Terana Hospital and Cloudnine Hospital
Navi Mumbai, Maharashtra, India

Dr Vidya Kharkar, MD, DVD
Professor and Head
Department of Dermatology
Seth G.S. Medical College & KEM Hospital
Mumbai, Maharashtra, India

Dr Kaleem Khan, MD
Consultant, Dermatology
Skin Indulgence Clinic, Wockhardt Hospital
    South Bombay, Surya Hospital
Mumbai, Maharashtra, India

Dr Niti Khunger, MD, DDV, DNB
Professor and Head
VM Medical College & Safdarjang
    Hospital
New Delhi, India

Dr Eswari L., MD, DVL, FRGUHS, FAADV
Associate Professor
Bangalore Medical College and Research
    Institute
Bangalore, Karnataka, India

Dr Krati Mehrotra, MD
Senior Research Associate
Department of Dermatology
Safdarganj Hospital
New Delhi, India

Dr Pragya Nair, MD, DVD
Professor
Department of Dermatology
Pramukh Swami Medical College, Bhaikaka
    University
Karamsad, Gujarat, India

Dr Sharmila Patil, MD
Professor and Head
Department of Dermatology, Venerology, and
    Leprosy
D.Y Patil University - School of
    Medicine
Navi Mumbai, Maharashtra, India

Dr Smitha Prabhu S, MD
Professor
Department of Dermatology & Venereology
Kasturba Medical College
Manipal Academy of Higher Education
Manipal, Karnataka, India

Dr Shreya Singh, DNB
Assistant Professor
Department of Dermatology, Seth G.S. Medical
    College & KEM Hospital
Mumbai, Maharashtra, India

Dr Archana Singal, MD, FAMS
Director and Head
Department of Dermatology & STD
University College of Medical Sciences &
    GTB Hospital
Delhi, India

Dr Anupkumar Tiwary, MD
Consultant, Dermatology
Yashoda Hospital and Research Centre
Ghaziabad, Uttar Pradesh, India

Dr Satish Udare, MD, DVD
Consultant, Dermatology
Sparkle clinic, Vashi, Disha Laser and
    Asthetic Clinic
Thane, Maharashtra, India

Dr Pavithra Vani, MD, DSBD
Consultant, Dermatology
Yashoda Hospital
Secunderabad, Telangana, India

ABOUT THE EDITOR

Dr Nina Madnani is a consultant dermatologist with 37 years of experience in clinical and hospital practice. She started the first Vulvar Clinic in India in 2008 and since then has successfully helped patients from across India, who often travel miles to consult her. With more than a decade of treating vulvar disease in patients across the country, she has immense clinical expertise and insights in dealing with darker skin types. She has amassed significant clinical material to serve as great reference material for any medical person interested in managing vulvar disease. Her accolades include being awarded several awards and orations, many for her work on vulvar disease in India. She has been instrumental in setting up the first "special interest group for female genital disease" (SIG FGD) for the Indian Association of Dermatology, Venereology, Leprology (IADVL), which holds regular CMEs across India. Dr Madnani runs charitable clinics twice a week, which include patients with vulvar disease. She is the first fellow from India of the International Society for the Study of Vulvovaginal Diseases (ISSVD), and is a regular speaker at National and International Conferences. Her dermatology passions are vulvar disease, hidradenitis suppurativa (HS), and acne.
COMP: Please add these two details.

Dr Kaleem Khan, MD, is a consultant Dermatologist, practicing in Mumbai since over a decade. After completing his M.D in Dermatology, he has received formal training at the National Skin Center in Singapore in the use of lasers and cold steel surgery. He has also completed a fellowship program in Advanced Medical Dermatology at the University of Toronto, Canada. In the last 10 years, he has 14 publications in indexed journals and has contributed chapters in 4 books. His key areas of interest include skin physiology and inflammatory dermatoses including psoriasis, atopic dermatitis, and acne.

Dr Nisha Chaturvedi (DNB,MD,DDVL) is a Consultant Dermatologist at Surya hospital and Dr Indu Child Care, Mumbai, India . She was awarded a Gold medal (Diploma in Dermatology) and has 15 years of clinical experience. She has a keen interest in vulvar dermatology and has gained vast experience in the same during her observership at P.D . Hinduja Hospital , Mumbai under Dr .Nina Madnani. She is an active member of the SIG- Female Genital Dermatosis since the last 3 years and has presented various lectures, published newsletters, and participated in social awareness programmes.

INTRODUCTION
Diversity: Need for This Atlas
Nina Madnani

Content

Introduction

Having traveled across continents attending various vulvovaginal disease conferences and symposiums, I was amazed at how little representation there was of a huge population of women with vulvar disease (women with darker skin tones or what is now termed as "skin of color"). In the real world, the same disease in a Fitzpatrick Type 1 and a Fitzpatrick Type 4 is so diverse in the play of colors that one may miss the diagnosis completely. As a result, management is naturally sub-optimal.

A few examples given below illustrate the clinical diversity of disease across the world. Notice that the Caucasian vulva has erythema as the marker of many diseases, while the darker skin types have more dyspigmentation (Figures 0.1–0.5).

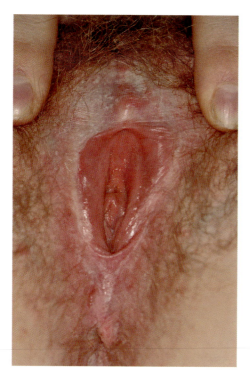 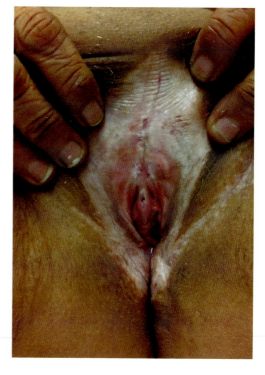

FIGURE 0.1 **(a and b)** Lichen sclerosus. (a – Photographs by Dr Lynette Margesson. b – Photographs by Nina Madnani.)

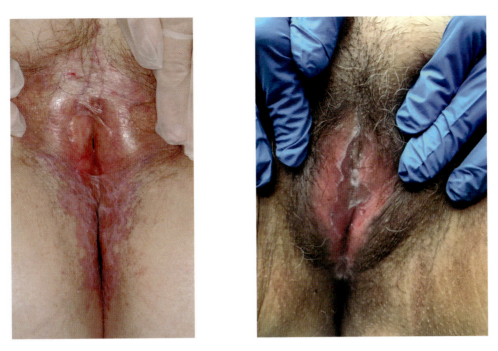

FIGURE 0.2 **(a and b)** Lichen planus. (a – Photographs by Dr Lynette Margesson. b – Photographs by Nina Madnani.)

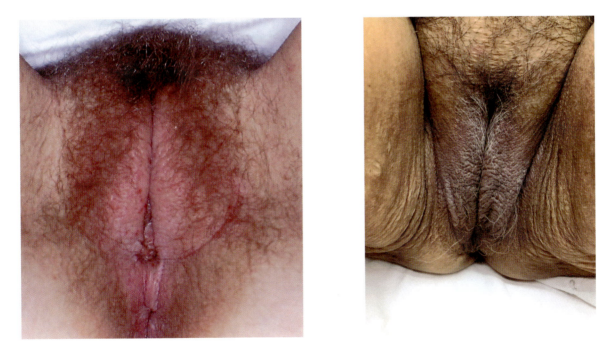

FIGURE 0.3 **(a and b)** Lichen simplex chronicus. (a – Photographs by Dr Lynette Margesson. b – Photographs by Nina Madnani.)

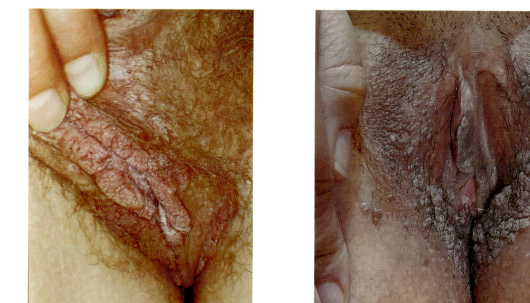

FIGURE 0.4 **(a and b)** Genital warts. (a – Photographs by Dr Lynette Margesson; b – Photographs by Nina Madnani.)

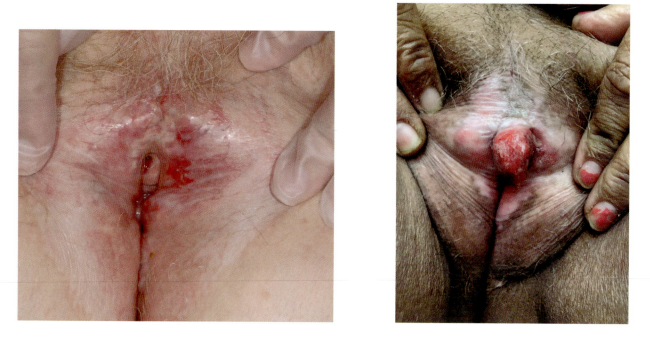

FIGURE 0.5 **(a and b)** dVIN. (a – Photographs by Dr Lynette Margesson; b – Photographs by Nina Madnani.)

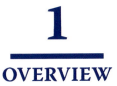

1

OVERVIEW

Pragya Nair and Nina Madnani

Contents

Female genital anatomy

Pragya Nair

Anatomy of vulva

The vulva lies in the perineum, which is a diamond-shaped region bounded anteriorly by the pubic symphysis, laterally by the left and right ischial tuberosities of the pelvic bones, and posteriorly by the coccyx. The perineum further subdivides into an anterior urogenital triangle with the vulva and a posterior anal triangle with the anus and its external sphincter.

The vulva consists of the female genital structures external to the vaginal opening (introitus) and is composed of mons pubis, labia majora, clitoris, labia minora, vulvar vestibule, vestibulovaginal bulbs, urethral meatus, hymen, Bartholin and Skene glands and ducts, vaginal introitus, posterior fouchette, perineum, and ventral part of the anus.

Mons pubis

The most *superficial* structure of the vulva is the mons pubis. It is a subcutaneous fat pad which is located anterior to the pubic symphysis and merges laterally on either side of the vestibular opening with the labia majora. The mons pubis is covered with terminal hairs (pubic hair).

Labia

The labia (lips) are folds of skin around the introitus. They can be short or long, wrinkled or smooth, and asymmetric. The labia can swell on sexual arousal.

Labia majora

Labia majora, called as outer lips, form the lateral boundaries of the vulva. They are longitudinal folds of adipose and fibrous tissue, which join anteriorly at the mons pubis and posteriorly at the commissure lying between the vaginal fourchette and the anus. They are embryologically derived from labioscrotal swellings. The mons pubis and labia majora are of ectodermal origin. Medial to the labia majora are the interlabial sulci, which separate the labia majora from the labia minora and mark a transition point where the skin becomes hairless. Histology of the labia majora shows the outer lining of stratified squamous epithelium, hair follicles, eccrine, apocrine, and sebaceous glands.

Labia minora

Labia minora embryologically derived from urethral folds are called nymphaea and consist of twofolds of connective tissue which contain little or no adipose tissue, are hairless, and lie within and are medial to the labia majora. They fuse anteriorly to form the hood (frenulum) of the clitoris and extend posteriorly to merge on either side of the introitus, creating a fold of skin known as the frenulum of the labia minora (vaginal fourchette). Posteriorly, they blend with the medial surfaces of the labia majora. The normal size of the labia varies between 2.5 and 3.5 cm with a wide variation ranging between 7 mm and 5 cm. Skin and mucosa of the labia minora are rich in sebaceous glands and seen as yellowish, smooth, pin-head papules (Fordyce spots). The deeper area contains dense

DOI: 10.1201/9781003284116-1

1

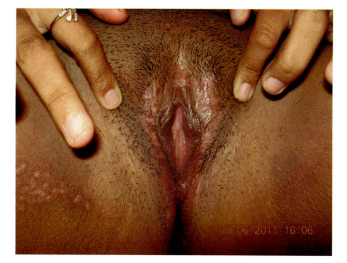

FIGURE 1.1 Normal anatomy of vulva. (Photograph by Dr Kaleem Khan.)

connective tissue. The labia minora surround the opening of the vestibule which contains the vaginal and urethral opening. Anteriorly, each labium minus bifurcates into a medial and lateral fold. The medial folds from each labia minora unite posterior to the clitoris to form the frenulum of the clitoris, whereas the lateral folds unite anterior to the clitoris to form the hood or prepuce of the clitoris. The labia minora has nonkeratinized stratified squamous epithelium.

Hart's line is an imaginary vestibular line defined anteriorly by the prepuce of the clitoris, laterally by the labia minora, and posteriorly by the vaginal fourchette. It demarcates the transition from keratinized to non-keratinized mucosa (Figure 1.1).

Hymen
The hymen is a thin elliptical/oval-shaped membranous ring made up of nonkeratinized stratified squamous epithelium found at the entrance to the vaginal orifice. It varies greatly in shape.

Hymenal caruncles are the remnants of this membranous ring in adult females. These are small thin elevations of the mucous membrane around the vaginal opening.

Clitoris
The clitoris is embryologically derived from the genital tubercle and is an erectile structure found beneath the anterior union of the labia minora.

The clitoris consists of a pair of crura, two erectile structures which attach to the ischiopubic rami.

Each crus converges to form the paired corpora cavernosa of the clitoris anteriorly, collectively called its body. Distally, the body is crowned by the glans (head) of the clitoris, a small tubercle of erectile tissue that arises from the junction of the vestibular bulbs.

The clitoris has an intimate relationship with the distal urethra and vagina.

Vestibule
Vestibule is an area between the hymen and Hart line, which is lined by nonkeratinized squamous epithelium, enclosed by the labia minora, which accommodates the opening of the vagina (external vaginal orifice, vaginal introitus) and urethra. It is demarcated anteriorly by the clitoral prepuce, laterally by the labia minora, and posteriorly by the fourchette.

Structures found in the vestibule include the major vestibular (Bartholin) glands, minor vestibular glands, periurethral (Skene) glands, and urethra.

The urethra is composed of membranous connective tissue with the length varying from 3.5 to 5.0 cm. It links the urinary bladder to the urethral meatus externally over the vestibule.

Vestibular bulbs
Vestibular bulbs are a pair of subcutaneous erectile tissues located on each side of the vestibule. They are covered with bulbospongiosus muscles and join in front of the urethral orifices under the vestibule of the vagina.

Vestibular glands
Bartholin glands (greater vestibular) are kidney, bean or pea-sized, located on either side of the vaginal orifice with a short duct and open into the vestibule. They are similar to the bulbourethral glands in the male. They secrete lubricating mucus into the vagina during sexual arousal.

Skene's glands (paraurethral) are comparable to the male prostate and open into the vestibule near the external urethral orifice. They act as sensory organs during sexual intercourse. They assist in micturition, by directing the flow of urine, thus protecting the female reproductive tract from infection (Figure 1.2).

Nerve supply
The vulva receives sensory and parasympathetic nervous supply (Figure 1.3).

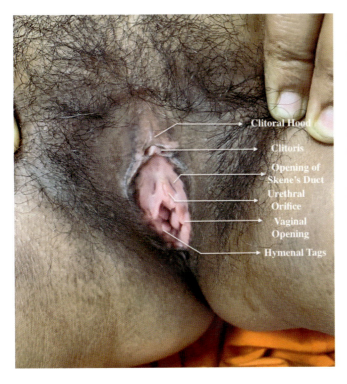

FIGURE 1.2 Normal anatomy – magnified view. (Photograph by Dr Kaleem Khan.)

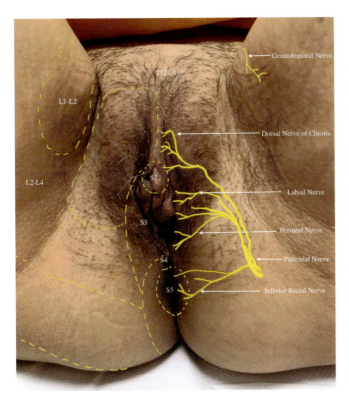

FIGURE 1.3 Nerve supply of vulva. (Photograph by Dr Kaleem Khan.)

Somatic innervation of the anterior vulva is largely via anterior labial nerves derived from lumber plexus. The Ilioinguinal (T12-L1) and genitofemoral nerves (L1-2) also serve the mons pubis and anterolateral labia majora.

The posterior vulva is supplied by the pudendal nerve and posterior cutaneous nerve of the thigh.

The internal pudendal nerve (S2-4) enters the perineum by coursing along the lateral wall of the ischioanal fossa within the pudendal canal formed by the fascia associated with the obturator internus muscle. The pudendal nerve gives rise to three major branches:

1. The inferior rectal nerve innervates the rectum and anus.
2. The perineal nerve provides motor innervation to the muscles of the perineum, sensory innervation via the posterior labial nerve, and sympathetic innervation to blood vessels and sweat glands.
3. The dorsal nerve of the clitoris passes through the perineal membrane just inferior to the pubic symphysis and courses along the dorsal body and glans of the clitoris to provide sensory innervation

The clitoris and vestibule receive parasympathetic innervation from the cavernous nerves which are derived from the uterovaginal plexus.

Vascular supply

The arterial supply to the vulva is from the paired internal and external pudendal arteries, which are branches of the internal iliac artery and femoral artery, respectively (Figure 1.4).

The femoral artery, which sends both superficial and deep external branches, supplies the mons pubis and anterolateral labia majora, respectively. The internal pudendal artery (terminal branch of internal iliac) supplies the rectum, anus, and perineal structures. It also supplies the vestibular bulb (artery to the vestibular bulb) and clitoris (the dorsal artery of clitoris).

The venous return is via the internal pudendal vein and vaginal venous plexus, which is anastomosed with the uterine venous plexus.

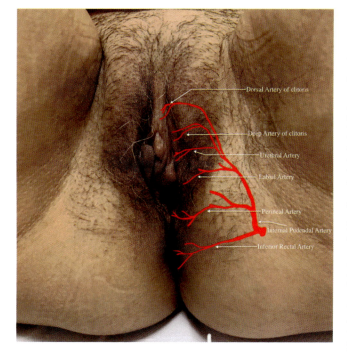

FIGURE 1.4 Blood supply of the vulva. (Photograph by Dr Kaleem Khan.)

Lymphatic drainage
Lymphatic drainage of the external female genitalia is through the superficial and deep inguinal lymph nodes (Figure 1.5).

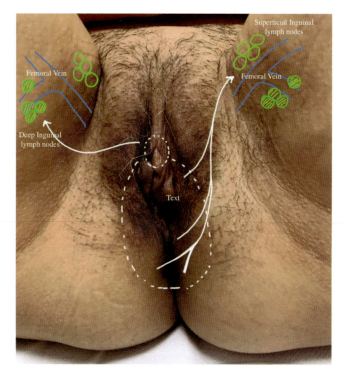

FIGURE 1.5 Lymphatic drainage of vulva. (Photograph by Dr Kaleem Khan.)

The superficial tissues of the labia majora and mons pubis go to the superficial inguinal nodes located superficial to the fascia lata near the emergence of the saphenous vein from the femoral vein.

The perineal deep structures follow the internal pudendal artery into the internal iliac nodes in the pelvis. The labia minora, clitoris, vestibule, and caudal-most vagina drain into deep inguinal nodes located deep to the fascia lata near the saphenous vein and external iliac nodes located along the external iliac artery. Lateral vulvar structures generally drain to the respective ipsilateral side, whereas medial structures drain centrally.

Normal anatomy according to age
The shape and appearance of the vulva change over the years. The most obvious changes are linked to hormonal changes occurring at puberty, during the menstrual cycle, in pregnancy, and around menopause.

Newborn
Female genitalia in a newborn is the result of maternal hormones acquired transplacentally. The labia majora appear full, the labia minora thickened, and the hymenal folds thick and redundant. The vaginal mucosa appears pink and moist, with an acidic pH and physiologic leucorrhea. The normal decline of maternal estrogen in the first week of life can cause vaginal bleeding, making parents anxious. With the decline of maternal hormones, the labia majora lose their fullness, and the labia minora and hymen become thinner and flatter.

Prepubertal girls
The labia decrease in size, leaving the vaginal vestibule less protected from bacteria and external irritants as the infant matures. The vaginal mucosa becomes thin and atrophic with a neutral or alkaline pH, and a scanty secretion.

The hymen becomes thin and translucent, with smooth edges, appears annular, crescentic, or fimbriated by the age of 18–24 months. The perineum, perivaginal tissues and pelvic supporting structures become rigid and inelastic with an increasing risk of tearing due to trauma. The shape of the vaginal orifice varies.

Peripubertal girls
During puberty, secondary sex characteristics are due to the effects of ovarian estrogen. The mons

pubis appears full, midline abdominal hair grows, and labia majora and labia minora thicken and become soft and more rounded. The clitoris enlarges slightly with the urethra becoming more prominent. The hymen thickens as its central opening enlarges. The vaginal mucosa also thickens, softens, and becomes pink. Vaginal secretions increase, making the mucosa moist and pH levels decrease. Perineal and pelvic tissues become more elastic, and the ovaries descend into the pelvis.

Pubertal
The first physical sign of puberty is breast development, followed by the growth of pubic hair which is due to an increase in androgens. Marshall and Tanner stages of pubertal development include short thin hair, which begin to grow on the labia majora around the age of 10 years (II). These become coarser and extend laterally in the next 3 years (III). They then extend across the mons pubis (IV) in the next 2 years and finally come onto the lateral thighs (V). Facial acne and body odor also develops.

Pregnancy
The labia majora and minora increase slightly in size and look puffy or swollen. The color of the inner and outer labia may temporarily darken to a bluish or purplish color due to increased blood flow. The outer lips may slightly retract, which makes the inner lips look bigger or expose them for the first time. Varicose veins are common during pregnancy over the vulva as increased blood flow throughout the body causes blood to pool in the pelvic region, dilating the blood vessels and leading to bluish, bumpy veins that get aggravated by standing, exercise, or sexual stimulation.

Post menopause
Due to the cessation of ovarian functions, female hormones such as estrogen and progesterone decline in the blood. Hair growth decreases. Pubic hairs lose their color and become gray. Skin becomes more friable and less elastic. The labia look smoother, less visible, indistinct in outline, and pale in color. Subcutaneous tissue begins to atrophy, and skin becomes thin and dry increasing the risk of chemical and irritant dermatitis.

Normal variations
Fordyce's spots

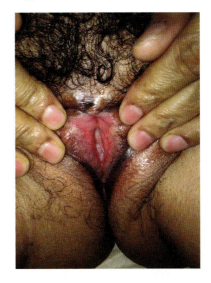
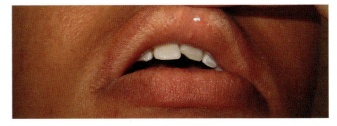

FIGURE 1.6 (a) Grouped, yellowish, pin-head-sized papules on both sides of the labia are typical for Fordyce's spots. (Photograph by Dr Nina Madnani.) (b) Lips are the common site for Fordyce's spots. (Photograph by Dr Bela Shah.)

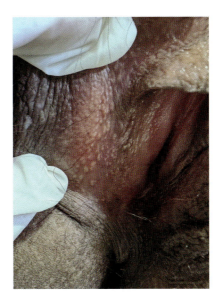

FIGURE 1.7 A closeup of the Fordyce's spots which are ectopic sebaceous glands. (Photograph by Dr Nisha Chaturvedi.)

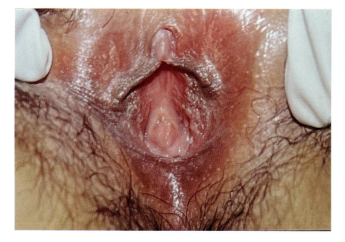

FIGURE 1.8 Often the Fordyce's spots may be larger and may resemble vestibular papillomatosis. (Photograph by Dr Nina Madnani.)

Vulvar papillomatosis

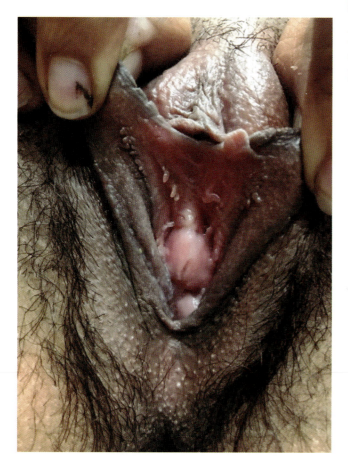

FIGURE 1.9 Vestibular papillomatosus are often mistaken for viral warts but are generally symmetrical in distribution on the labia minora. (Photograph by Dr Nina Madnani.)

Labial variations

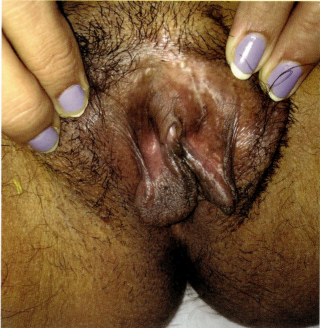

FIGURE 1.10 Rarely, the labia minora may be enlarged, thick, and fleshy. (Photograph by Dr Nina Madnani.)

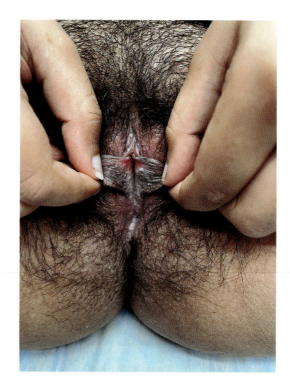

FIGURE 1.11 In this lady, the labia minora were thin and elongated and resembled butterfly wings. (Photograph by Dr Nina Madnani.)

Vulvar anomalies

Clitoromegaly or macroclitoris is an abnormal enlargement of the clitoris. It is congenital or acquired and is due to exposure to an excess of androgens in fetal life, infancy, and adolescence.

Imperforate hymen is at the extreme spectrum of variations in hymenal configuration. Variations in the embryologic development of the hymen are common and result in fenestrations, septa, bands, micro-perforations, anterior displacement, and differences in rigidity and elasticity of the hymenal tissue.

Labial fusion also called as labial adhesion or agglutination is a condition where the two flaps of skin are joined together on either side of the opening to the vagina (the labia minora).

Recommended reading

1. Yeung J, et al. Obstet Gynecol Clin North Am (2016). PMID: 26880506.
2. Yavagal S, et al. Semin Plast Surg (2011). PMID: 22547969.
3. Adams JA, et al. Arch Pediatr Adolesc Med (2004). PMID: 14993089.
4. Clerico C, et al. Aesthetic Plast Surg (2017). PMID: 28314908.
5. Bendtsen TF, et al. Reg Anesth Pain Med (2016). PMID: 26780419.

Normal vulvovaginal flora

Nina Madnani

The "normal" vaginal flora varies from woman to woman and is difficult to define. It also varies depending on the pH and the various stages of life. The vagina is sterile at birth, but within the first 24 hours, enterococci, diphtheroids, and micrococci are identified. Lactobacilli production starts few days before puberty. Estrogen production during the reproductive stage is responsible for stimulating glycogen production in the cells. This glycogen is metabolized to lactic acid which reduces the vaginal pH to < 4.5, favorable for the growth of lactobacilli. *Candida* species can also survive in this pH. An alkaline pH is encountered during pre-menarche, menstruation, and post-menopausal, and favors the growth of aerobic streptococci and coliforms. An "asymptomatic" vagina may have a normal flora, coliforms (*Escherichia coli*), mycoplasma (*Mycoplasma hominis, Ureaplasma urealyticum*), bacilli (*E. coli*, diptheroids, bacteroid species, *Propionibacterium* species), *Gardnerella vaginalis*, lactobacilli (*Lactobacillus crispatus, L. gensenni, L. gasseri*), virus (human papilloma virus), and yeast (*Candida albicans*). This flora gets altered during menstruation, sexual activity, intrauterine device (IUD) insertion, etc.

The proximity of the urethra and rectum/anal orifice contributes to the mixed flora of the vagina.

Vulvar hygiene

Nina Madnani

Introduction

Vulvar cleansing habits are not uniform across the world. They are often influenced by the local cultural practices, education status, awareness, economics of the community, religious norms, and familial habits gone down through generations. The diversity in practices also depends on rural or urban life, and the facilities available there.

Women use various home remedies on the vulva and inside the vagina including yogurt, cooking oils, garlic clove suppositories, etc. for indications like lubrication, soothing, anti-itch, or sexual stimulation. Infections, vaginal burns, and contact dermatitis are some of the complications often encountered with these practices. Women need to be educated about safe genital hygiene practices.

Vulvar hygiene includes genital hygiene, menstrual hygiene, sexual hygiene, and vulvar grooming.

Vulvar hygiene

The vulva has an inherent ability to protect itself by virtue of the acidic pH, physiological discharges, and local flora. The microbial flora diversity is influenced by the proximity to the anal canal, the urethra, and the intertriginous areas. And include micrococci, staphylococci, diptheroids, yeast, lactobacilli, gram-negative rods, and coliform species.

Vulvar hygiene products available in the market include washes, douches, wipes, deodorant sprays, suppositories, moisturizers, and serums.

Recommendation for Vulvar hygiene

Genital hygiene

1. Washing with plain water once or twice a day is adequate.
2. It is important to dry after washing or after a bladder or bowel movement.
3. Washing from front to back is important to prevent the flow of fecal organisms onto the vulva.
4. Specialized pH-balanced washes may be used during disease states, and in the presence of a vulvovaginal discharge.
5. Mechanical scrubbing with sponges, loofahs, scrubs, and wet wipes are strongly discouraged, as the vulvar skin has an inherently weak barrier function and is prone to further breakdown.
6. Shower baths are preferable to tub baths. Community baths are discouraged. Bubble baths and other bath salts may trigger contact dermatitis in atopic individuals and need to be avoided.
7. Douches are strongly discouraged for use as the process can push infection higher into the genital tract. Medical douches are sometimes performed in clinics by the care provider as a case-based need.
8. Hand-held hygiene showers are useful, but the showerhead should not touch the vulvar or anal skin.

Menstrual hygiene

1. Absorbent sanitary pads are generally used and should be changed frequently, including through the night.
2. Sanitary pads are generally disposable. Re-usable pads are available and can be washed after every use.
3. In low socioeconomic families where sanitary towels are unaffordable, strips of cotton fabric are commonly used. A clean cloth is recommended for each use.
4. Patients with dermatitis on and around the vulva should avoid synthetic pads/liners. And an allergic contact dermatitis (ACD) should be suspected. The use of cotton or organic pads is recommended in such patients.
5. In such individuals, tampons or menstrual cups may also be useful.

6. Tampons should be changed regularly, and a single tampon should not be left in for more than 5 hrs.
7. Menstrual cups should be cleaned as per the manufacturer's recommendation, stored in a clean receptacle when not in use, and not be shared.
8. The vulva can be washed with water or a wash before each pad change.
9. Bathing daily is essential during menstruation, unlike the notion that bathing needs to be avoided.

Efforts are ongoing in India to educate women on menstrual hygiene, and hygienic sanitary towels are being provided to women in villages or of lower socioeconomic status, either gratis or at the cost of Rs 1/per pad (8 cents).

Sexual hygiene

1. Cleansing the vulva before sexual intercourse, either with water or a vulvar wash, is recommended.
2. Post which the bladder needs to be emptied.
3. Physician-recommended vaginal lubricants may to be used.
4. Persistent irritation post sexual intimacy could be due to an ACD (condoms/spermicidal jelly/lubricants). A patch test is recommended to detect the allergen.

Vulvar grooming

1. The pubic hair has the function of buffering the vulva against injury and does not need removal for hygiene purposes.
2. If the patient desires hair removal, the following procedures need to be discussed with her, viz. shaving, sugar waxing, depilatory creams, and laser hair reduction.
   a. Shaving with a razor cuts the hair at the skin surface. Wet shave with the use of a lubricating shaving gel is preferred to a dry shave where no intermediate medium is used, as skin injury/scrapes/nicks are minimized. Folliculitis, abrasions, and nicks are some of the complications encountered.
   b. Sugar waxing is a process by which a sticky mixture made of water, sugar, and lemon, is applied to the skin and pressed down with

the help of a cloth or plastic strip. The hairs get stuck to the mixture. Subsequently, the strip is rolled out or abruptly pulled out to remove the hairs. Waxing burns and folliculitis are complications seen.

c. Depilatory creams dissolve the hair shaft at the skin level. Contact dermatitis is a complication in predisposed individuals.

d. Laser hair reduction is now a popular modality. Several lasers are available, and the Q-Switched Nd:YAG laser is most suitable for use in darker skin types. Laser burns, dyspigmentation, and folliculitis are often seen as complications.

3. 'Fur oil' is used by some women on the pubic hair to smoothen them down, akin to hair gels used on the head.

International bodies have formulated guidelines for vulvar hygiene which are published in various journals:

- The Middle East and Central Asia (MECA) Guidelines on Female Genital Hygiene
- Royal College of Obstetricians & Gynecologists Guidelines

Recommended reading

1. Sharma S, et al. Int J Environ Res Public Health (2020). PMID: 31963862.
2. MacRae ER, et al. PLoS One (2019). PMID: 31369595.
3. Chen Y, et al. Womens Health (Lond) (2017). PMID: 28934912.
4. Torondel B, et al. BMC Infect Dis (2018). PMID: 30241498.
5. American College of Obstetricians and Gynecologists' Committee on Practice Bulletins—Gynecology. Diagnosis and Management of Vulvar Skin Disorders: ACOG Practice Bulletin, Number 224. Obstet Gynecol. 2020. PMID: 32590724.
6. Arab H, Almadani L, Tahlak M, et al. The Middle East and Central Asia guidelines on female genital hygiene. BMJ Middle East 2011; 19: 99–106.

Rational use of topical medication in vulvar disease

Nina Madnani

Topical applications are often used either alone or in combination with systemic treatments in the management of several vulvar dermatoses. Generally, ointments are preferred to creams as they are "vulvar-friendly" and do not contain ingredients like propylene glycol which often irritate or produce an ACD. The vulvar skin inherently has a defective skin barrier and allows rapid absorption of ingredients. Its location, and constant pressure and friction via clothes and day-to-day activities, compounds this defect.

A guide to the use of some of the common topicals is given below: corticosteroids (Cs), calcineurin inhibitors, antifungals, imiquimod, 5-fluorouracil, and Vit-D analogues.

1. **Topical corticosteroids** are very effective in managing inflammatory disorders such as eczemas, psoriasis, lichen planus etc. The vulva, surprisingly, tolerates prolonged use of potent topical corticosteroids for several weeks to months without developing steroid side effects like telangiectasia and striae/atrophy. Conversely, if the ointment is applied to the genito-crural folds or inner thighs, atrophy is seen with striae. Commonly, super-potent Cs ointments (clobetasol propionate (0.05%) or potent Cs Mometasone furoate (0.1%) are used initially for few weeks to control the disease, and then the frequency is reduced or the strength changed to one of lower potency. A half-fingertip amount is sufficient for one application to the entire vulva. Combination creams containing an anti-fungal with a super-potent Cs cream are misused by patients for several months to years. Dyspigmentation to almost a vitiligoid appearance is the outcome of this misuse (Figures 1.12 and 1.13).

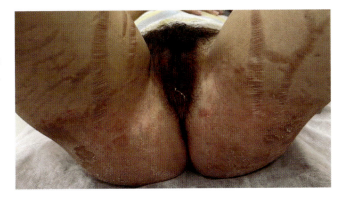

FIGURE 1.12 Extensive straie following gross abuse of topical corticosteroid application. (Photograph by Dr Nisha Chaturvedi.)

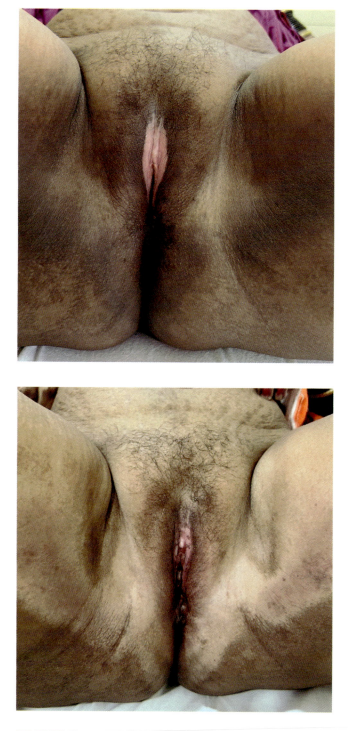

FIGURE 1.13 (a and b) Prolonged, unsupervised application of a super-potent corticosteroid may lead to depigmentation, mimicking vitiligo. (Photograph by Dr Nisha Chaturvedi.)

2. **Calcineurin inhibitors** (tacrolimus 0.03%, 0.1%, pimecrolimus 1%) are immunomodulators, with anti-inflammatory action, used as a step-down from topical corticosteroids in the management of inflammatory disorders and vitiligo. They are used twice a day for several weeks. Some patients seem intolerant to tacrolimus ointment and complain of stinging and burning. Refrigerating the tube occasionally before use may help in improving tolerance. Somehow, in the author's experience, this did not provide any benefit.

3. **Antifungals** are available as solutions, gels, creams, ointments, and vaginal pessaries or troches. Tinea cruris and vulvovaginal candidiasis (VVC) are common especially in obese, diabetics, and immunocompromised individuals. Clotrimazole 1%, miconazole 1%, ketoconazole 2%, eberconazole 1%, terbinafine 1% and luliconazole are the molecules commonly used. The duration for VVC depends on the chronicity of the condition (refer to chapter). Vaginal pessaries are useful in delivering the active ingredients deep into the vagina. Boric acid pessaries 600mg are compounded for patients with complicated VVC. Topical clotrimazole and miconazole creams are safe in pregnancy and lactation.

4. **Vit D analogues**: Calcitriol ointment used twice a day has shown good results in genital psoriasis, matching that of topical tacrolimus 0.1% ointment. Calcipotriene has also been used. Hands should be washed after application, and contact with the eyes should be avoided. Combinations with betamethasone valerate are also available, but caution needs to be exercised as long-term use could result in steroid side effects. Irritation and high cost are some of the disadvantages.

5. **Imiquimod** is an immune modulator, which causes apoptosis of the diseased cells. It stimulates immune responses (acquired and innate). It is available as sachets, each containing 0.25g of 5% imiquimod. Application is recommended 3 times a week for 12 to 16 weeks. An eczematous reaction is often seen necessitating temporary discontinuation, hand holding, and use of a mild topical steroid preparation. It has shown efficacy in vulvar intraepithelial neoplasia (VIN), extramammary Paget's disease, and human papillomavirus (HPV) infections (Figure 1.14).

6. **5FU (fluorouracil)** acts on rapidly proliferating tissue, and has been used for urogenital

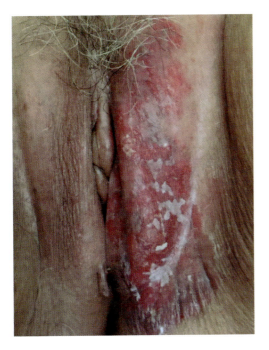

FIGURE 1.14   A severe eczematous reaction in a case of extra-mammary Paget's disease following the application of 5% imiquimod cream. (Photograph by Dr Nina Madnani.)

cancers. It is available in 1%, 2%, and 5% concentration, but 5% is most commonly used. It is applied twice a week for 16 weeks. Application results in edema, erosion, ulceration, and necrosis of the lesion. 5FU has been used for high-grade squamous intraepithelial lesion (HSIL) when surgery is not an option, and for recurrences.

7. **Topical estrogen** creams are useful in women with premature ovarian failure or in menopausal women with genitourinary syndrome of menopause (GUSM). These creams are usually provided with an applicator, and a half to one applicator is adequate to be inserted vaginally, on alternate nights for 2 to 4 weeks. Response is usually seen in 4 weeks. Treatment may be required to be maintained intermittently. Breast tenderness, burning, and irritation are some of the side effects experienced.

8. **Coconut oil** and **petroleum jelly** are cheap and effective barriers for broken skin and can be used as protection until the skin heals. Coconut oil is also used as a lubricant in GUSM, and often facilitates as a lubricant during sexual intimacy.

9. **Topical anesthetics** like Xylocaine 5% jelly can be used for patients suffering from dyspareunia. It can be applied prior to penetration. Topical eutectic mixture of lidocaine-prilocaine can be used as a topical anesthetic half hour before a vulvar biopsy to reduce the pain of the injectable local anesthetic.

Recommended reading

1. Farr A, et al. Mycoses (2021). PMID: 33529414.
2. Carton I, et al. J Gynecol Obstet Hum Reprod (2021). PMID: 32828871.
3. Lee A, et al. Am J Clin Dermatol (2018). PMID: 29987650.
4. Kapila S, et al. J Low Genit Tract Dis (2012). PMID: 22968059.

Bedside diagnostic procedures
Nina Madnani

The following bedside procedures may help in clinching a diagnosis. The simplicity of these tests with minimum tools makes diagnosis quick and cost effective for the patient.

1. **pH strip**: This is a useful test which indicates the pH of the vaginal secretions. An acidic pH favors a candidial infection, while an alkaline pH favors the growth of trichomonads and bacterial vaginosis (BV). Sexually active women have an acidic pH, while in menopausal women, the pH is alkaline (Figure 1.15).

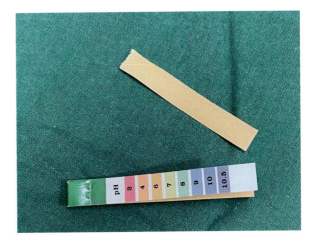

FIGURE 1.15   pH strip is the simplest and cheapest test which should be performed by all vulvar care specialists. (Photograph by Dr Nina Madnani.)

2. **Woods lamp examination**: This is a UV lamp with a peak of 365nm. The examination room is darkened, and the lamp is switched on while holding it about 6 inches from the area to be examined. Various different colors of fluorescence indicate specific diseases: bright white (vitiligo), coral-red (erythrasma), pityriasis versicolor (yellowish-white), and trichomycosis axillaris (yellow).

3. **Dermoscopy**: A hand-held or a video dermoscopy can be used. Sterility may be maintained by using a glass slide/cellophane paper/cling film between the contact plate and the area to be examined. This procedure is useful for diagnosing inflammatory and pigmented lesions. A polarizing setting allows visualization of structures in the dermis.

4. **Vulvovaginal swab**: This is taken with the patient in the lithotomy position under speculum examination. A sterile swab stick is introduced into the posterior fornix, and any discharge is picked up. This swab should be directly sent for culture before it dries out for evaluating bacterial/fungal/viral infection.

5. **Wet mount**: It is useful to identify the infectious agent in discharges. The discharge is collected with a gloved finger, plastic spatula, a dacron swab, or a brush used for Pap smears. Cotton swabs need to be avoided. Touching the posterior fornix and the cervix is not recommended during collection. A drop of normal saline is added, and the fluid is spread evenly on a glass slide. It is then examined under the microscope with phase contrast. This remains a popular test to diagnose trichomoniasis (jerky movement of the oval to pear-shaped T. vaginalis), BV (clue cells, decreased or absent lactobacilli), and candida (refractile pseudo-hyphae and budding yeast cells).

6. **Whiff test**: This test is useful for diagnosing BV. A swab is taken from the posterior fornix, and a drop of potassium hydroxide (KOH) 10–20% is placed on it. A fishy odor indicates BV. This test may not be necessary if a fishy smell is already perceived during the examination. The KOH alkalization releases volatile amines, which give the characteristic odor.

7. **Gram stain**: This test is useful to diagnose the infective organism from a smear of the discharge. Kidney-shaped gram-negative mirror-image organisms (N. gonorrhea), gram-positive rods and cocci (vulvitis/vaginitis), and gram-positive budding yeast cells (candidiasis)

8. **KOH mount**: This test is used when suspecting fungal infection on keratinized skin. The KOH serves to dissolve the keratin to expose the fungal elements. The suspicious area is gently scraped with a sterile blade, and debris is mounted on a glass slide with a drop of 10% KOH. After 5 min, the slide is examined for pseudohyphae and spores (candidiasis), and branching hyphae (dermatomycosis).

9. **Cellophane tape stripping**: A piece of cellophane tape is stuck onto the perianal area and pulled off. It is then placed sticky side down on a glass slide and examined for the eggs of E. vermicularis (elongated with one side convex and the other flattened). This method can also be used to identify fungal infections.

10. **Mineral oil mount**: This is useful for detecting a scabietic infection. The suspicious area is scraped with a sterile blade, and the debris was placed on a glass slide with a drop of mineral oil. The scabietic mite/scybala/eggs may be visualized.

11. **Tzanck smear**: This is an important test to diagnose vesiculo-bullous disorders and viral infections. The blister is de-roofed, the base scraped with a No 15 blade, and the material is then smeared onto a slide. This is fixed with alcohol and then stained with Giemsa stain. Multinucleated giant cells are seen in herpes, while acantholytic cells are seen in pemphigus vulgaris.

12. **Patch test**: This test is indicated in women with vulvar pruritis not responding to treatment, where an ACD is suspected. One of the following kits can be used: The Indian Standard Series (ISS) or European Standard Series or American Academy Patch-Test kit or the TRUE TEST. The back between the scapulae is the favored site for testing. The patches are removed in 48hrs and observed for any reaction. The area is evaluated again in 5 to 7 days. Erythema, edema, or vesiculation indicate a test positivity.

Recommended reading

1. Amrin SS, et al. Indian J Sex Transm Dis (AIDS). 2021. PMID: 34765936.
2. Micheletti RG, et al. J Am Acad Dermatol (2017). PMID: 28711083.
3. Eryılmaz A, et al. Int J Dermatol (2014). PMID: 23557278.

Vulvar biopsy: Tips and tricks

Nina Madnani

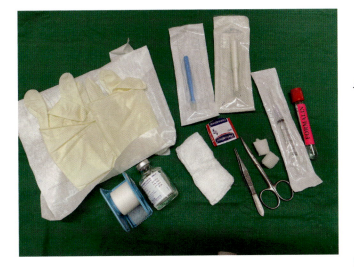

FIGURE 1.16 Setup cart for skin biopsy. (Photograph by Dr Nina Madnani.)

When to perform?

A vulvar biopsy is required when

a. The diagnosis is in doubt or needs to be confirmed.
b. For most blistering disorders (except herpes simplex and zoster).
c. The lesion is not responding to treatment as expected?
d. To rule out VIN or malignancy.
e. When the patient requires validation for the diagnosis made.

Site selection

a. The biopsy should be taken from the area which represents the most typical changes.
b. The edge of an ulcer including the normal skin.
c. The edge of the blister includes the normal skin.

d. A hyperkeratotic plaque, an indurated area, or a non-healing erosion/ulcer in a lesion of Lichen sclerosus (LS).
e. The clitoris and fourchette area should be avoided for this procedure, as post-biopsy healing and pain are a concern.

Pre-biopsy concerns

a. Valid consent needs to be taken from the patient after giving her a detailed brief on the procedure and complications.
b. Blood thinners, garlic, ginko biloba, and green tea to be discontinued as per the guidance of their primary physician.
c. Consent for photography if relevant.

Anesthesia?

a. A topical anesthetic may be applied to the vulva under occlusion, half an hour prior to injecting the local anesthetic agent. Remember, the vulvar area is an extremely pain-sensitive area, and this blunts the discomfort of the hypodermic needle.
b. 2% lidocaine with/without adrenaline, 1–2 cc under the site.

Punch biopsy or scalpel biopsy?

a. A Keye's punch of diameter 3 or 4 is generally used.
b. A scalpel biopsy may be required if a larger section is needed or an excision biopsy of the entire lesion when necessary.
c. A 3 to 4 mm punch biopsy does not need sutures unless there is prolonged oozing.
d. The biopsy is sent to the laboratory in 10% formalin or in Michel's medium when immunofluorescence is required.

Biopsy procedure

a. The area is cleansed with betadine solution.
b. The area to be biopsied is identified and marked with a disposable marker or 1% GV (gentian violet) lotion.
c. Local anesthesia (1–2%) lidocaine is infiltrated.
d. The skin is stretched between the thumb and index finger of the non-dominant hand.
e. The Keyes punch of the required size is held vertically with the sharp edge in contact with the skin, and rotated downwards with firm pressure until you reach the hub of the punch.

f. The punch is removed, the base of the cylindrical sample is snipped off, and the sample is put in the required medium (either 10% formalin, saline or Michel's medium) and sent to the histopathologist.

g. Biopsy mapping is recommended when multiple biopsies are taken, and sent to the histopathologist together with the sample.

h. When larger samples are required, excision and suturing can be performed.

Biopsy labeling

a. When multiple biopsies are taken, each is placed in a separate container and correctly labeled.

b. A requisition slip should contain the name, age, sex, site of biopsy, differential diagnosis, and previous biopsy details if relevant.

Hemostasis

a. Pressure with a wad of gauze for 3 to 5 min

b. Monsel's solution (ferric subsulfate solution) application

c. Silver nitrate stick touched the site

d. Absorbent gel cut to the appropriate size and pressed firmly onto the wound

e. Simple suture

Complications

a. Bleeding
b. Pain
c. Infection
d. Scarring

Post-care

a. The area can be wetted.

b. A topical vaseline-based antiseptic applied 3 times a day for the next few days is sufficient. Or simple Vaseline jelly.

c. A non-steroidal anti-inflammatory drug (NSAID) may be prescribed to alleviate the pain if present.

Caveats

a. More than one area may need to be biopsied if the lesion is multifocal.

b. A clinic-histopathological correlation is required as often the biopsy result may not match your clinical diagnosis.

c. The sample may be inadequate or not representative of the disease.

2

DISORDERS OF PIGMENTATION

Satish Udare

Contents

Introduction

Almost all pigmentary conditions involving the extra-genital skin and mucosa can affect the vulva and perineum. These often cause stigmatization, social isolation and ostracization. These psychosexual implications hamper interpersonal relations. Vulvar pigmentation is ultraviolet light independent. Post-inflammatory hyperpigmentation is the karma of skin types 4–6, especially on frictional areas such as the axillae, vulva, groins and inner thighs. This is especially common in Asians, Hispanics and African-Americans. Also, inflammatory processes stimulate the activity of the melanocytes to increase the production and distribution of eumelanin. Increase in dermal melanophages renders a bluish hue to the skin, the Tyndall effect. This is seen as intense pigmentation in certain vulvar inflammatory conditions, which may be mistaken as melanomas. In contrast, the vaginal mucosa generally has no melanocytes, and any pigmented area needs to be investigated. Complete or partial loss of pigmentation, resulting in depigmentation or hypopigmentation, is more evident in the skin of color. Important causes of vulvar dyspigmentation are listed in Table 2.1.

Hyperpigmentary disorders

Pigmentary vulvar lesions have been reported in 10–15% of the Caucasians population. This number is higher in darker skin types, but exact statistics are unknown. The lesions may be melanocytic or non-melanocytic.

Hyperpigmentation of the vulva often presents as a diagnostic dilemma. Physiological hyperpigmentation is usually symmetrical, asymptomatic

TABLE 2.1: Causes of Dyspigmentation in the Vulvar Area

Hypo or Depigmentation in Vulvar Area	Hyperpigmentation in Vulvar Area
Post-inflammatory hypo or depigmentation	Physiologic hyperpigmentation
Vitiligo	Acanthosis nigricans
Lichen sclerosus	Vulvar melanosis
Vitiligoid LS	Post-inflammatory hyperpigmentation
Nevus depigmentosus	Fixed drug eruption
Contact depigmentation	Lentigines
Fordyce's Spots	Nevi
	VIN
	Melanoma
	Vascular lesions which appear deeply pigmented e.g. angiokeratoma, bruises

and without any textural changes. It occurs in dark-skinned individuals more marked on the labia, introitus and upper inner thighs. Pregnancy, obesity and B12 deficiency enhance pigmentation.

Acanthosis nigricans (AN)

Skin under the influence of insulin excess gets thick, velvety and appears hyperpigmented. This may be seen in all folds including genitocrural folds, vulva and inner thighs (Figures 2.1 and 2.2). The face, neck, axillae and infra-mammary folds are the other sites involved. Vulvar AN maybe associated with obesity and diabetes mellitus. Dermoscopy of AN shows linear crista cutis and sulcus cutis, corresponding to the papillomatosis

DOI: 10.1201/9781003284116-2

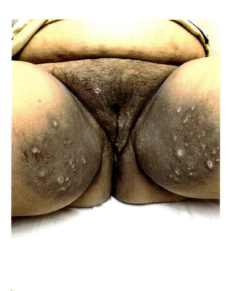

FIGURE 2.1 Thick velvety hyperpigmented patched of acanthosis nigricans on the vulva and inner thighs in a patient of HS.

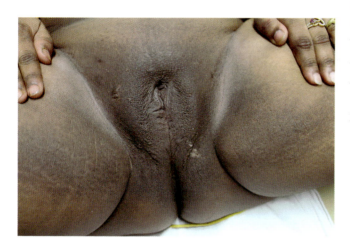

FIGURE 2.2 Selected velvety pigmented plaques of acanthosis nigricans involving the vulva and inner thighs. (Photographs by Dr Nina Madnani.)

and interspersed sulci, with well-defined black or brown dots of pigmentation. Insulin-sensitizing drugs over several months, together with significant weight loss, may bring about a reduction of acanthosis. AN is commonly associated with polycystic ovarian syndrome (PCOS).

Recommended reading

1. Grasinger CC. Vulvar acanthosis nigricans: a marker for insulin resistance in hirsute women. Fertil Steril (1993). PMID: 8458461.

Vulvar melanosis

Melanotic macules are a benign condition commonly seen on the non-keratinized mucosa and sometimes on the keratinized skin of the vulva, in women of reproductive age with a median age of 40–44 years. Also known as idiopathic lenticular mucocutaneous pigmentation. This is usually asymptomatic, but picked up during a self-examination or during a routine gynecological check-up (Figure 2.3). The pigmented area involved is more than 4 mm in diameter, is usually dark brown and occurs mainly on non-keratinized mucosae of the lower vagina, vestibule, perineum, labia majora or minora as single or multiple patches with irregular borders. The lesions are flush with the surrounding skin. Brownish reticular, parallel or honeycomb pattern may be seen on dermoscopy. Histopathology shows basal cell hyperpigmentation, with no increase in melanocyte numbers or epidermal hypermelanosis (Figure 2.4). Malignancy (melanoma and pigmented vulvar intraepithelial neoplasia (VIN)) is the most important differential diagnosis in vulvar melanosis. An adequate and prompt biopsy is required for a correct diagnosis.

Counselling and reassurance about the benign nature of the condition is necessary.

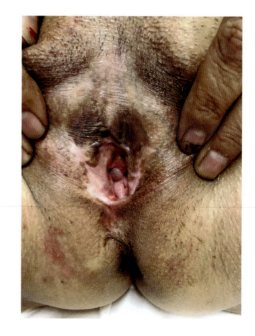

FIGURE 2.3 Asymptomatic patches of vulvar melanosis on either side of the clitoris. (Photograph by Dr Nina Madnani.)

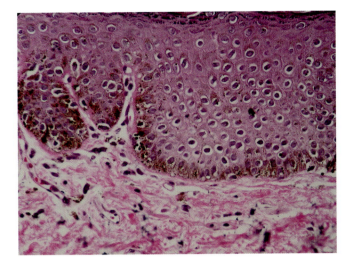

FIGURE 2.4 H & E, 400×, prominent melanin in basal layer with pigmented dendrites in spinous layer. (Photograph by Dr Rajiv Joshi.)

Recommended reading

1. De Giorgi V, et al. JAMA Dermatol (2020). PMID: 32785609.

Post-inflammatory hyperpigmentation

In skin types 4–6, the tendency to intense post-inflammatory hyperpigmentation lasting over months to years is a common phenomenon. Most injuries or dermatoses can elicit this (Figure 2.5). Detailed history and tell-tale signs of inflammation may give clues to the primary inciting condition. Controlling the inciting agents and use of

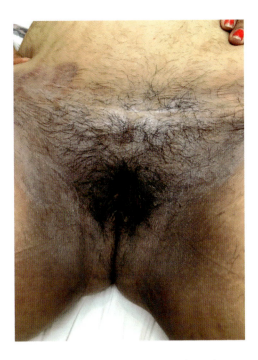

FIGURE 2.6 Deep pigmentation in areas of past dermatophyte infection. (Photograph by Dr Nina Madnani.)

topical medications containing kojic acid, arbutin and botanicals are helpful. Often, the pigmentation fades off over weeks/months/years, once the inflammatory process has settled. Post-inflammatory pigmentation of dermatomycosis is a classic example of this phenomenon (Figures 2.6 and 2.7).

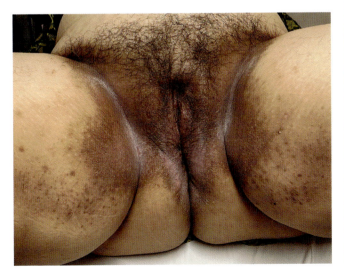

FIGURE 2.5 Many inflammatory disorders can result in hyperpigmentation upon resolution. (Photograph by Dr Nina Madnani.)

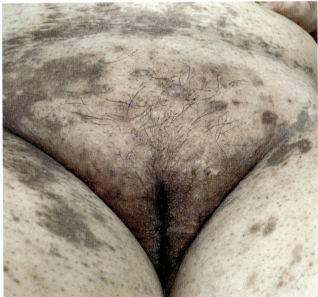

FIGURE 2.7 Grayish black pigment with follicular involvement in a case of lichen planus pigmentosus. (Photograph by Dr Nina Madnani.)

Fixed drug eruption

This is a common, distinct cutaneous allergic reaction resulting from exposure to some medication and characteristically recurring at the same sites on re-exposure.

On keratinized skin, it presents as a single, well-defined, round or oval dusky red patch which may later blister or ulcerate to heal with intense, brown-black pigmentation. Non-pigmented variants have been reported on the mucosa. Fixed drug eruption (FDE) reported on the vulva is usually bilaterally symmetrical and presents as an erosive vulvitis, unresponsive to treatment until the offending drug has been identified and stopped. It is observed most commonly on mucocutaneous junctions. Non-steroidal anti-inflammatory drugs (NSAIDS), anti-epileptics and anti-microbials are commonly implicated in this reaction. Others implicated are griseofulvin, fluconazole, ibuprofen, COX2-inhibitors and metronidazole. Once the culprit drug is discontinued, topical mid-potency corticosteroids are useful. In severe cases, systemic corticosteroids may be administered. The use of depigmenting agents and lasers may hasten the resolution of the post-reaction pigmentation.

Recommended reading

1. Fischer G. J Reprod Med (2007). PMID: 17393766.
2. Drummond C et al. Australas J Dermatol (2009). PMID: 19397565.
3. Abril-Pérez C, et al. Am J Obstet Gynecol (2022). PMID: 34610321.

Nevi

These are common in darker skin types and are often asymptomatic but cause considerable anxiety to the patients. They are uniformly colored, have a regular border and are small in size (Figure 2.8). These mainly present on the labia majora, minora and clitoral hood. Those on the non-keratinized surface need to be kept under observation for any changes.

Dermoscopic findings include globular and uniform reticular pigment pattern (Figure 2.9). A biopsy may be required in equivocal cases, wherein histopathology examination will give a definitive diagnosis (Figure 2.10).

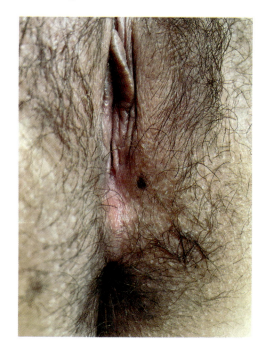

FIGURE 2.8   Well-defined, dark brown, flat papule. (Photograph by Dr Nina Madnani.)

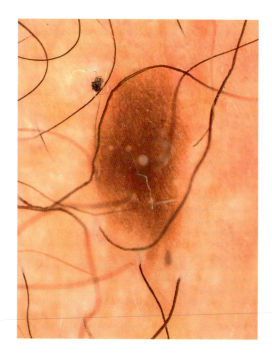

FIGURE 2.9   Dermoscopic image of the nevus. Dinolite Digital Microscope WF-20_polarized 10×. (Photograph by Dr Nina Madnani.)

Recommended reading

1. Allbritton JI. Obstet Gynecol Clin North Am (2017). PMID: 28778635.
2. Venkatesan A. Dermatol Clin (2010). PMID: 20883921.

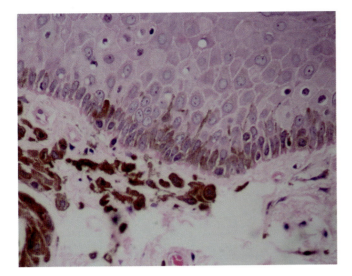

FIGURE 2.10 Vulvar Melanocytic Nevus 4: H & E, 400×, pigmented melanocytes in the dermis and pigmented dendritic processes in epidermis. (Photograph by Dr Rajiv Joshi.)

Hypopigmentory disorders

Post-inflammatory hypo or depigmentation

A prior injury or an inflammatory disorder may be sufficient to damage/destroy melanocytes leading to hypo or depigmentation. On the vulva, conditions like psoriasis, seborrheic dermatitis, candidiasis, pityriasis versicolor or topical steroid misuse can resolve with a clinical situation resembling vitiligo. The trend for genital lightening with procedures/lasers/cosmetics may result in unwanted permanent hypo or depigmentation (Figures 2.11 and 2.12).

The woman may notice a lightening of color at the areas of pre-existing skin rashes either as they settle or following the excessive and prolonged use of high-potency topical corticosteroids. The hypo/depigmentation may be asymptomatic, or be itchy due to the persistent activity of the pre-existing event/disease. Without eliciting a careful history, the patches can often be mistaken as vitiligo. These may involve any part of the vulva including the groins and often the upper parts of the thighs. There is no fluorescence on Wood's lamp examination, unlike that seen with vitiligo. The presence of striae may be indicative of topical steroid abuse.

Vitiligo needs to be differentiated mainly due to the stigmatization associated with it. Vitiliginous

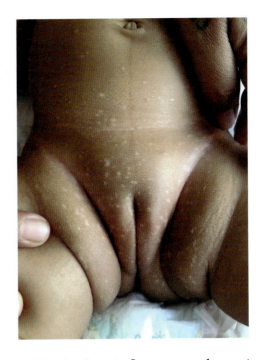

FIGURE 2.11 Post-inflammatory hypopigmentation secondary to resolving guttate psoriasis in a child. (Photograph by Dr Nisha Chaturvedi.)

patches are usually symmetrical, asymptomatic and fluoresce under the wood's lamp.

Late stages of lichen sclerosus may appear depigmented, but sclerosis and agglutination of vulvar parts clinch the diagnosis.

Spontaneous re-pigmentation is possible. Topical emollients, calcineurin inhibitors (pimecrolimus 1% or tacrolimus 0.1%) used twice a day may hasten the recovery.

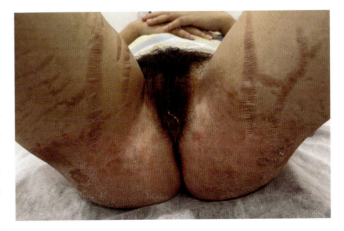

FIGURE 2.12 Misuse of steroids in the treatment of dermatophyte infection resulting in hypopigmentation and extensive striae. (Photograph by Dr Nisha Chaturvedi.)

Recommended reading

1. Gutierrez P, et al. Case Rep Womens Health (2020). PMID: 32642448.
2. García-Montero P, et al. Actas Dermosifiliogr (2017). PMID: 27912903.

Vitiligo

Vitiligo is a chronic, acquired disease characterized by depigmented macules and patches with loss of functional melanocytes. Although familial clustering of cases is seen, the exact cause is still an enigma.

The global incidence of vitiligo has been reported between 0.5 and 2%. The statistics reported for India range from 0.45% to 4%, and in China, 0.093%. Exact statistics of genital involvement in women is difficult to obtain as many do not reveal their problem due to fear of stigmatization by family and society.

The autoimmune theory, the neurohumoral theory, free-radical theory and defective melanocyte adhesion are some of the hypotheses put forth to explain the complex pathogenesis. Although a purely cosmetic concern, vitiligo may be associated with other autoimmune disorders like pernicious anemia, alopecia areata, thyroiditis etc., symptoms and signs if which should be looked out for.

The condition is usually asymptomatic, but the itching has been a complaint in patients where the disease is actively evolving. The vitiliginous patches are depigmented, sharply demarcated, usually symmetrical on the labia majora, minora and sometimes involving the pubis and the groins. These may be associated with leukotrichia, which signifies an unfavorable prognosis. The patches are accidentally discovered by the patient, significant other, or a caregiver (Figure 2.13).

Bright white area, perilesional follicular pigmentation, telangiectasias and reverse pigment network have been described on dermoscopy. Perifollicular depigmentation is seen in unstable lesions. A Woods lamp examination gives bright bluish-white fluorescence. Biopsy of a depigmented area shows absent melanocytes in a normal epidermal architecture, mild lymphocytic infiltrate at the junction between pigmented and non-pigmented areas.

Vitiligo needs to be differentiated from other conditions like contact depigmentation (h/o contact

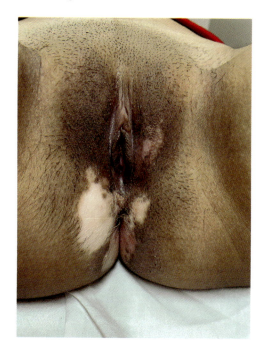

FIGURE 2.13 Milky-white, well-demarcated depigmented patches on the vulva and buttocks with leucotrichia vitiligo. (Photograph by Dr Nina Madnani.)

with latex, rubber, condom use), vitiligoid lichen sclerosus (a non-itchy condition, often mistaken for vitiligo, where the macules on biopsy show typical changes of lichen sclerosus) and lichen sclerosus (severe itching, with "missing" anatomical parts of the vulva. Also, LS involves the clitoris and clitoral hood, while vitiligo may spare it).

The course is unpredictable. Trichrome vitiligo, koebnerization and confetti-like macules indicate an unstable disease. Re-pigmentation occurs from the periphery or around pigmented hairs.

When localized purely to the genitals, topical treatment is recommended. Judicious use of moderately potent topical corticosteroids and topical calcineurin inhibitors, tacrolimus (0.03–0.1%) or pimecrolimus 1% twice a day for several months is required. Targeted narrow-band UVB (NBUVB) and excimer lasers are useful for vitiligo on hairy areas in patients (mucosal areas need to be treated cautiously) in those who have a poor response to topicals.

Recommended reading

1. Veronesi G, et al. Pediatr Dermatol (2021). PMID: 34561885.

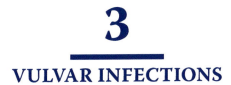

3

VULVAR INFECTIONS

Nisha Chaturvedi, Nina Madnani, and Kaleem Khan

Contents

Herpes genitalis

Nisha Chaturvedi

Introduction

Herpes genitalis is a common genito-ulcerative disease, generally sexually transmitted, and endemic across the world.

Epidemiology

The infection is caused by a large DNA virus, the herpes simplex virus (HSV) type 2, with humans as the only host. More than 400 million people have genital herpes caused by HSV2, although the incidence of primary genital infection occurring with HSV-1 has also increased. Seroprevalence studies suggest that all HSV 2 infections are acquired between 15 and 40 years of age.

Pathophysiology

Primary HSV infections are acquired from close contact with someone who is actively shedding the virus from skin or secretions. This may occur even in the absence of active lesions (asymptomatic shedding) and is the primary mode of disease transmission. Upon contracting the virus, the incubation period varies from 5 to 14 days.

During the initial infection, viral DNA travels via the axon to the spinal cord sensory ganglion, where it persists for life. Reactivation of the virus causes migration back through the axon, its branches or contralateral axons to the skin and mucosa, resulting in clinical disease.

Presenting complaints

Symptoms may range from totally asymptomatic to severe genital disease. Women with primary infections may present with severe pain, burning, dysuria, fever, myalgia or headache. In others, milder symptoms are present. Recurrent herpetic episodes are accompanied with mild local symptoms, and a prodrome of burning and itching is common.

Clinical examination

Patients with a primary attack, on examination, may have grouped papulo-vesicles on an erythematous base, which rapidly rupture to form coalescing

DOI: 10.1201/9781003284116-3

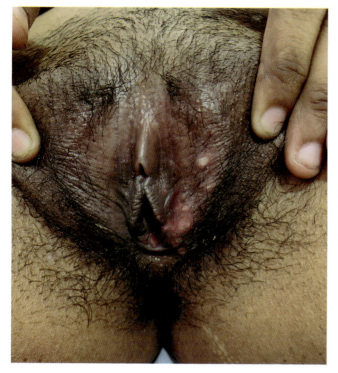

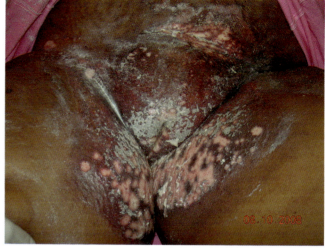

FIGURE 3.3   Involvement of extensive areas in an immunocompromised female. (Photograph by Dr Nina Madnani.)

FIGURE 3.1   Notice the scalloped border of the large ulcer on the left inter-labial sulcus. (Photograph by Dr Nisha Chaturvedi.)

round ulcers with a scalloped border (Figure 3.1). Occasionally, in severe attacks, there may be labial edema. The lesions are extremely tender, and the patient may be uncooperative for examination (Figure 3.2). Local enlarged, tender lymph nodes

may be palpable. The lesions can involve all parts of the vulva and can encroach onto the vaginal mucosa. Atypical manifestation of herpes genitalis includes tiny erosions or fissures on the genitalia.

In immunocompromised patients, hemorrhagic, hypertrophic verrucous, ecthyma like and deeply ulcerated lesions can be seen (Figure 3.3).

Systemic findings
Aseptic meningitis, sacral radiculopathy and autonomic dysfunction may occur especially during the primary episode of primary HSV infection.

Laboratory examination
Tzanck smear helps in the rapid diagnosis of genital herpes (presence of multinucleate giant cells), but it is less sensitive than viral culture. Immunofluorescence staining increases the sensitivity and specificity of a Tzanck smear preparation.

Viral culture is the "gold standard" for HSV diagnosis. Primary infections have a higher chance of isolation (80%) as compared to recurrent infections (25–50%).

Serological tests include enzyme-linked immunosorbent assay (ELISA), complement fixation test and the Western blot. These tests detect antibodies to HSV in the blood. Serology can rule out a previous HSV infection.

Advanced tests include HSV direct detection (electron microscopy), HSV antigen detection (immune-peroxidase tests, immunofluorescence,

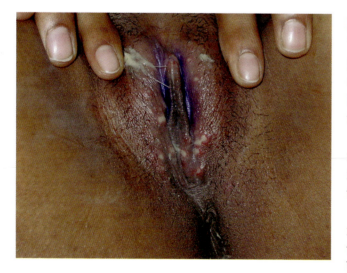

FIGURE 3.2   Active herpetic infection with secondary bacterial infection. Note the purple staining with 1% Gentian violet lotion. (Photograph by Dr Nina Madnani.)

enzyme immunoassay), HSV-DNA detection (DNA hybridization) and HSV-polymerase chain reaction (PCR).

Histopathology

Histopathology findings characteristic of HSV infections are ballooning of epidermal keratinocytes and intra-epidermal vesicles with multinucleated giant cells.

Differential diagnosis

Differential diagnosis of herpes genitalis includes varicella zoster, aphthous ulcers, Crohn's disease, syphilis and chancroid.

Varicella zoster presents with clusters of vesicles and pustules arranged in a dermatomal pattern associated with pain in the affected dermatome.

Aphthous ulcers are extremely painful, usually larger, single or multiple, well-defined punched out, usually seen in girls and younger women.

Crohn's disease usually presents with a linear knife cut ulcers in the inter-labial sulci, vulvar skin fold or gluteal cleft, accompanied with labial edema, and with or without gastrointestinal involvement.

Chancre seen in primary syphilis classically presents as a painless, indurated, clean ulcer seen on the labia, around the clitoris, fourchette or cervix with non-tender firm rubbery lymphadenopathy.

Chancroid ulcers are classically painful ulcers with a purulent dirty gray base, undermined edges, located on the fourchette, labia minora, vestibule and clitoris, and often associated with painful inguinal lymphadenitis.

Course and prognosis

Untreated primary infections may spontaneously resolve in 10–14 days. Occasionally, impetiginization occurs with increased pain and crusting. In immunocompromised patients, lesions can persist for several weeks (Figure 3.4).

Treatment

Sexual intimacy is to be avoided during the active phase. Systemic antiviral drugs are recommended for the treatment of herpes genitalis. However, these drugs do not eradicate the latent virus. Acyclovir, valacyclovir and famciclovir are approved for the treatment.

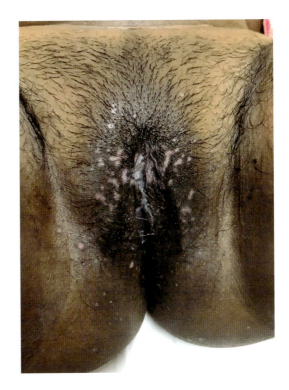

FIGURE 3.4   Healed, scarred lesions with post-inflammatory depigmentation. (Photograph by Dr Nina Madnani.)

For primary infections, acyclovir 400 mg three times a day or famciclovir 250 mg thrice a day or valacyclovir 1 gm orally twice a day can be given for a period of 7–10 days.

Recurrent episodes of herpes genitalis can be treated with acyclovir 400 mg twice a day for 5 days or famciclovir 125 mg twice a day for 5 days or valacyclovir 500 mg orally twice a day for 3 days. Suppressive therapy is given in patients who have more than 6 episodes per year. Acyclovir 400 mg twice a day or valacyclovir 500 mg once a day or famciclovir 250 mg twice a day is recommended. Valacyclovir appears to be better than famciclovir for the suppression of herpes genitalis. Topical antivirals have not been so effective. Systemic antibacterial and anti-inflammatory medications are useful adjuvants.

Pearls

Viral shedding may occur even in the absence of the lesions. The period of asymptomatic shedding and recurrence rates are unpredictable.

Clinically severe infections should prompt the search for an immune-suppressed state.

Recommended reading

1. Groves MJ. Am Fam Physician (2016). PMID: 27281837.
2. Jaishankar D, et al. Microb Cell (2016). PMID: 28357380.
3. Sauerbrei A. Infect Drug Resist (2016). PMID: 27358569.
4. Workowski KA, Bolan GA, Centers for Disease Control and Prevention. Sexually transmitted diseases treatment guidelines, 2015. MMWR Recomm Rep 2015; 64(RR-03):1–137.

Herpes zoster

Nisha Chaturvedi

Introduction

Herpes zoster (HZ), commonly known as shingles, is caused by reactivation of the varicella-zoster virus (VZV).

Epidemiology

It is seen in adults, the elderly and in those with immunocompromised conditions such as leukemia, lymphoma, transplant recipients and HIV. The commonest dermatomes involved are the thoracic, ophthalmic and cervical. Only 5% are sacral. Vulvar involvement is rare.

Pathophysiology

Varicella zoster occurs in individuals with past varicella infection. This virus persists and remains dormant in the posterior root ganglion. Reactivation occurs at a later stage with a drop in immunity. Triggering factors are trauma, stress, old age and immunosuppression. The lesions appear on the vulva if the S2 or S3 dermatome is involved.

Presenting Complaints

Patients present with unilateral pain, burning sensation and severe discomfort with difficulty in walking or sitting (Figure 3.5). This may be accompanied with fever and malaise. Some patients may present with urinary retention.

Clinical examination

The affected dermatome will have grouped vesicles on an erythematous base (Figure 3.6). The vesicles rupture within a few days and heal with scarring. Local lymphadenopathy is frequent. In immunocompromised patients, the presentation may be florid with multi-dermatomal involvement, hemorrhagic, necrotic or bullous lesions.

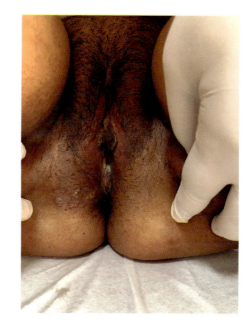

FIGURE 3.5 Scattered grouped vesicles in a dermatomal pattern. (Photograph by Dr Kaleem Khan.)

Dermoscopy

Dermoscopy shows central brown dots and multiple white lobulated structures with surrounding erythema. These findings change as per the stage of the eruption.

Laboratory examination

Tzanck smear from the base of a new vesicle demonstrates the presence of multinucleated giant cells. Direct fluorescent antibody (DFA) testing or PCR

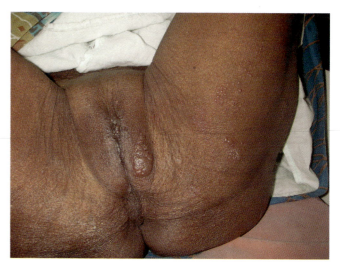

FIGURE 3.6 Clustered vesicles in a dermatomal pattern involving left labia majora and left thigh posteriorly. (Photograph by Dr Nisha Chaturvedi.)

test can also be done, both of which have greater sensitivity and specificity than the Tzanck smear and allow for differentiation between HSV and VZV infections. Biopsy is rarely done.

Histopathology

Histopathology shows ballooning degeneration and acantholysis of keratinocytes and multinucleated giant cells.

Differential diagnosis

HZ must be differentiated from herpes genitalis, bullous impetigo and bullous pemphigoid.

Herpes genitalis presents with a localized cluster of vesicles that form superficial well-demarcated erosions, which often cross the midline, whereas HZ is unilateral along a dermatome.

Bullous impetigo presents with thin-walled, vesicles and bullae which quickly break down to erosions with honey-colored crusting. Cultures demonstrate *Staphylococcus aureus*.

Bullous pemphigoid presents with thick-walled bullae on a normal or erythematous skin. Other sites are also involved.

Course and prognosis

Most patients recover from HZ without any complications within 2–3 weeks. Postherpetic neuralgia (persistence or recurrence of pain in the affected area for more than a month even after the lesions have healed) can be disabling, especially in the elderly.

Treatment

Antiviral drugs used for the treatment of HZ are acyclovir, valacyclovir and famciclovir. Acyclovir is given in a dose of 800 mg orally five times a day, valacyclovir 1 gm thrice a day and famciclovir 500 mg thrice a day for 7–10 days. Early diagnosis and treatment can reduce the duration of HZ and the risk of developing post-herpetic neuralgia.

The varicella-zoster vaccine (Zostavax) is FDA approved for people over 60 years of age. The vaccine can reduce the occurrence and severity of HZ and post-herpetic neuralgia. A new vaccine (Shingrix) seems to have better efficacy and is safe in immunosuppressed individuals.

Pearls

Multi-dermatomal herpes zoster is seen in immune-compromised individuals.

Patients with HZ can cause varicella in contacts who have never had varicella or varicella vaccine.

Recommended reading

1. Martins MM, et al. BMJ Case Rep (2021). PMID: 34972780.
2. Koshy E, et al. Indian J Dermatol Venereol Leprol (2018). PMID: 29516900.

Molluscum contagiosum

Nisha Chaturvedi

Introduction

Molluscum contagiosum (MC) is a contagious dermatosis caused by the Pox virus. Both children and adults can contract the infection.

Epidemiology

The virus is a double-stranded DNA virus of the poxvirideae family with four different subtypes: mcv1, mcv2, mcv3 and mcv4. It is transmitted by direct contact, sexual or non-sexual with infected skin, and via fomites like towels and sponges, or by autoinoculation. Humans are the only host for the virus. The incubation period varies between 14 and 50 days

MC is seen in children especially atopics, sexually active adults and immunocompromised individuals.

Pathophysiology

The virus infects only the epidermis where it replicates in the cytoplasm producing cytoplasmic inclusions and enlargement of infected cells.

Presenting complaints

Patients accidentally notice "boils" during self-examination, or during a hair-removal procedure. Itching or pain is rare.

Clinical examination

The lesions are pearly-white, sub-centimeter, smooth, firm, dome-shaped papules with a central umbilication (Figure 3.7). The papules may be single, multiple or clustered, located on the lower abdomen, pubis, inner thigh and genitalia (Figure 3.8). Lesions can get eczematized (molluscum dermatitis). Children can have florid lesions on the labia, inner thighs and perianal area. Molluscum in children should raise suspicion for sexual abuse.

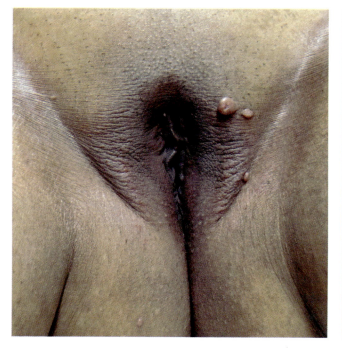

FIGURE 3.7 Classical discreet dome-shaped papule with central dell. (Photograph by Dr Nina Madnani.)

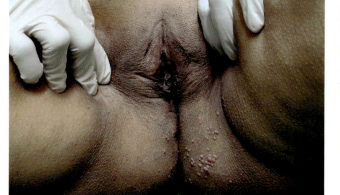

FIGURE 3.8 Molluscii can often involve areas beyond the vulva. (Photograph by Dr Nina Madnani.)

Dermoscopy

Characteristic findings include a central pore or umbilication, poly-lobular white-to-yellow amorphous structures and peripheral crown vessels (Figure 3.9). They can also have rosettes when seen under polarized light.

Laboratory Examination

Giemsa or Grams stain from the cheesy material demonstrates cytoplasmic molluscum bodies.

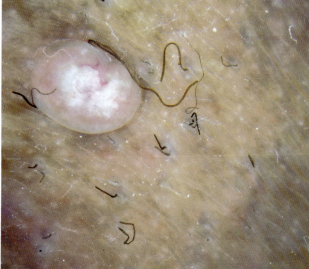

FIGURE 3.9 Dermoscopy reveals a central whitish area surrounded by vessels resembling a crown. Dinolite Digital Microscope WF-20, polarized, 10×. (Photograph by Dr Nina Madnani.)

Histopathology

The histopathology shows the presence of large intracytoplasmic eosinophilic inclusion bodies with a small peripheral nucleus, the Henderson-Paterson bodies, in the hyperplastic epidermis (Figure 3.10).

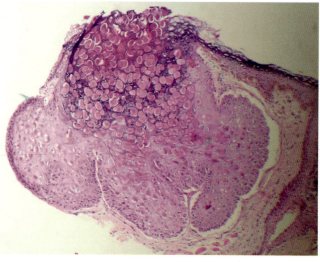

FIGURE 3.10 H & E, 100×, bulbous follicular infundibular proliferation with numerous molluscum bodies in mid and upper spinous layers. (Photograph by Dr Rajiv Joshi.)

Differential diagnosis

Differential diagnosis includes genital warts and syringoma. In an immunocompromised patient, it must be differentiated from cryptococcosis, histoplasmosis and penicillosis.

Genital warts (condyloma accuminata) are single or multiple papules with a rough, warty surface ranging from pink to red to brown in color.

Vulvar syringoma are multiple, discrete, firm dark brown papules seen on the inner surface of the labia majora. They can be pruritic. Peri-orbital syringoma may co-exist in some patients.

Cryptococcosis, Histoplasmosis and penicillosis are fungal infections that clinically present as umbilicated papules with central necrosis or hemorrhagic crusts. These papules usually have a generalized distribution. Associated findings like fever, weight loss and cough may exist.

Course and prognosis

MC is a self-limiting disease, but lesions may take months or years to regress. It is not uncommon for new lesions to develop before they disappear.

Treatment

Patients should avoid shaving, waxing or sharing towels and beddings. Several topical and systemic treatment modalities are in use but with variable results.

Lesions can be curetted with a molluscum curette or enucleated with a needle or chemically cauterized with trichloroacetic acid or potassium hydroxide at 1–2 weekly intervals. Cryotherapy with a fine applicator tip and electrodessication are other alternatives. Immunomodulatory therapy with the application of imiquimod can be used, but an irritant reaction can be a deterrent.

Pearl

Genital molluscum in children is mainly due to autoinoculation, but sexual abuse must be considered and investigated.

Recommended reading

1. Meza-Romero R, et al. Clin Cosmet Investig Dermatol (2019). PMID: 31239742.
2. Ianhez M, et al. An Bras Dermatol (2011). PMID: 21437525.
3. Edwards S, et al. J Eur Acad Dermatol Venereol (2021). PMID: 32881110.

Genital warts

Nisha Chaturvedi

Introduction

Human papillomavirus (HPV) causes various diseases like condyloma acuminata (genital warts), vulvar intraepithelial neoplasia and squamous cell carcinoma affecting the anogenital area depending on the viral type, host factor and local environmental factors.

Epidemiology

HPV is a double-stranded, non-enveloped DNA virus with icosahedral symmetry. It has more than 120 genotypes of which 40 subtypes can infect the anogenital area. Genotypes 6 and 11 are found in 90% of anogenital warts and are considered low-risk subtypes. HPV 16 and 18 are high-risk types and can induce vulvar intraepithelial neoplasia. HPV infections have been increasing across the world, but the exact incidence is unknown as many are asymptomatic or unreported. Genital HPV is transmitted primarily through sexual contact, although auto-transmission via warts on fingers has been reported. It is highly contagious with the rate of infectivity estimated at 60%.

Risk factors for genital warts include unprotected intercourse, multiple sexual partners, smoking, history of other sexually transmitted diseases, use of oral contraceptives and immunosuppression including pregnancy.

The incubation period ranges anywhere from 1 to 8 months with an average of 3 months.

Pathophysiology

HPV has an affinity to epithelial cells. Upon entry into the cell, HPV may remain dormant without any replication for prolonged periods of time (latent infection), or the virus may replicate, causing the clinical disease. Several studies estimate the rate of subclinical infection as high as 40%.

Presenting complaints

Women usually present with asymptomatic "boils" or growth/bumps on the vulva (Figure 3.11). Some may have symptoms of pruritus, burning, soreness and rarely pain. Larger lesions may emanate a foul smell.

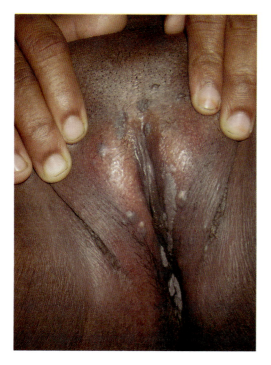

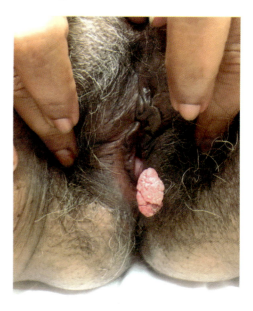

FIGURE 3.11 Skin colored to pigmented flat-topped papules with an irregular surface. (Photograph by Dr Nisha Chaturvedi.)

FIGURE 3.12 Single pedunculated polypoidal pinkish growth arising from the left labia resembling a verrucous carcinoma. (Photograph by Dr Nina Madnani.)

Clinical examination

The common sites involved are the introitus, labia majora, labia minora, posterior fourchette and perianal area. They can also occur intravaginally, on the cervix, or involve the urethral meatus.

Genital warts can vary in size and presentation. Some may be small, ranging from 1 to 4 mm papules or grow several inches in diameter, especially in pregnancy. Others may be pedunculated, cauliflower shaped, dome shaped or flat (Figure 3.12). They are frequently seen in clusters but can also present as a solitary keratotic papule or plaque. When present on the mucosa, they may vary in color from white to pink, purple or red, and on keratinized skin, they may be brown, gray or black. Giant condyloma accuminata of Buschke and Löwenstein (HPV subtypes 6 and 11) clinically presents as a large exophytic cauliflower-like mass (Figure 3.13). It is a low-grade, locally invasive tumor which rarely metastasizes.

Dermoscopy

Dermoscopy depends on the morphology of genital warts. Sessile lesions show dotted vessels and a whitish network (mosaic pattern), while

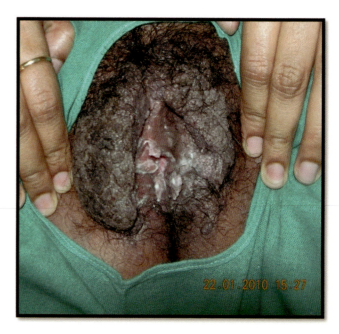

FIGURE 3.13 Tumor-like verrucous growth obliterating both labia. (Buschke-Lowenstein tumor). (Photograph by Dr Nina Madnani.)

Systemic findings

Warts may be seen in other mucosal areas like oral, laryngeal, rarely conjunctival and nasal. Digits should always be examined for peri-ungual warts.

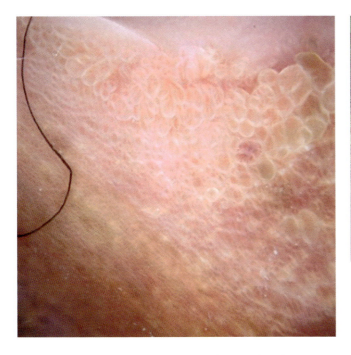

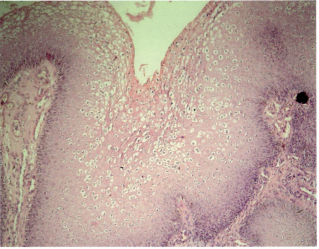

FIGURE 3.15 H & E, 100×, papillated epidermal hyperplasia with numerous vacuolated cells in upper spinous layers.

FIGURE 3.14 Dermoscopy shows closely aggregated, digitate and knob-like projections with a single dotted vessel within. Dinolite Digital Microscope WF-20, polarized, 10×. (Photograph by Dr Nina Madnani.)

pedunculated/cauliflower-like lesions show whitish finger-like projections with elongated dilated vessels within (finger-like pattern) (Figure 3.14). Knob-like, brain-like and nonspecific patterns have also been described.

Laboratory examination

In the majority of the patients, clinical history and careful examination is adequate for the diagnosis. A speculum examination must be done in all women with anogenital warts to identify the presence of co-existing vaginal and/or cervical warts. Mild or subclinical cases can be identified by the use of a 3–5% acetic acid solution (acetowhite test) in which the suspected lesion turns grayish white. A biopsy is indicated only when malignancy is suspected or to distinguish it from vulvar papillomatosis.

Detection and typing of HPV are currently not recommended for the diagnosis and management of genital warts.

Histopathology

The epidermis shows papillomatosis, acanthosis with thick elongated rete ridges (Figure 3.15), and

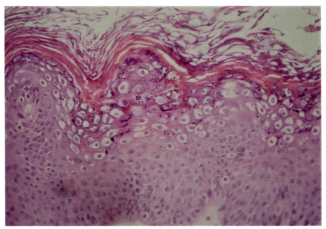

FIGURE 3.16 H & E, 200×, Owl's eye cells characteristic of verruca seen in the upper spinous zone. (Photograph by Dr Rajiv Joshi.)

moderate granulomatosis with the characteristic presence of koilocytes (HPV-infected epithelial cell) (Figure 3.16). Increased vascularization with the presence of thrombosed capillaries may be seen in the dermis.

Differential diagnosis

Genital warts must be differentiated from various conditions like vestibular papillomatosis, MC, seborrheic keratosis, fordyce spots, lichen planus, condyloma lata, skin tags and rarely, linear epidermal verrucus nevus (Figure 3.17).

Vestibular papillomatosis are uniformly arranged, symmetrical, monomorphic, soft pink papillae seen

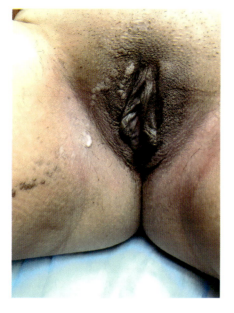

FIGURE 3.17 Linear epidermal verrucus nevus mistaken for vulvar warts. (Photograph by Dr Nina Madnani.)

on inner labia and vestibule and are considered as a normal variant of the vulvar epithelium (Figure 3.18).

MC are dome-shaped, pearly white, umbilicated papules.

Fordyce's spots (enlarged sebaceous glands) are small, grouped yellowish papules seen on the labia minora.

Seborrheic keratoses appear as single or multiple verrucous, well-circumscribed, brown to black pigmented papules ranging from 2 to 10 mm in size. Some lesions may have a stuck-on appearance.

Acrochordon (skin tags) are soft, single or multiple, brown or skin-colored, pedunculated growths particularly seen on inguinal folds or the labia majora.

Papules of lichen planus are flat-topped, and violaceous, seen on the labia majora and mons pubis. Lesions on the inner surface of the labia minora look whitish. Similar lesions can be seen elsewhere.

Condyloma lata are cutaneous lesions of secondary syphilis characteristically seen as pale, broad, flat whitish papules seen in the perianal area, vulva and cervix. Similar papules can also be seen in other areas like the angle of mouth, nose, inframammary region and axillae.

Course and prognosis

HPV infections can clear spontaneously, but in 10–20% of women, these infections persist, and they are at risk for progression to grade 2/3 cervical intraepithelial neoplasm and, in which if left untreated, can eventually develop into an invasive cancer of the cervix. Very often HPV infections may co-exist with other bacterial or fungal infections (Figure 3.19).

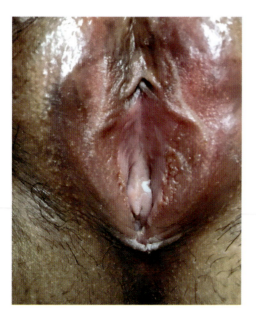

FIGURE 3.18 Pink, smooth, digitate projections on the mucosa of left labia minora. Often mistaken for vestibular papillomatosis. (Photograph by Dr Nina Madnani.)

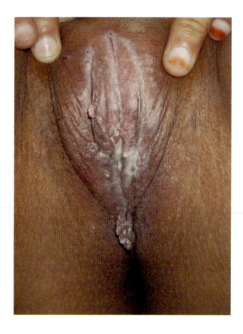

FIGURE 3.19 Patient with co-existing verrucae and vulvovaginal candidiasis. (Photograph by Dr Nisha Chaturvedi.)

Treatment

A wide range of therapeutic options are available for the treatment of genital warts such as cyto-destructive methods (surgical excision, cryotherapy, laser therapy, electrosurgery, podophyllotoxin, podophyllin, trichloroacetic acid), immunomodulation (imiquimod, sinecatechins), antivirals (cidofovir, interferons) and 5-fluorouracil. The choice of treatment is dictated by many factors including size, location, extent of the lesion, cost of treatment and patient preference.

Cryotherapy, electrosurgery and surgical excision can be used to treat warts in pregnancy

The success rate of each modality is very variable and recurrences are almost a norm. Multiple treatments and use of multiple methods may be required.

Gardasil (Quadrivalent) and Cervirax (bivalent) are two vaccines approved by the USFDA. Gardasil is approved for females and males, 9–26 years of age, to prevent anogenital warts, anogenital dysplasia and cancers.

Pearls

Biopsy should be deferred for a few weeks after podophyllin application as histopathologic changes may resemble vulvar intraepithelial neoplasia and lead to a false diagnosis.

Recommended reading

1. Yanofsky VR, et al. J Clin Aesthet Dermatol (2012). PMID: 22768354.
2. Chatterjee M, et al. Indian Dermatol Online J (2021). PMID: 33768019.

Tinea cruris

Nina Madnani

Introduction

Tinea has become endemic in India. Recurrences and frequent relapses are the norm, in spite of proper dosing of anti-fungal medications for adequate periods.

Epidemiology

Tinea Cruris (Jock's itch or Dhobi's itch) is a superficial fungal infection caused by dermatophytes. The three genera include *Trichophyton* (T), *Epidermophyton* (E) and *Microsporum* (M).

In the last decade, there has been a change in the spectrum of dermatophytes and while *T. mentagrphytes* is common in the northern parts of India, *T. rubrum* remains the culprit in southern parts of India. The exact incidence is not known, but there has been an alarming increase in the number of cases in the past decade. This condition is generally seen post puberty and some predisposing factors include hot humid environment, excessive sweating, tight clothing, diabetes, immunosuppressive medications, topical corticosteroid use and infection in other family members (common cause in infants and children). Intimate contact with a partner suffering from tinea genitalis may transfer infection.

Pathophysiology

Dermatophytes produce keratin-digesting enzymes which allow them to grow on the skin and hair. Their spread is restricted to the epidermis, and clinical features are seen due to the inflammatory response to this infection. External factors and local host immune response produce a varied clinical presentation. This is especially true if hair removal procedures are done prior to sexual intimacy.

Presenting complaints

Patients complain of a severely itchy rash, which distracts them from doing day-to-day activities. The itch may worsen in the evening and upon removing clothes when back from work. In severe cases, it may cause sleep disruption. Some may complain of unsightly dark patches.

Clinical examination

Characteristic presentation is of a hyperpigmented scaly plaque with central clearing (Figure 3.20). The advancing border has erythematous papules and pustules with varying degrees of inflammation. The plaque may be annular, polycyclic or geographic (Figure 3.21).

Sites generally involved are the genito-crural folds, upper medial thighs (Figure 3.22). Post-inflammatory hyperpigmentation is seen on areas which have cleared and may extend onto the mons pubis and buttocks (Figure 3.23).

This presentation is significantly different in patients who have used topical steroids.

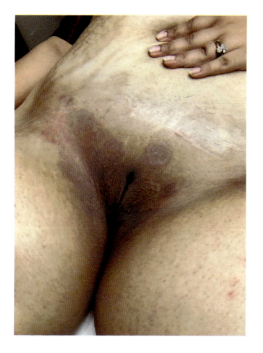

FIGURE 3.20 Typical annular pigmented plaque with active border on the pubis. (Photograph by Dr Nina Madnani.)

In steroid-modified tinea (Tinea incognito), there is minimal or no scaling; the inflammation is subdued and extends much beyond the site of initial infection. Other signs of steroid abuse

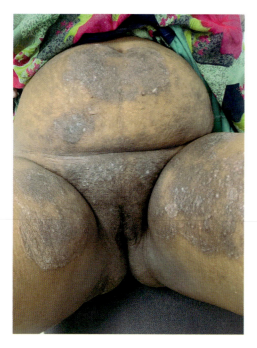

FIGURE 3.21 Extensive, intensely pigmented scaly patches with polycyclic border. (Photograph by Dr Nisha Chaturvedi.)

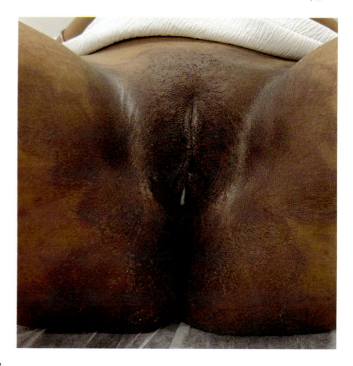

FIGURE 3.22 This obese lady has extensive involvement of her vulva, upper medial thighs going back to involve the buttocks. (Photograph by Dr Nisha Chaturvedi.)

may be noted including hypopigmentation, atrophy and striae formation (Figure 3.24). A pseudo imbricata pattern (Tinea indecisiva) may be seen and an increased incidence of Majocchi's granuloma has been described.

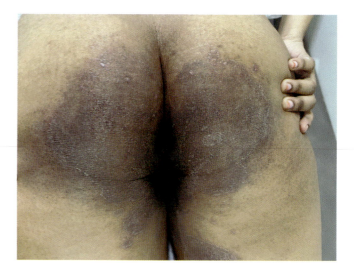

FIGURE 3.23 The Same patient with involvement of the buttocks. (Photograph by Dr Nisha Chaturvedi.)

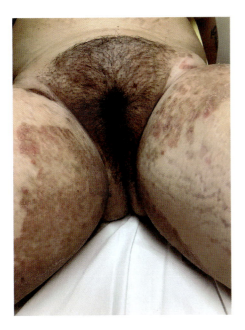

FIGURE 3.24 Many patients apply triple combination creams containing super-potent corticosteroids as a therapy for their tinea, resulting in extensive striae. (Photograph by Dr Nisha Chaturvedi.)

Systemic findings

Other body parts must be examined for tinea including face, truck and other body folds (especially in steroid-modified tinea) (Figure 3.25). Always check for nail and feet involvement.

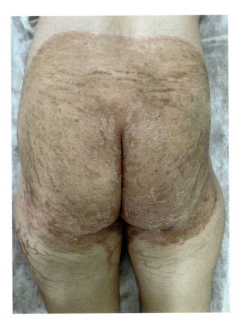

FIGURE 3.25 Examination of buttocks is important in a woman with vulvar tinea. (Photograph by Dr Nisha Chaturvedi.)

Dermoscopy

Dermoscopy findings differ based on the duration of the disease rather than age or site of involvement. Early lesions have red, reddish-brown dots and globules corresponding to exudate and extravasated red blood cells. Older lesions have brown-black dots and globules due to post-inflammatory changes. Scales are much more abundant in older lesions than in newer lesions (except in steroid-modified tinea) (Figure 3.26).

Laboratory examination

Diagnosis is based on clinical features, but in resistant tinea, steroid-modified tinea and for species identification, skin scraping and fungal cultures can be done.

Direct microscopy of skin scraping mounted in 10% KOH shows branched septate hyphae. Arthrospores may or may not be seen.

Selective culture media should include Emmons' modification of Sabouraud's dextrose agar and dermatophyte test medium.

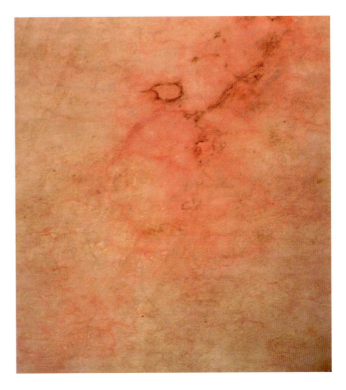

FIGURE 3.26 Dermoscopy of the steroid-modified tinea shows evidence of atrophy, telangiectatic vessels and irregular scales. Dinolite Digital Microscope WF-20, polarize 10×. (Photograph by Dr Nina Madnani.)

Histopathology

An hematoxylin and eosin (H & E) section of a well-established lesion shows parakeratotic foci, acanthosis and dermal edema with a chronic inflammatory infiltrate. A periodic acid-Schiff (PAS) stain reveals septate hyphae in the stratum corneum

Differential diagnosis

Differential diagnosis includes eczema, seborrheic dermatitis, inverse psoriasis, Hailey-Hailey disease, intertrigo and extra-mammary Paget's disease.

Eczema usually involves the genitocrural folds and may extend onto the labia majora or perianal areas as erythematous to scaly patches.

Inverse psoriasis is often difficult to differentiate from a tinea but tends to be more erythematous, very well demarcated and restricted in the inguinal folds. There is characteristic absence of scales with a glazed appearance. Similar lesions may be seen in other body folds.

Seborrheic dermatitis shows well-defined erythema with greasy yellow scales within the folds extending onto the labia majora. Non-genital sites such as scalp, eyebrows, naso-labial folds, chest and upper back may be involved.

Intertrigo is commonly seen in the body folds of obese or geriatric individuals and can start as mild erythema and evolve into a red plaque. Satellite pustules help to make the diagnosis.

Patients with Hailey-Hailey disease may present with erosions, flaccid lesions or crusts in the crural folds, giving a wet-tissue appearance. There is no central clearing.

Very rarely, vulvar porokeratosis can be mistaken for tinea infection (Figure 3.27).

Extramammary Paget's disease, a rare disease, can present with a well-defined erythematous, crusted scaly plaque in the groin, extending onto the labia majora, minora, clitoris and clitoral hood. Eczematous patches not responding to topical corticosteroid treatment are a clue to the diagnosis.

Course and prognosis

Untreated genital tinea can persist for months or years, gradually enlarging to involve extensive areas and distant sites by contiguous spread

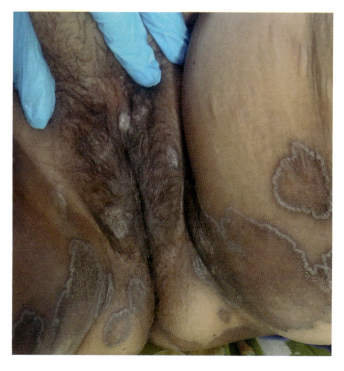

FIGURE 3.27 Vulvar porokeratosis with classical annular lesions, central clearing and a raised border. Note the absence of scaling. (Photograph by Dr Dipti Desai.)

or autoinoculation. Secondary bacterial infection may be seen in patients with poor hygiene or reduced immunity. Chronic infections lasting for more than 6 months, frequent relapses and recurrences, and resistant infections have been reported due to topical steroid use.

Treatment

General measures are as important as a pharmacological treatment to improve outcomes and prevent recurrences. It is advisable to wear loose cotton clothes and avoid synthetics. Clothes are to be washed daily and sun-dried if possible. Ironing also adds to the sanitization of fomites. Soaps, towels and personal clothes should not be shared and should be washed separately. Weight loss is encouraged in obese and over-weight individuals. Strict sugar control in diabetics is recommended. All infected members of a family should be treated together.

Topical antifungals are recommended mainly in infants and children with limited lesions. These may not suffice for extensive infection, especially that which is steroid-modified. Azoles (miconazole, clotrimazole, ketoconazole and econazole) applied twice a day for 2–3 weeks and an additional 1–2 weeks post-clearing are effective. Topical terbinafine and ciclopirox olamine have an added advantage by virtue of their anti-inflammatory effect. The addition of creams and lotions containing paramoxine hydrochloride gives better relief from itching. These applications are applied in a circular motion starting 1 cm beyond the active margins up to the center.

Extensive infection, especially steroid-modified, requires systemic antifungals. The standard dosing may not be sufficient to eradicate the infection and increasing the dose and/or duration may be required like terbinafine 250 mg twice daily, fluconazole 150–300 mg bi weekly, for 6–8 weeks or itraconazole 200–400 mg daily for 2–4 weeks.

In India, a popular local application called Sapat Malam (contains salicylic acid and tolnaftate) often causes an irritant reaction (Figure 3.28).

Pearls
Tinea in darker skin types results in prolonged post-inflammatory hyperpigmentation, which is distressing for the patient

Proper disinfection of the fomites plays an important role in preventing recurrences.

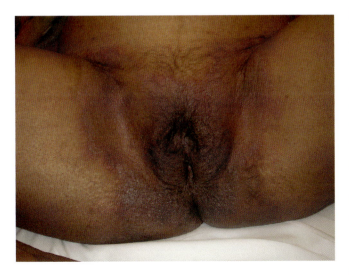

FIGURE 3.28 Topical applications of salicylic acid used on this tinea infection have resulted in an irritant reaction. The polycyclic border is evident at the periphery. (Photograph by Dr Nisha Chaturvedi.)

Recommended reading
1. Thakur R, et al. Clin Cosmet Investig Dermatol (2020). PMID: 33061514.
2. Luchsinger I, et al. Sex Transm Infect (2015). PMID: 26071391.
3. Ankad BS, et al. Indian Dermatol Online J (2020). PMID: 32477979.

Vulvovaginal candidiasis
Nina Madnani

Introduction
Vulvovaginal candidiasis (VVC) is the second-most common cause of vaginal discharge in a woman.

Epidemiology
VVC usually occurs in the child-bearing age when estrogen levels are high, and the vaginal pH is acidic i.e. < 4.5. It may rarely occur in infants due to maternal hormones. VVC affects the skin and mucous membranes. Ninety percent of cases are caused by *Candida albicans*. The remaining are caused by *C. tropicalis, C. krusei, C. parapsilosis, C. pseudotropicalis* and *C. glabrata*. The non-candida species are often non-pathogenic or cause mild symptoms. *C. albicans* is a normal commensal of the vulva in 20% women, and frequently colonizes the moist, warm, intertriginous folds.

Pathophysiology
The woman has to be genetically predisposed to develop VVC. Skin barrier damage with tight clothing, diapers sweating, and endocrine disorders like hypothyroidism, Cushing's disease, Addison's disease and diabetes are some of the predisposing factors. Topical and systemic corticosteroid use aggravates the issue. Antibiotic treatment, high-dose estrogen-containing contraceptives, obesity, anemia, malnutrition and HIV can also be contributory (Figure 3.29).

Presenting complaints
The woman usually complains of intense vulvovaginal itching, burning, soreness or dyspareunia, with or without a vulvovaginal discharge. Often she reports a premenstrual flare with each cycle. Rarely, the woman may have a colorless discharge.

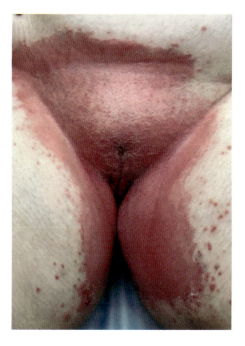

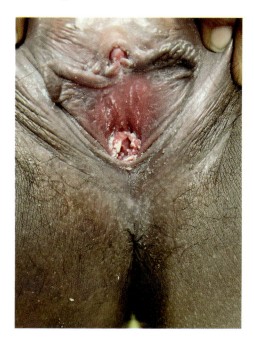

FIGURE 3.29 Obese patients with lighter skin types can manifest as intense erythema. (Photograph by Dr Nina Madnani.)

Clinical examination
Gentle separation of the labia reveals an erythematous vulva with thick curdy-white discharge adherent to the vaginal walls (Figures 3.30 and 3.31).

FIGURE 3.31 Thick yellowish curdy discharge seen at the introitus resembling cottage cheese. (Photograph by Dr Nina Madnani.)

Satellite papulo-pustules may be seen (Figure 3.32). Fissures or edema complicate the condition in severe cases. A per-speculum examination is painful and often not allowed by the patient in view of

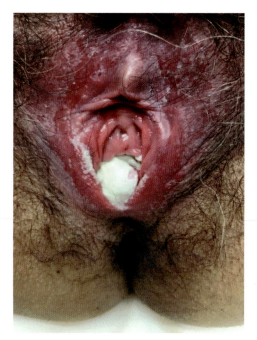

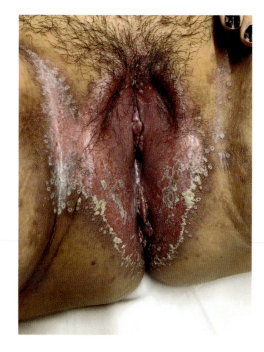

FIGURE 3.30 Profuse, creamy discharge with intense erythema. (Photograph by Dr Nina Madnani.)

FIGURE 3.32 Extensive VVC involving the genito-crural fold with characteristic satellite pustules. Erythema, satellite pustules and scaling can mimic psoriasis. (Photograph by Dr Nina Madnani.)

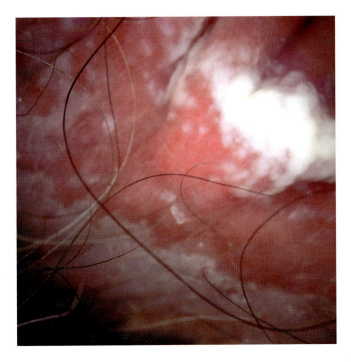

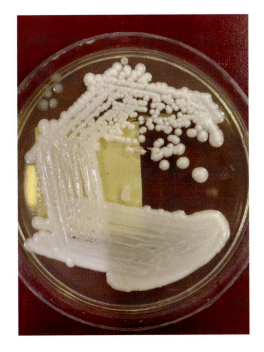

FIGURE 3.33 Structureless white area corresponding to the candida colonies and erythematous background with blurred blood vessels. (Photograph by Dr Nina Madnani.)

FIGURE 3.34 Creamy, grayish-white colonies of *Candida albicans* on Sabourauds medium. (Photograph by Dr Nina Madnani.)

her pain. A simple pH strip evaluation reveals an acidic pH, which corroborates the diagnosis.

Dermoscopy
Dermoscopy of candidial infection has been described as whitish areas corresponding to the colonies of the yeast and blurred vessels on an erythematous background (Figure 3.33).

Laboratory Examination
A KOH mount from a vaginal swab shows highly refractile budding yeasts forming pseudohyphae (100% specific). The species are gram positive.

Culture on Sabourauds medium shows grayish moist colonies (Figure 3.34). Reconfirmation is done with smears stained with lactophenol which show budding yeast and pseudohyphae.

Histopathology
Biopsies are only done when the diagnosis is in doubt. PAS stains will show pseudohyphae in the upper stratum corneum (Figure 3.35).

Differential diagnosis
Candidial vulvitis is commonly confused with inverse psoriasis, intertrigo, seborrhoeic dermatitis and Hailey-Hailey disease.

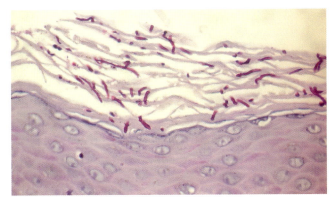

FIGURE 3.35 H & E, 400×, PAS-positive, vertically oriented pseudohyphae of Candida in the stratum corneum. (Photograph by Dr Rajiv Joshi.)

Flexural psoriasis typically has a bright pink color, with no or minimal scales. The involved skin is well-demarcated. Other body folds may be involved.

Seborrheic dermatitis has typical yellowish, greasy, adherent scales. Other seborrheic sites such as the scalp, nasolabial folds, chest and back may be involved.

Intertrigo is usually seen in obese individuals as a result of friction, well demarcated with maceration or fissuring.

Lesions in Hailey-Hailey disease are moist with flaccid vesicles involving the body folds, as also the inner surface of the labia and perianal area. Itching is a prominent complaint. Patients complain of a musty odor from their lesions.

Course and prognosis

Untreated, VVC can persist, causing the severe quality of life issues. Sexual intimacy becomes almost impossible. Women may have a single episode or multiple episodes depending upon their genetic susceptibility.

Treatment

The treatment depends on the number of infections per year. More than 4 per year are denoted as recurrent VVC. Uncomplicated cases do well with topicals. Clotrimazole 1% or miconazole 1% or fenticonazole 2% or butoconazole 2% or terconazole 5%, 5 g local application daily for 1–2 weeks, is usually curative. Vaginal pessaries are another option. Clotrimazole 100 mg intravaginally daily for 7 days or 200 mg every night for 3 nights or 1200 mg single dose. When systemic medication is required, fluconazole 150 mg single dose or ketoconazole 200 mg bid or 400 mg single dose or itraconazole 200 mg bid or 400 mg single dose is prescribed. For recurrent or complicated cases, systemic treatment needs to continue for 6 months and includes fluconazole 150 mg weekly, or ketoconazole 100 mg daily or itraconazole. If these fail, compounded boric acid pessaries 600 mg for day 1–5 of the periods for 6 months. Oteseconazol and Ibrexafungerp are new fungicidal drugs in the pipeline for resistant *C. albicans*.

Pearls

Candidiasis is not a sexually transmitted infection (STI).

Sexual partners may contract candidial balanitis only if genetically susceptible or with co-morbid conditions.

A vaginal pH < 4.5 helps to corroborate the diagnosis.

Recommended reading

1. Farr A, et al. Mycoses (2021). PMID: 33529414.
2. Mtibaa L, et al. J Mycol Med (2017). PMID: 28314677.
3. Kalia N, et al. Ann Clin Microbiol Antimicrob (2020). PMID: 31992328.

Pityriasis versicolor

Nina Madnani

Introduction

Pityriasis versicolor (adj. of various colors) gets its name from the various colors seen in clinical presentation. In dark-skinned individuals, it tends to be either hypo or hyperpigmented. Vulvar involvement is uncommon and may be seen in women with extensive infections or in the immunocompromised.

Epidemiology

It is caused by a dimorphic fungus, Malassezia, and is almost ubiquitous in hot tropical countries. These exist as normal flora, in the individuals, waxing and waning over the various seasons. The most commonly identified species include *Malassezia furfur, Malassezia Globosa* and *Malassezia sympodalis*. Seen more commonly in adolescent and young adults, other predisposing factors include genetics, excessive sweating, a hot humid climate, diabetes, systemic corticosteroids or other immunosuppressants, and malnutrition.

Pathophysiology

Under favorable conditions (humidity, sweating, oil application etc) in genetically susceptible individuals, the dimorphic, lipophilic yeast changes from spore form to the pathogenic mycelial form. In this form, it produces azelaic acid, which causes discoloration and hence the varied colors.

Presenting complaints

The patient may be unaware, and the infection may be detected during a casual examination. Patients are asymptomatic but occasionally complain of itch. Most patients will notice dark or discolored spots and seek help for cosmesis.

Clinical examination

The characteristic lesion is a well-defined hypopigmented/erythematous/brown or hyperpigmented, macule covered with fine scales (Figure 3.36). The scales become accentuated upon scratching with a glass slide (scratch test). The macules coalesce to form larger patches.

There is no distinct distribution pattern and lesions can be seen on the thighs, buttocks, groins and pubic areas.

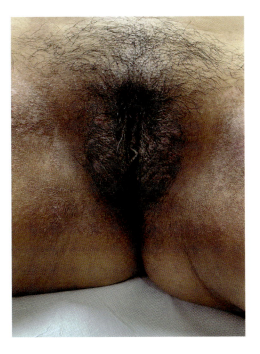

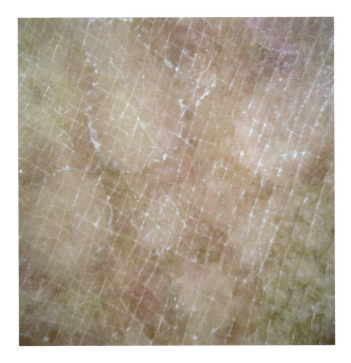

FIGURE 3.36 Areas of hypopigmented scaly lesions on both thighs in an obese lady with Lichen simplex. (Photograph by Dr Nina Madnani.)

Systemic findings
Similar scaly patches may be seen on the face (esp children), chest, shoulders and upper back.

Dermoscopy
Non-uniform pigmentation, perilesional or marginal hyperpigmentation and mild patchy scaling are some of the dermoscopic features described in literature. Wire-Fence pattern (fine scaling along the skin markings) may be a clue to the diagnosis (Figure 3.37).

Laboratory examination
Wood's lamp examination reveals a yellow-orange fluorescence characteristic of a *M. furfur* infection.

A skin scraping mounted in 10% KOH or tape-stripping stained with Parker-Q ink will show characteristic spores and mycelia describes as the "spaghetti-meatballs" appearance.

Specialized media like Sabourauds dextrose-agar + chloramphenicol + olive oil will yield yellowish colonies within a week.

Histopathology
A biopsy(rarely required) from the lesion shows an orthokeratotic stratum corneum with bluish spores and hyphae. These stain pink with the PAS stain and are easy to identify.

FIGURE 3.37 Selected PV-dermoscopy showing the fish-net pattern of scaling along skin crease, altered pigment network and hyperpigmentation around areas of hypopigmentation. Dinolite Digital Microscope WF-20, polarized, 10×. (Photograph by Dr Nina Madnani.)

Differential diagnosis
Seborrheic dermatitis has characteristic yellowish-greasy scales limited in the inguinal folds. Patients tend to be itchy and involvement of other areas like the scalp, naso-labials, chest and back may provide additional clues.

Vitiligo patches are depigmented, well defined and usually larger with no scaling. Woods lamp reveals bright white fluorescence due to the lack of pigment.

Erythrasma tends to be more confluent, involving the inguinal folds and inner thighs. There is bright red fluorescence under the woods lamp.

Course and prognosis
If untreated, the infection persists with no additional symptoms.

Treatment
Topical antifungals including terbinafine 1%, ciclopirox olamine 1% or miconazole cream, applied twice daily for 2 weeks, should be used. Systemic itraconazole 200 mg od for 7 days or fluconazole 400 mg single dose is also effective.

Pearls

Infection due to non-obligatory Malassezia species may not fluoresce under Woods Lamp.

Selenium sulfide or ketoconazole shampoo application is not recommended on the genitals due to the potential of irritation

Recommended reading

1. Gupta AK, et al. J Fungi (Basel) (2015). PMID: 29376896.
2. Mathur M, et al. Cosmet Investig Dermatol (2019). PMID: 31118732.

Folliculitis and furunculoses

Kaleem Khan

Introduction

The vulva, by virtue of its follicular density, is prone to the development of infections which track along the hair follicle. This is especially true for women living in hot humid climates. Depending upon the depth of infection, it may be superficial (folliculitis) or deep with intense inflammation (furuncle). Two or more confluent furuncles constitute a carbuncle but are rarely seen in the perineum.

Epidemiology

Vulvar folliculitis is seen in post-pubertal women and is frequently caused by *S. aureus* but occasionally by *Pseudomonas aeruginosa* (hot tub folliculitis) or other gram-negative organisms. Non-bacterial causes include dermatophyte and candidial infection. Furuncles are seen in the adolescent age group, in obesity, diabetics or immunocompromised individuals. *S. aureus* is the commonest causative organism.

Pathophysiology

Compromised skin integrity allows *S. aureus* infection to track deeper into the skin along the hair follicle, causing an intense inflammation in the subcutaneous tissue. Factors which compromise the skin integrity include pressure, friction, increased sweating and hair-removal procedures. Persistent scratching in diseases like atopic dermatitis, dermatophyte infection and lichen simplex chronicus can cause superficial erosions, which allow entry of the bacteria. Wearing tight thick trousers aka jeans in a hot humid environment is also a major contributing factor.

Presenting complaints

Patients complain of an abrupt onset of tiny painful pustules, some of which rupture to form raw areas. This sometimes follows a hair-removal procedure like waxing or shaving. Sometimes, the deeper infection presents as a painful hard lump, which rapidly enlarges only to become soft with a central point of pus discharge. Upon rupture, there is a dehiscence of pain.

Clinical examination

In folliculitis, the primary lesion is a small, dome-shaped pustule around the follicular ostia with a rim of surrounding erythema. The pustule ruptures easily to leave a superficial erosion. Lesions tend to be grouped together in the hair-bearing areas viz pubis, labia majora, inner thighs and buttocks.

A furuncle presents as a well-defined, erythematous, firm, tender nodule with a pus point at the summit (Figure 3.38). These may be seen anywhere on the perineum but are more common on the pubis and inner thighs.

Systemic findings

Systemic features such as fever and increased respiratory rate are usually absent, but if present, they are ominous signs and suggest systemic bacteremia.

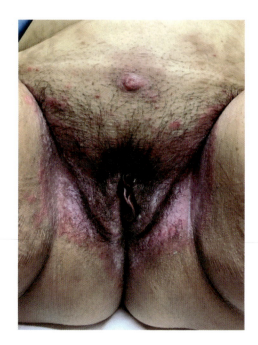

FIGURE 3.38 A large furuncle with multiple folliculitides in the suprapubic region is seen in this patient with poorly controlled inverse psoriasis. (Photograph by Dr Nina Madnani.)

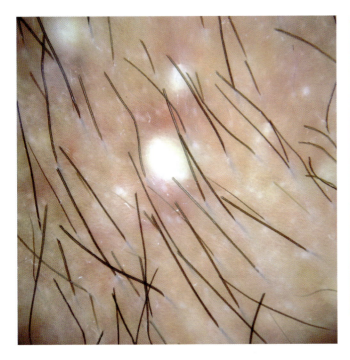

FIGURE 3.39 Dermoscopic image showing yellowish-white amorphous material with follicular localization and surrounding pinkish background. Dinolite Digital Microscope, WF-20, polarized, 10×. (Photograph by Dr Nina Madnani.)

Dermoscopy

Folliculo-centric, homogenous yellow area with linear and dotted vessels in seen is folliculitis (Figure 3.39).

Laboratory examination

A gram-stained smear from the pustule will demonstrate gram-positive cocci. Pus swabs for culture and antibiotic sensitivity must be done to identify the causative organism and dictate the correct choice of antibiotic to be used, especially in recurrent cases.

Differential diagnosis

Other diagnoses to be ruled out include:

Pseudo-folliculitis is due to ingrowing hairs and presents as firm papules with a coiled hair piercing through it. Itching and discomfort are the presenting complaints.

Lesions of MC are asymptomatic, firm and pearly white, with a central divot.

Infected dermoid cysts will have a punctum and a long-standing history of swelling before developing into an inflamed nodule.

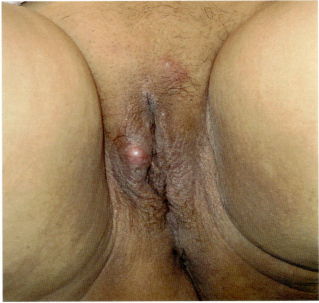

FIGURE 3.40 A large furuncle on the right labia majora which could be mistaken for a Bartholin cyst. Multiple small follicular pustules are also seen on the pubis. (Photograph by Dr Nina Madnani.)

An inflamed Bartholin gland should be suspected based on the location of the swelling i.e. junction between the middle and lower 1/3rd of the labia majora (Figure 3.40).

Lesions of hidradenitis suppurativa (HS) can be recognized by the presence of comedones, fibrous tracts, nodules and sinuses in the perineum, groins or similar lesions in the axilla or other body folds.

Course and prognosis

Untreated, most cases of folliculitis may spontaneously heal with post-inflammatory hyperpigmentation in darker skin type. Very rarely, keloidal scarring can occur in a genetically prone individual. A furuncle eventually ruptures with immediate relief of symptoms but only to recur at a different spot (Figure 3.41).

Treatment

Topical therapy is helpful in most cases. Twice daily application of mupirocin, fusidic acid or clindamycin is curative for superficial folliculitis. To prevent recurrences, the nasal carriage must be addressed. Prophylactic use of benzoyl peroxide or chlorhexidine washes has been recommended. Tight and occlusive clothing is to be avoided. Systemic treatment for furuncles must include

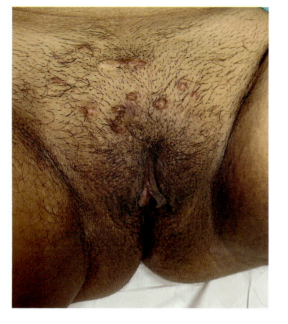

FIGURE 3.41 Notice the keloidal scarring over the pubis, following repeated episodes of folliculitis/furuncles. (Photograph by Dr Nina Madnani.)

first-generation cephalosporins (cefadroxil, cephalexin) up to 1–2 g per day. If no response or a resistant strain is suspected, appropriate antibiotics as per the sensitivity report should be administered. Warm compress helps in faster resolution.

In recurrent furunculosis, rifampicin and clindamycin combination should be considered.

Pearls
Suspect MRSA (methicillin-resistant *S. Aureus*) if unresponsive to conventional antibiotic treatment.

Recommended reading
1. Durupt F et al. Br J Dermatol (2007). PMID: 17916211.

Cellulitis
Kaleem Khan

Introduction
Cellulitis, an inflammation of the subcutaneous tissues, is seen in adults with increasing age. As with most bacterial infections, obesity, diabetes or an immunocompromised state are predisposing factors. Cellulitis in the vulvar area could be complicated by organisms from the urethra and the anal canal. MRSA has also been reported in acute vulvar infections.

Epidemiology
Streptococcus pyogenes (Group A streptococcus – GAS) is the causative organism in most cases, and *S. aureus* in a smaller number, though, in some, it may be a polymicrobial infection.

Pathophysiology
The pathogenic organism enters through a breach in the skin barrier caused by trauma or subclinical microinjuries, e.g. post hair-removal procedures. The infection rapidly spreads along the lymphatics (erysipelas) or into the deeper subcutaneous tissues (cellulitis).

Presenting complaints
The patient complains of a painful red-hot swelling accompanied with fever and constitutional symptoms. The skin feels tight and stretched, which makes walking difficult.

Clinical examination
Cellulitis can present as an ill-defined, erythematous plaque with induration (Figure 3.42). Usually, it is unilateral, involving the labia majora but can extend upwards to the groin or lower abdominal wall along the fascial planes. The overlying skin may have a "peau-d'-orange" appearance. Local

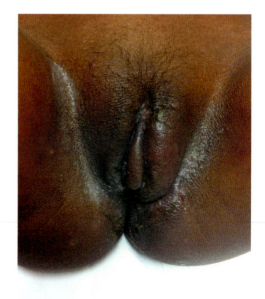

FIGURE 3.42 Erythema of cellulitis may not be evident in darker skin types. (Photograph by Dr Nina Madnani.)

draining lymph nodes may be tender and palpable. The affected area will be warm to touch and tender to touch.

Systemic findings
The patient may have constitutional symptoms like fever, malaise, tachycardia and lethargy.

Laboratory examination
There is leukocytosis with neutrophilia, elevated erythrocyte sedimentation rate (ESR) and C-reactive protein.

Differential diagnosis
Vulvar cellulitis must be differentiated from an abscess and early necrotizing fasciitis. Sometimes contact dermatitis and bite reactions may also pose a diagnostic dilemma.

A vulvar abscess or an infected Bartholin cyst can present in a similar way, but an abscess may be fluctuant, and a Bartholin cyst diagnosed by its location in the lower 1/3 of the labia (Figure 3.43).

Early-onset necrotizing fasciitis will have a history of penetrating trauma and the infection rapidly progresses from red to blue back within 24–48 hours. Anesthesia of the involved area is characteristic.

Acute irritant contact dermatitis is usually well-demarcated, erythematous or oozing, with a history of the application of a strong detergent/chemical usually for cleansing.

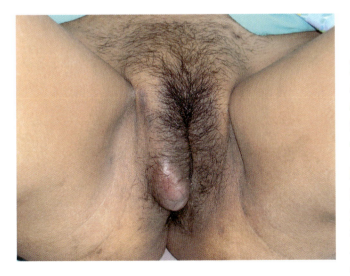

FIGURE 3.43 Cellulitis of the right labia majora showing a tense erythematous swelling. (Photograph by Dr Janak Maniar.)

Arthropod bites are usually multiple, and the bitten area may be identifiable.

Course and prognosis
Cellulitis requires immediate administration of appropriate systemic antibiotics in order to bring about resolution.

Treatment
Patients should be advised to avoid prolonged sitting or wearing tight clothes. Pus swabs and anti-bacterial sensitivity are ideally recommended for targeted therapy. Penicillins (amoxicillin + clavulanic acid) and first-generation cephalosporins (cephalexin, ceftriaxone, cefazolin) are most effective in uncomplicated cellulitis. Occasionally, tetracyclines (doxycycline, minocycline) and clindamycin can be used. Linezolid and vancomycin should be used when suspecting MRSA infection.

Pearl
A sharp 'cut-off' border is seen in erysipelas, whereas an indistinct border is suggestive of cellulitis.

Recommended reading
1. Raff AB, et al. JAMA (2016). PMID: 27434444.
2. Kim TH, et al. J Menopausal Med (2016). PMID: 27617247.

Streptococcal vulvovaginitis
Kaleem Khan

Introduction
Although streptococci *(Greek: streptos = chain, kokhos = berry)* are a part of the normal vaginal flora, it can cause severe infections with significant morbidity.

Epidemiology
Streptococcal vulvovaginal infection is seen in pre-pubescent girls (between 2 and 7 years of age), immunocompromised adults and post-pregnancy. *S. pyogenes* (GAS) is the most frequent causative organism. In immunocompromised adults and in pregnant women, *Streptococcus agalactiae* (GBS – Group B Streptococcus), a commensal in the vaginal mucosa, may also be the culprit organism.

Pathophysiology

Most patients have a history of (streptococcal) pharyngitis or of a streptococcal infection in a family member. Autoinoculation is the usual mode of transmission.

Presenting complaints

Most children cannot really voice their discomfort but may cry incessantly on passing urine. Associated perianal involvement may give rise to constipation, bleeding on passing stools, anal fissures and skin tags. Adults complain of irritation, soreness or dyspareunia and vaginal discharge.

Clinical examination

On separating the labia, a well-defined erythema can be noticed, with peripheral scaling (Figure 3.44). The vulvar erythema may extend backwards and become confluent with the perianal rash.

In adults, there may be a copious vaginal discharge which is watery, yellow-green or rarely purulent.

Systemic findings

Children may have associated pharyngitis and tonsillitis.

Laboratory examination

A swab for gram stain reveals purple coccoid bacteria in pairs or in chains. Culture (blood agar or Streptococcal Selective Media) shows the growth of translucent or white-gray opaque colonies surrounded by a zone of beta hemolysis.

Differential diagnosis

Important differentials include contact dermatitis, candidal vulvovaginitis and seborrheic dermatitis.

Contact dermatitis usually has a triggering allergen/irritant agent.

Seborrheic dermatitis has greasy scales with symptoms of itching. Lesions elsewhere help to confirm the diagnosis.

Candidiasis will have characteristic satellite pustules, bordering a bright red, sore vulva.

Course and prognosis

If untreated, the infection persists with severe discomfort.

Treatment

Topical application of mupirocin/fusidic acid multiple times a day effectively clears the rash (Figure 3.45). Second-generation cephalosporin (cefuroxime) should be the drug of choice at 20–30 mg/kg/day in two divided doses for 7 days, in cases not responding to topical treatment.

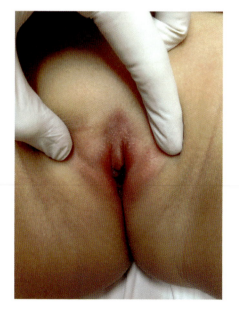

FIGURE 3.44 Bright red patch on the vulva extending onto the perianal area. (Photograph by Dr Nina Madnani.)

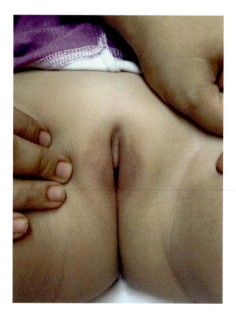

FIGURE 3.45 Same patient as earlier (Figure 3.44), showing complete resolution after topical therapy. (Photograph by Dr Nina Madnani.)

Pearls

Keeping the vulva and perianal area clean and dry can prevent recurrent episodes.

A seasonal exacerbation of streptococcal vulvitis in children is often seen in winter when pharyngitis is common.

Recommended reading

1. Kim TH, et al. J Menopausal Med (2016). PMID: 27617247.
2. Mirowski GW, et al. J Low Genit Tract Dis (2012). PMID: 22460276.

Erythrasma

Kaleem Khan

Introduction

Erythrasma is a non-itchy or mildly itchy condition seen usually in patients living in hot and humid climates and often associated with hyperhidrosis, poor hygiene, obesity and diabetes. It is uncommon in children and elderly.

Epidemiology

Erythrasma is caused by a gram-positive rod, *Corynebacterium minutissimum*, which is a normal skin commensal. The organism lives in the body folds, on the soles and in between the toes, but can affect the upper inner thighs and crural folds.

Pathophysiology

Excessive moisture in the genitocrural folds results in overgrowth of this commensal in the upper layers of the stratum corneum. The organism produces coproporphyrin III, and this may be used to identify the infection under a woods lamp.

Presenting complaints

This infection is usually asymptomatic but can occasionally be itchy. Patients complain of a dark patch in the groin fold or inner thighs.

Clinical examination

Well-defined, tan-colored or pinkish patch with fine scaling distributed in the inguinocrural folds, inner thighs or the perineum area. The skin appears wrinkled and is described as cigarette paper.

Systemic findings

Similar patches may be seen in the axilla, inframammary area or in the 4th toe webspace.

Laboratory examination

Woods Lamp examination reveals coral pink fluorescence due to the coproporphyrin III produced by the bacteria.

Differential diagnosis

Erythrasma must be differentiated from commonly encountered fungal infections in the inguinal folds including tinea cruris, intertrigo and pityriasis versicolor.

Tinea cruris also presents as scaly, pigmented plaques but has an inflamed active border. It is associated with intense pruritis.

Candidial intertrigo presents as a moist, macerated patch with erythema and satellite pustules.

Pityriasis versicolor has a remarkably similar presentation, but it is folliculo-centric and presents with fine branny scales which become prominent on scratching (scratch test positive).

Course and prognosis

This asymptomatic condition persists until treatment is initiated or there is a change in predisposing factors. In immunocompromised individuals, granuloma formation following deeper invasion into the tissue has been described.

Treatment

Topical applications of erythromycin, clindamycin, mupirocin, fusidic acid or miconazole are effective. Benzoyl peroxide washes are helpful adjuncts. Oral erythromycin 500 mg three times a day for 7–14 days usually clears the infection. A single dose of 1 gm clarithromycin is curative.

Pearls

Erythrasma has been seen to co-exist in at least 45% of inverse psoriasis lesions and can be detected by wood's light fluorescence.

If the affected area has been washed recently – there may not be any fluorescence on Woods lamp examination.

Patients of erythrasma can have co-existent trichomycosis pubis and pitted keratolysis.

Recommended reading

1. Forouzan P, et al. Cureus (2020). PMID 33145138.
2. Pinto M, et al. Indian Dermatol Online J (2016). PMID 27294050.
3. Janeczek M, et al. J Clin Aesthet Dermatol (2020). PMID 32308789.

Vulvar tuberculosis
Kaleem Khan

Introduction
India has the world's largest burden of tuberculosis (TB) with an incidence of 2.64 million at the rate of 193 per 100,000 population.

Epidemiology
Tuberculosis is caused by *Mycobacterium tuberculosis*, an aerobic bacillus. The incidence of genital TB in India varies from 1 to 26%, while in the USA, it is 1% (from infertility clinics). Vulvar TB makes up 2% of these cases. The incidence is higher in children and in women in the reproductive age group who may present with infertility. Predisposing factors for TB include endemic areas, poor living conditions, malnutrition and immune suppression due to HIV or medication. A resurgence is being seen due to a new class of drugs, the biologics.

Pathophysiology
Genital TB is most often due to hematogenous or lymphatic spread from a primary focus in the lungs or a distant organ. Vulvar involvement may be a direct extension from the uterus/cervix or urinary system, or from a sexual partner with active genitourinary TB. The host's immune response and prior exposure to the bacteria are responsible for the clinical presentation.

Presenting complaints
The patients may present with painless vulvar edema, ulceration or vaginal discharge. The patient, on further interrogation, may disclose a history of menstrual abnormalities or infertility.

Clinical examination
Primary inoculation lesion (following trauma, body piercings, tattoos) begins as a skin-colored/reddish nodule which enlarges slowly over 4–6 weeks and breaks down to form an ulcer (tuberculous chancre). The draining lymph nodes are enlarged. In a previously sensitized individual with high immunity, the nodule may become hyperkeratotic and enlarge without breakdown to form a verrucous plaque (tuberculosis verrucose cutis, TBVC).

Erosions and ulcers around the urethra extending up to the labia may be an extension of genitourinary TB (peri-orificial TB). Similarly, rectal TB may present with perianal fistulas.

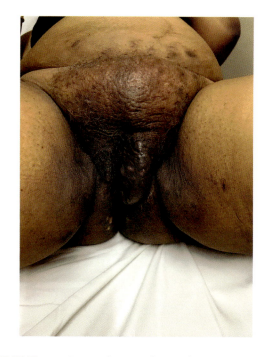

FIGURE 3.46 Vulvar tuberculosis esthiomene can mimic HS or Vulvar Chron's. (Photograph by Dr Nina Madnani.)

If the lesion is in the perineum or upper thighs, the draining inguinal lymph nodes will be enlarged and may suppurate to form discharging sinuses (scrofuloderma). They have a distinctly firm feel and are surprisingly painless (*cf* abscess); hence, also called as a cold abscess (Figure 3.46). The patient may present with a gradually enlarging asymmetric firm swelling, which may become woody hard. Separating the labia may reveal a foul-smelling discharge and granularity of the surfaces.

Systemic findings
If pulmonary TB is the primary focus of infection, the patient may have persistent cough and/or weight loss.

Dermoscopy
Dermoscopy findings consist of yellowish-white globules on a pinkish-red background. These are suggestive of dermal granulomas which are not specific to the tuberculous etiology.

Laboratory examination
X-ray chest should be done to rule out a pulmonary focus, while ultrasonography of the pelvis helps to rule out internal organ involvement.

An ESR may be elevated. HIV serology is recommended. A Mantoux test may have limited value in an endemic country like India, but when done along with interferon-γ release assays (IGRAs) e.g. QuantiFERON TB Gold, false-negative results are less than 2%.

A pus swab for acid-fast bacillus (AFB) staining may be helpful in suppurative lesions. Exudate or tissue culture is helpful only in 50% of the cases and may take up to 6 weeks for results. Running PCR assays or GeneXpert MTB on the samples provides faster and reliable results. TruNat TB test can diagnose TB within 1 hour. A biopsy is mandatory, and a fine needle aspiration cytology (FNAC) of any enlarged lymph nodes may reveal inflammatory cells.

Histopathology

A biopsy from the advancing edge of an ulcer or a nodule will provide a high yield for the diagnosis. Classic findings include epithelioid-cell granulomas with or without Langerhans giant cells in the upper and mid dermis. These have a variable mantle of lymphocytes (cf sarcoidosis) with a tendency to coalesce. Areas of caseation are seen but are not a norm. The overlying epidermis may show changes of hyperkeratosis and hyperplasia (TBVC) or may be thin, atrophic, ulcerated (Lupus vulgaris, scrofuloderma, orificial TB). AFB may have to be looked for but the lack of AFB does not rule out the diagnosis.

Differential diagnosis

Many genito-ulcerative diseases may have a similar presentation as genital TB and a high index of suspicion is required to make the correct diagnosis.

Most sexually transmitted disease like chancroid and herpes present as ulcers that are painful and have a history of short duration.

Crohn's disease and Hidradenitis suppurativa can also present with vulvar edema and discharging sinuses.

Cutaneous malignancies like squamous cell carcinomas present as slow-growing, painless ulcers, and a biopsy is the only definitive way to exclude them.

The ulcers of granuloma inguinal are painless and tissue smear showing Donovon bodies is diagnostic.

Course and prognosis

If untreated, the disease progresses to involve the surrounding skin and deeper structures. The lesions enlarge and ulcerate to form non-healing ulcers which may be secondarily infected, leading to scarring and disfigurement. Persistent sinus tracts and organized vulvar edema may be a consequence of the disease.

Treatment

With the availability of drug susceptibility testing (DST), WHO- formulated categories have been abandoned. Patients are grouped into "drug-susceptible" or "drug-resistant" TB. For drug susceptible TB, a combination of 4 drugs (isoniazid, rifampicin, ethambutol and pyrazinamide) is given for 2 months (intensive phase) followed by only 2 drug (isoniazid and rifampicin) for another 4–7 months(continuation phase). Bedaquiline and delamanid are newer drugs approved for treatment, especially in drug-resistant TB. Surgical excision should be considered only in cases of isolated lesions or in scrofuloderma.

Pearls

Women with infertility in the reproductive age group must be evaluated for genital TB.

Vulvar TB is an important differential in women with chronic vulvar edema.

Recommended reading

1. Ankad BS, et al. Indian Dermatol Online J (2020). PMID: 33344345.

Scabies

Kaleem Khan

Introduction

Scabies is a common, contagious infestation seen worldwide with the disease burden being highest in the tropical regions of the world.

Epidemiology

Scabies is caused by the infestation of an obligate, ecto-parasite *Sarcoptes scabiei* var. *hominis*. Prolonged skin-to-skin contact rather than fomites is the main mode of transmission. There is a bimodal peak, with infestations common in children less than 10 years and in the elderly. Sexual transmission, though uncommon, may be the reason in young adults. Overcrowding in an institutional setup, poverty, malnutrition and bed sharing are some of predisposing factors. Reduced pruritus in hemiplegics, immunosuppressed and those applying topical steroids are at a higher risk of extensive infestation.

Pathophysiology

The scabies mites are capable of surviving in the environment outside the human body for 24–36 hours and are capable of transmission during this time. The mite has an affinity for thin skin areas and fewer predilections for pilosebaceous-rich areas, which can explain the classical distribution of the rash. Most clinical symptoms are due to humoral and delayed hypersensitivity to the mite. Hence, clinical symptoms tend to appear early in previously sensitized individuals.

Presenting complaints

Patients complain of intense vulvar pruritus with nocturnal exacerbation. The itch may be localized initially but quickly becomes generalized.

Patients may also complain of rash on the body with some water-filled boils in the webspaces of the hand, the periumbilical area, and buttocks and groin.

Clinical examination

Vulvar examination reveals excoriation marks and scattered erythematous papules (Figure 3.47a and b). Unlike the male genital disease, the vulva seems to be spared of the typical burrows. The natal clefts, as also the place where the buttock joins the thigh, are the favored spots and must be examined for burrows (Figure 3.48).

The burrow is identified as a short, serpiginous gray or white line and represents the tunnel dug by the mite. Usually, there is a small papule or vesicle on the "blind" end of the burrow and is suggestive of a live mite. Previously sensitized individuals may present with nodular or vesiculobullous lesions. Secondary bacterial infection may complicate with pustules, crusts and eczematization.

The vulva may be involved as part of a generalized infection in Norwegian scabies and may present as thick plaques with scales. Burrows can be seen at the periphery of these plaques.

Systemic findings

There may be a generalized papular eruption in the disease of longer duration. The distribution

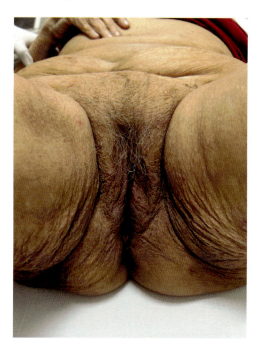

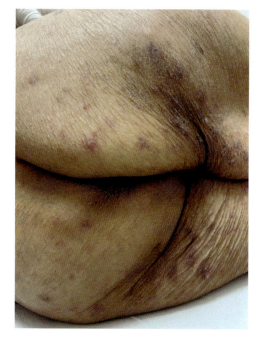

FIGURE 3.47 **(a and b)** Intensely pruritic, erythematous papules scattered over the vulva and the buttocks in this elderly patient. (Photographs by Dr Nisha Chaturvedi.)

may be around the nipples, anterior axillary folds, volar aspect of wrist, inter-digital web spaces, periumbilical skin and ankles (Circle of Hebra) (Figure 3.49). Bacterial sepsis and acute post-streptococcal glomerulonephritis have been described.

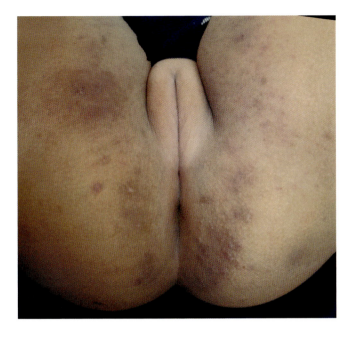

FIGURE 3.48 Excoriated papules in an eleven years old child with scabies. (Photograph by Dr Kavitha Athota.)

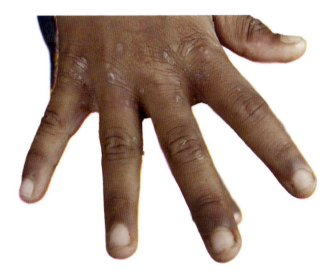

FIGURE 3.49 Webspace involvement is classical for scabies. (Photograph by Dr Nisha Chaturvedi.)

Dermoscopy

It helps in better identification of the burrows. A triangular dot (hand glider sign) corresponds to the head and front legs of the mite, while the S-shaped burrow which it has dug is described as a 'jet with condensation trail' sign. Video-dermoscopy provides higher magnification and helps in better identification.

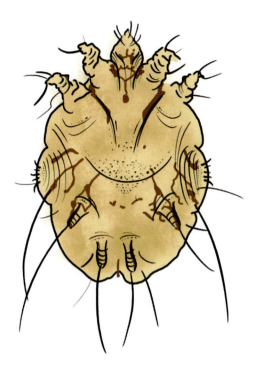

FIGURE 3.50 Diagrammatic representation of a scabies mite. (Photograph by Aashka Mehta.)

Laboratory examination

Direct identification of the mite from the skin scrapings is diagnostic. Staining the suspected area with a drop of ink and wiping the excess delineates the burrow and helps for easy identification. The skin scrapings are placed on a glass slide with mineral oil or potassium hydroxide or soaked in saline and observed under low-power microscopy. The mite is easily identified from its morphology (Figure 3.50).

Epiluminescence microscopy and reflectance confocal microscopy have been used in research settings.

Histopathology

A papulo-vesicular lesion or a burrow should be biopsied. The epidermis shows eosinophilic spongiosis. Bizarre pink structures corresponding to eggs, larvae, mites and excreta may be seen in the stratum corneum. The dermis has mild lymphocytic infiltrate with few eosinophils. Biopsy from a nodule may reveal a dense inflammatory infiltrate and a pseudo-lymphoma reaction pattern. Clinically evident hyperkeratosis correlates with massive orthokeratosis on histopathology in Norwegian scabies. There is psoriasiform hyperplasia with spongiosis and eosinophils, but more importantly, the stratum corneum is studded with mites in various stages of development.

Differential diagnosis

Intense vulvar pruritus may be seen in many diseases, and the burrow may be difficult to identify, so a high index of suspicion is required to diagnose scabies.

Atopic dermatitis has a long-standing history and other body areas like flexures may be involved.

Patients with delusional parasitosis may present with generalized itching but have no papulo vesicular rash as seen in scabies. Family members are not affected.

Prurigo mitis presents as excoriated papules on the exposed areas in children and young adults.

Course and prognosis

If untreated, the infestation increases with a more generalized rash and intense pruritus. There may be secondary bacterial infection. More importantly, the patient may cause a local outbreak of scabies.

Treatment

Topical application of permethrin 5% is the treatment of choice. The application should be used all over the body below neck, left overnight and washed off the following morning. A repeat application is recommended after 1 week. All family members need to be treated simultaneously, and it is recommended all fomites which include towels, bedding etc need to be laundered. It is safe for young children, pregnant or lactating women. Oral ivermectin (0.2 mg/kg) as a single dose repeated after 2 weeks is safe for use in adults and children weighing more than 15 kg. Combining with topical permethrin improves outcomes. Antihistamines provide immediate relief from pruritus. Post-scabietic itch may need treatment with oral antihistaminics, topical or intralesional steroids.

Pearls

Norwegian (crusted) scabies has minimal to no pruritus.

Recommended reading

1. Thomas C, et al. J Am Acad Dermatol (2020). PMID: 31310840.
2. Srinivas S, et al. Indian J Paediatr Dermatol (2019). DOI: 10.4103/ijpd.IJPD_25_18.

Pediculosis pubis

Introduction

Pediculosis pubis is an infectious disease caused by infestation with *Pthirus pubis (crab louse)*. With almost 70–80% population practicing some form of pubic hair removal, the number of cases has gone down significantly in the recent past.

Epidemiology

P. pubis is an obligate ectoparasite with humans as the only host. Pediculosis pubis is a disease affecting approximately 2% of the world population, most commonly seen in sexually active adults across all socio-economic strata. Fomites have a limited role in disease transmission.

Pathophysiology

P. pubis is morphologically distinct from other pediculosis and is extremely sedentary. It clings to the terminal hair of the pubic region, and hence the mode of transmission is through sexual contact or prolonged close physical contact. It is not a known vector for any other infections.

Presenting complaints

The patients present with severe, intractable itching in the pubic region, which may be socially embarrassing and disrupting day-to-day life activities. The itching may extend to the groin, thighs, buttocks and/or the perianal region.

Clinical examination

Diligent examination will reveal the pubic louse clutching the pubic hair. Nits, egg casts or even fecal matter may be visible. Usually, there are accompanying excoriations on the vulva, thighs, buttocks or perianal area. Blue or slate color macules (maculae cerulae) seen on the inner thighs represent altered blood pigments secondary to scratching.

Small blood stains on the patient's underwear are a testament to the intense itching due to this infestation.

Systemic findings

It is important to examine other areas likely to be affected including the axillae, chest, back, beard and rarely scalp. Eyebrows and eyelashes must be evaluated in children.

Dermoscopy

Helps in better visualization of the parasite.

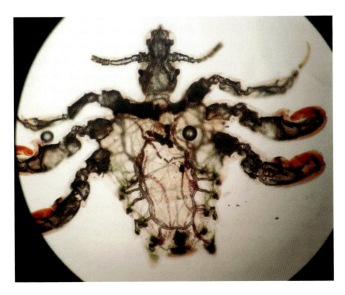

FIGURE 3.51 Pthirus Pubis resembles a crab and is found attached to the pubic hair. (Photograph by Dr Rajiv Joshi.)

Laboratory examination

Direct identification of the pubic louse is definitive. Better visualization can be achieved with a magnifying glass or dermatoscopy. The ectoparasite has a distinctive appearance as the body is wider than longer (resembling a crab) (Figure 3.51). Claws on the 2nd and 3rd pairs of legs help in grasping the curled, widely spaced pubic hair.

Differential diagnosis

Scabies is the closest differential diagnosis of pediculosis. The presence of burrows, papulo-vesicle nocturnal itch and multiple family members affected are points in favor of scabies.

Eczema or atopic dermatitis usually has a long-standing history and may be present on other parts of the body.

Course and prognosis

If untreated, the infestation spreads to other body parts with a severe impact on quality of life due to the intense pruritus. The excoriations can get secondarily infected.

Treatment

Shaving off the pubic hair is curative.

For other body parts, a single application of 1% permethrin lotion is recommended with a repeat application after 7–10 days. Oral ivermectin at the dose of 250 mcg/Kg body weight, repeated at 1 week has also been recommended.

Pearls

Patients diagnosed with pediculosis pubis must be screened for all sexually transmitted diseases.

Pubic lice in children (even on eyebrow/eyelash) must raise the possibility of sexual abuse.

Recommended reading

1. Clin Exp Dermatol (2021). PMID: 33811771.
2. Veraldi S, et al. Int J STD AIDS (2018) PMID: 29130406.

Pinworm infestation

Introduction

Enterobiasis (pinworm/threadworm/seatworm infestation) is the most commonest intestinal parasite in humans, having affected nearly 70% population at some time.

Epidemiology

Enterobiasis is caused by *Enterobius vermicularis*. It is more common in children between 4 and 15 years of age, where uncontrolled anus-finger-mouth contact is frequent. Other predisposing factors include nail biting and poor basic hand hygiene. Fomites also play an important role in disease transmission.

Pathophysiology

Humans get infected by direct or indirect ingestion of the pin-worm eggs. Upon hatching, the parasite undergoes its life cycle and the gravid female reaches the anal canal by active migration. It crawls out at night and lays its eggs in the perianal area. The migratory movements of the worms often cause uncomfortable pruritus, which promotes the child to scratch the perianal region. Mechanical dislodging results in the release of eggs in the clothes and surrounding area.

Presenting complaints

The child complains of perianal itching, which is worse in the evening and night. There may also be vulvar or perineal itching. Patients may complain of a burning micturition or, rarely, nocturnal enuresis.

Clinical examination

Direct visualization of the worm is rare. There may be signs of excoriation on the labia with occasional erythema and petechiae. Long-standing cases may have lichenification.

Systemic findings

A large majority have no systemic complaints, but occasionally, patients may complain of pain in the abdomen and anorexia. Extraintestinal infestation has been described.

Laboratory examination

Demonstration of the worm or its egg is diagnostic.

The worm is identified by its eponymous "thread-like" appearance. It is pale white in color and moves with a vigorous worm-like crawling motion.

The Scotch tape test: Commercially available scotch tape is cut 10 by 2 cm and is put sticky side down on the perianal area several times after spreading the buttocks apart and in the morning before the child passes stools. The tape is then stuck with the adhesive side down and observed under a microscope to observe the eggs. No medium is needed. To increase the sensitivity of the test, this is repeated on 3 consecutive days (from 50% if done once to 90% on 3 consecutive days).

A cotton swab is used on the perianal area and then mounted on a saline slide also helps see the eggs under the microscope.

Differential diagnosis

With no active features, all causes of vulvar pruritus in children should be excluded.

In scabies, lesions are seen in the webspaces of the fingers, axilla and other sites where papules and vesicles maybe visible.

In atopic dermatitis, the rash is visible on the other flexor aspects of the body.

Course and prognosis

The disease can be self-limiting due to the short life span of the worm. The cure rates are very high, but recurrences are common.

Treatment

Hand care and personal hygiene are the cornerstones of therapy. Hand hygiene practices must be taught and followed. Fomites (clothes, towels) must be washed in hot water (40°C)

Albendazole and mebendazole (100–200 mg single dose, repeated after 14 and 28 days) are curative.

In the case of chronic recurrent infection, simultaneously treating all members of a household has proved a successful approach (a single dose of mebendazole every 14 days for a period of 16 weeks).

Pearls

Stool examination is generally not helpful as the eggs are deposited outside of the intestine.

Humans are the only species that can transmit the parasite

The eggs of *E. vermicularis* can stay alive 2–4 weeks under the fingernails and lead to repeated infections, and hence special emphasis has to be given to maintaining hand hygiene.

Recommended reading

1. Wendt S, et al. Dtsch Arztebl Int (2019). PMID: 31064642.

4

SEXUALLY TRANSMITTED INFECTIONS

Eswari L. and Sowmya Aithal

Contents

Syphilis

Introduction

Syphilis is a sexually and vertically transmitted infection (STI) caused by the spirochaete *Treponema pallidum* subspecies *pallidum* (order Spirochaetales).

Epidemiology

The estimated prevalence and incidence of syphilis varies substantially by region or country, with the highest prevalence in Africa and >60% of new cases occurring in low- and middle-income countries. It is common in high-risk sub-populations, such as female sex workers (FSWs) and significant other. Syphilis is associated with high-risk sexual behaviors and substantially increased HIV transmission and acquisition. Infection with or treatment for HIV alters the natural history of syphilis. Mother to child transmission (MTCT) of syphilis continues to cause perinatal and infant mortality.

Pathophysiology

Transmission of venereal syphilis occurs during sexual contact with an actively infected partner. Spirochetes directly penetrate mucous membranes or enter through abrasions in the skin, which is less heavily keratinized in perigenital and perianal areas than skin elsewhere. Once below the epithelium, organisms multiply locally and begin to disseminate through the lymphatics and bloodstream. The infection rapidly becomes systemic. Penetration of the blood–brain barrier, occurring in as many as 40% of individuals with untreated early syphilis, can cause devastating neurological complications

Presenting complaints

A painless ulcer appearing 2–3 weeks after exposure is a characteristic presentation. Patients may also complain of swelling in their groins or other body parts. Sometimes, they may complain of fleshy, moist growths on the vulva or the perianal region. Similar lesions may be present in the oral cavity. There can be a concurrent, no-itchy skin rash (Figures 4.1 and 4.2).

Clinical examination

Initial lesions appear as painless, usually solitary, with 'button-like' induration, clean-based ulcers

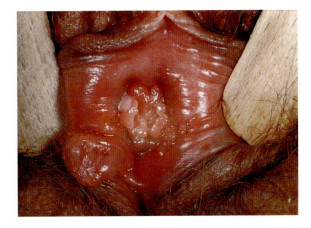

FIGURE 4.1 Button-like, solitary, syphilitic ulcer with a clean base on the labia minora. (Photograph by Dr Janak Maniar.)

DOI: 10.1201/9781003284116-4

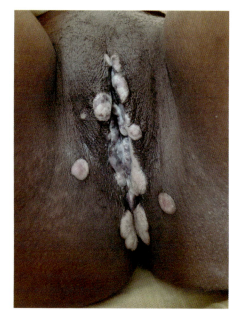

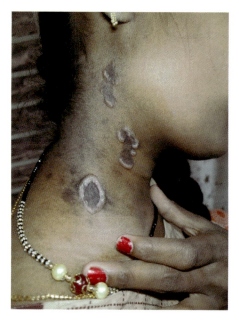

FIGURE 4.2   Flat, grouped, grayish white, plaques of condyloma lata on the vulva, extending to the perianal area. (Photograph by Dr Kavitha Athota.)

FIGURE 4.3   Annular pigmented plaques of secondary syphilis. (Photograph by Dr Kavitha Athota.)

(primary chancre), on the vulva, in the vagina and cervix, in and near the rectum, and in the mouth, as well as on other potentially exposed body parts such as fingers and neck. This ulcer can be accompanied by tender or non-tender regional lymphadenopathy. The rash of secondary syphilis can be widespread or localized; annular, macular, papular, scaly or

pustular in appearance. In lighter skin types, the rash may be reddish or copper colored, whilst it is deeply pigmented in the skin of color. Lesions on the palms and soles are characteristic. The mucous membrane lesions on the vulva can be exuberant or verrucous, grayish white and tend to resemble flat warts (condyloma lata) (Figures 4.3 and 4.4).

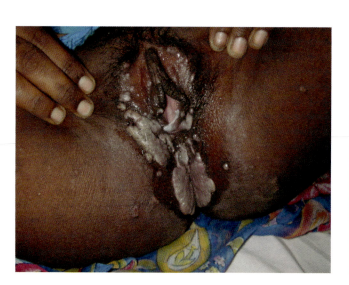

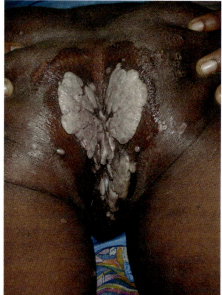

FIGURE 4.4   **(a & b)** Condyloma lata lesions when exuberant can mimic Condyloma accuminata. (Photograph by Dr Nisha Chaturvedi.)

Systemic findings

Symptoms such as malaise, myalgia, sore throat, headache or low-grade fever are commonly detected. In addition to cutaneous manifestations, the presentation of secondary syphilis can also include diffuse lymphadenopathy, hepatosplenomegaly, hepatitis and nephrotic syndrome.

Laboratory examination

Identifying T. pallidum by dark field microscopy gives a definite diagnosis. It is useful for smears from chancres, condyloma lata and other mucous lesions. However, this test is not available easily. Non-treponemal tests like VDRL (venereal disease research laboratory test) and RPR (rapid plasma reagin) are useful but may give false-negative results. Also, high dilutions are required to diagnose secondary syphilis. If the above tests are positive, re-confirmation can be done by TPHA (treponema pallidum hemagglutination test), FTA-ABS (fluorescent treponemal antibody absorption test) and MHA-TP (microhemagglutination assay– treponema pallidum).

Histopathology

Perivascular infiltration of lymphocytes, histiocytes and plasma cells with endothelial cell swelling and proliferation are characteristic histopathological findings in all stages of syphilis and can progress to frank endarteritis obliterans.

Differential diagnosis

The primary chancre needs to be differentiated from other STIs like chancroid, granuloma inguinale, aphthous ulcer, herpetic ulcers and traumatic ulcer.

- Chancroid ulcers are multiple and painful.
- Granuloma inguinale ulcers are fleshy with a beefy-red appearance.
- Aphthous ulcers are extremely painful unlike a chancre and may be recurrent.
- Herpetic ulcers are grouped, multiple, and painful with a polycyclic border.
- A history of trauma may suggest a traumatic ulcer which will be painful, and not indurated.

Course and prognosis

When primary syphilis goes undetected because of the unidentified painless chancre, there is progression to secondary syphilis. Once the diagnosis is made and appropriately treated, the outcome is good. Untreated, complications of late syphilis can develop, particularly those involving the eyes, central nervous system and cardiovascular system, causing lifelong disability and even death.

Treatment

Important factors in managing syphilis are early detection, prompt treatment and treatment of sex partners of a person with infectious syphilis. The WHO 2021 guidelines for the treatment of early syphilis include intramuscular benzathine penicillin G 24 lakh units (single dose) or intramuscular procaine penicillin (daily doses for 10–14 days). If penicillin-based treatment cannot be used, oral doxycycline (twice daily doses for 10–14 days) or intramuscular ceftriaxone (daily doses for 10–14 days) are used.

Pearls

Even after adequate treatment, the TPHA may remain positive for several months to years and does not warrant re-treatment.

Multiple primary syphilitic chancres may be seen in immunocompromised individuals.

The Centre for Disease Control and Prevention (CDC) recommends desensitization for those who are allergic to penicillin.

Recommended reading

1. Peeling RW, et al. Nat Rev Dis Primers (2017). PMID: 29022569.
2. Bond SM, et al. J Midwifery Womens Health (2021). PMID: 34101969.

Chancroid

Introduction

Chancroid has become a very rare STI globally. It is called as soft sore, soft chancre and ulcus molle, which is clinically characterized by one or more non-indurated genital ulcers with inguinal lymphadenitis.

Epidemiology

Hemophilus ducreyi which is a gram-negative rod is the causative organism of chancroid. It is a significant factor in the acquisition and transmission of HIV infection because of the interrupted mucosal surface caused by genital ulceration.

HIV, in turn, will alter the clinical presentation of chancroid, causing a delay in healing and treatment failures.

Pathophysiology

The bacterium enters via a breach in the mucosa, produces a toxin which causes irreversible cell death of epithelial cells and may lead to the development of skin breakdown and subsequent ulcer development.

Presenting complaints

Patients typically present with lesions which develops in the genital area typically 4–10 days after experiencing a minor trauma or microabrasion during sex. They complain of severe pain in the lesions with the discharge of pus or even bleeding.

Clinical examination

Initially, the lesion develops as an erythematous papule which evolves into a pustule and subsequently ruptures to form an extremely painful ulcer with irregular non-indurated margins called as 'soft chancre'.

Ulcers can be found on the fourchette, labia, vestibule, clitoris, vaginal wall, cervix and perianal skin. Extragenital lesions can occur on the breasts, fingers, thigh and oral mucosa. Kissing ulcers occur in two adjacent areas due to direct contact. Multiple ulcers develop with a size varying from 1 to 2 cm, with yellowish-gray exudate on a friable base that bleeds easily on touch. Classic chancroid triad consists of undermined ulcer edge, purulent dirty gray base and moderate to severe pain. These ulcers can be associated with tender inguinal lymphadenopathy, which may form suppurative buboes. These buboes may rupture and get secondarily infected, leading to deep tissue destruction of the external genitalia. Vaginal fistulae can complicate subclinical vaginal ulceration in females (Figures 4.5–4.7).

Laboratory examination

Since there is a potential similarity to other genital ulcers like syphilis and herpes, diagnostic tests to rule out such infections need to be done. Gram stain of the exudate shows gram-negative rods arranged in 'school of fish' or 'rail road track appearance'. As per the CDC recommendations,

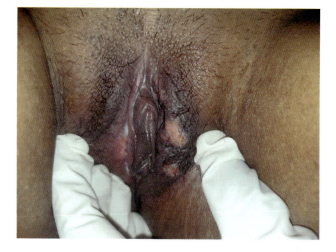

FIGURE 4.5 Large ulcers with irregular margins and purulent base. (Photograph by Dr Eswari L.)

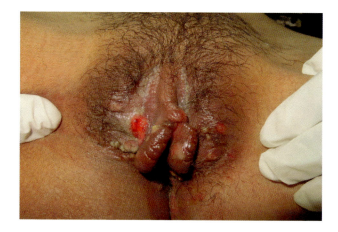

FIGURE 4.6 Multiple chancroid ulcers which may be mistaken for genital herpes. (Photograph by Dr Pragya Nair.)

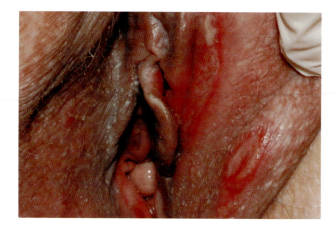

FIGURE 4.7 In immune-suppressed females, chancroid ulcers are much larger and deeper. (Photograph by Dr Janak Maniar.)

definitive diagnosis requires identification of *H. ducreyi* on special culture media. This culture media is neither widely nor consistently available to general public health entities and when used has a sensitivity of less than 80% when compared to polymerase chain reaction (PCR).

Isolation of causative agent, H. ducreyi is obtained from the undermined edge of the anogenital ulcer, after removing the superficial pus with a cotton-tipped swab, plated directly onto culture medium and incubated at 33°C, in high humidity with 5% carbon dioxide for a minimum of 48–72 hours.

Several serologic tests have been developed, including adsorption enzyme immunoassay (EIA) and lipooligosaccharide (LOS) EIA, to detect H. ducreyi infection.

There is also no FDA-approved PCR test available.

Histopathology

Characteristic 3 zones have been described in the histopathology of chancroid ulcer viz

a. A narrow superficial zone of necrotic tissue, red cells, some fibrin and degenerate polymorphonuclear leucocytes
b. A broader middle zone of oedematous inflamed tissue with numerous prominent small dilated vessels and strands of endothelial cells which approach the surface
c. The third, deep zone merges with the middle zone and shows a fairly dense infiltrate of plasma cells and lesser numbers of lymphocytes.

Differential diagnosis

This includes other STI ulcers like syphilis, genital herpes and granuloma inguinale.

Genital herpes: doing a simple tzanck smear will help. The serology of herpes simplex virus (HSV) antibodies will also confirm the diagnosis.

A syphilitic ulcer is usually painless and indurated. Serological tests like VDRL and TPHA can help in diagnosis.

Granuloma inguinale presents with painless beefy red ulcers which bleed easily on touch. Lymphogranuloma venereum (LGV) should also be considered when there is the presence of inguinal bubo.

Course and prognosis

There is full recovery after appropriate antibiotic therapy. Lesions also subside without treatment but may take a longer time which may also lead to inguinal lymphadenopathy. When there is no response to treatment, coinfection with HIV should be suspected.

Treatment
CDC recommended regime 2021

Azithromycin 1 gm orally in a single dose or ceftriaxone 250 mg IM in a single dose or ciprofloxacin 500 mg orally 2 times/day for 3 days or erythromycin base 500 mg orally 3 times/day for 7 days.

The 4 Cs of managing STIs should be followed i.e. counseling, compliance, condom usage and contact treatment.

Regardless of whether disease symptoms are present, sex partners of patients with chancroid should be examined and treated if they had sexual contact with the patient during the 10 days preceding the patient's symptom onset.

Pearls

All patients of chancroid must be tested for HIV.

Recommended reading

1. Irizarry L et al. Chancroid. StatPearls Publishing; 2021. PMID: 30020703.
2. Roett MA. Am Fam Physician (2020). PMID: 32163252.
3. Fuchs W, et al. J Dtsch Dermatol Ges (2014). PMID: 24889293.

Lymphogranuloma venereum

Introduction

LGV is an STI caused by specific serovars of *Chlamydia trachomatis* (L1, L2, L3). It is transmissible by vaginal, oral or anal sex.

Epidemiology

Chlamydia is a ubiquitous obligate intracellular bacterium. LGV can occur at any age; however, the highest prevalence of LGV is in the sexually energetic populace between 15 and 40 years. LGV affects both sexes equally, although it is more commonly reported in men because early manifestations of LGV are more apparent in men. LGV is endemic in regions of Africa, Southeast Asia,

India, the Caribbean and South America. An incidence of 0.2–11% has been reported in some parts of India.

Pathophysiology

The organism enters through a breach in the skin, impacts the lymphatic system, and causes lymphangitis, lymphatic obstruction, edema and elephantiasis. *Chlamydia trachomatis* serovars amplify from the primary infection site to the nearby (regional) lymph nodes and lead to a lymphoproliferative reaction. The lymph nodes eventually swell, form buboes, and rupture, resulting in scarring.

Presenting complaints

Patients present with painful swelling in the groin or, if long standing, with permanent edema of the vulva. Long-standing cases can also have chronic constipation. Very rarely, they may present with an ulcer. They manifest as an asymptomatic, evanescent ulcer or painful swellings in the groin. They might also additionally present with fever, chills and malaise.

Clinical examination

Within the first month of exposure, women present with a small, painless papule/pustule that could erode to form a small, asymptomatic herpetiform ulcer which normally heals rapidly without scarring. This often goes unnoticed by the patient. Common sites of infection include the posterior vaginal wall, posterior cervix, fourchette, and vulva.

At a later stage, enlarged, painful matted lymph nodes adherent to the overlying skin are seen, which finally breakdown and ulcerate. Ulcerations around the introitus including the clitoris, labia minora and posterior fourchette constitute the anogenitorectal syndrome seen in a very later stage of the disease. Progressive lymphatic obstruction results in esthiomene (Figures 4.8 and 4.9).

Systemic findings

Constitutional signs and symptoms include fever, chills, myalgias and malaise. Long-standing disease may have other manifestations like arthritis, ocular inflammation, cardiac and pulmonary involvement, aseptic meningitis, hepatitis or perihepatitis.

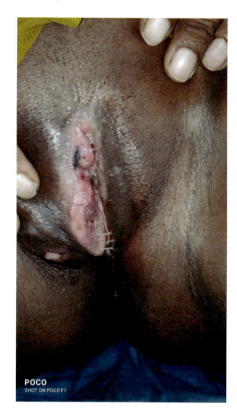

FIGURE 4.8 Notice the large ulcer, involving the entire clitoris, right labia minora, up to the perineum. A small ulcer on the labia majora indicates a possible discharging sinus. (Photograph by Dr Eswari L.)

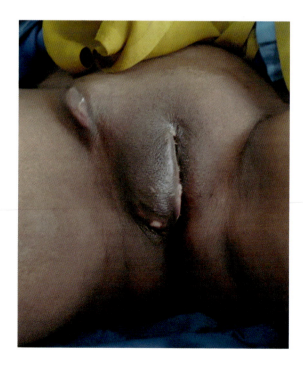

FIGURE 4.9 Esthiomene with inguinal bubo. (Photograph by Dr Eswari L.)

Laboratory examination

The best method to obtain tissue for culture is needle aspiration of an involved bubo. *Chlamydia trachomatis* can be identified in genital, rectal and lymph node specimens by culture, nucleic acid amplification test (NAAT) or direct immunofluorescence. A NAAT can detect both LGV strains and non-LGV C. trachomatis strains, so it is the preferred test. Even though the culture of C trachomatis is definitive diagnostically, it is technically demanding and expensive and yields an isolate only 30% of the time. Serological tests like complement fixation or micro-immunofluorescence are also diagnostic and comparatively easily available in laboratories.

Histopathology

Earliest microscopic change is characterized by tiny necrotic foci infiltrated by neutrophils. These enlarge and coalesce to form the stellate abscess, which is the hallmark of this disease. In subsequent stages, epithelioid cells, scattered Langerhans' giant cells and fibroblasts are seen lining the walls of the abscess. The healing stage is characterized by the presence of nodules with dense fibrous walls surrounding amorphous material.

Differential diagnosis

In LGV, ulcers are rarely seen, and the differentials include diseases which cause inguinal swelling (bubo). These include granuloma inguinale, TB lymphadenitis, secondary syphilis and non-Hodgkin lymphoma. Fine needle aspiration cytology (FNAC) and/or biopsy may be definitive in making the right diagnosis. Differentials for esthiomene include other diseases like filariasis, metastatic vulvar Crohn's disease and pelvic tumors with lymphatic obstruction.

Course and prognosis

The prognosis is fair if recognized and treated early. Complications may occur when the disease is left untreated, like necrosis and rupture of the lymph nodes, anogenital fibrosis, strictures and anal fistulae. Elephantiasis of the genital organs may arise in longstanding cases. Systemic complications like pneumonia and hepatitis have also been reported.

Treatment

The CDC 2021 Guidelines recommend treating with doxycycline 100 mg twice daily orally for 21 days. An alternate regimen is erythromycin 500 mg orally four times a day for 21 days (safe in pregnancy). Azithromycin 1 gm orally once a week for 3 weeks is also an effective alternative regimen. Aspiration of fluctuant or pus-filled abscess in the node provides symptomatic relief, although incision and drainage of the nodes are not recommended as it can delay the healing process and leave behind a sinus.

Pearls

Although classically described in LGV, the groove sign can also be seen in pelvic tuberculosis and non-Hodgkin's lymphoma.

Aspiration of the bubo must be done from the non-dependent part to avoid the risk of sinus formation.

Recommended reading

1. Collins L, et al. BMJ (2006). PMID: 16410560.
2. O'Byrne P, et al. Can Fam Physician (2016). PMCID: PMC4955081.

Granuloma inguinale

Introduction

Granuloma inguinale is a rare chronic destructive granulomatous disease that primarily affects the genitalia. It is also known as serpiginous ulcer of groin, ulcerating granuloma of pudenda and granuloma venereum.

Epidemiology

The disease is rare with sporadic cases described in South Africa and South America. In India, donovanosis is prevalent in states like Orissa, Tamil Nadu, Himachal Pradesh and Puducherry. The incubation period is variable, and it may range from 3 days to 3 months. The average incubation period is 40–50 days. The genital region is involved in 90% of cases and the inguinal region in 10% cases.

Pathophysiology

The disease is caused by gram-negative bacteria called *Klebsiella granulomatis* (formerly known as *Calymmatobacterium granulomatis*). It is seen in tissue as intracellular organisms in vacuoles that resemble closed safety pins, with denser staining at the ends than in the center. The organism enters through a breach in the epithelium and causes granulomatous changes in dermis.

Presenting complaints

The lesions are usually painless, but the patient may complain of a foul smell, discharge, a vulvar swelling or hematuria.

Clinical examination

Early lesions start as a painless papule or nodule in the vulvar area which erodes to form progressive ulcerative lesions without regional lymphadenopathy. Lesions are highly vascular with a beefy red appearance and can bleed easily (Classic type). Other variants include hypertrophic/verrucous, necrotic/phagedenic or sclerotic/cicatricial type.

The anatomical areas affected are the labia minora, fourchette. The involvement of deeper parts of the vagina and cervix are usually associated with vulvar lesions. Lesions appearing in the groin i.e. subcutaneous granulomas may mimic lymphadenopathy and have been referred to as pseudo buboes.

Laboratory examination

Diagnosis can be done by demonstrating the organism by direct microscopy of crushed tissue smear stained by Giemsa stain. Donovan bodies are seen within macrophages that have a bipolar appearance as a small safety pin. It is difficult to culture. DNA-detecting molecular assays might be useful (Figures 4.10 and 4.11).

Histopathology

Biopsy from the ulcerated lesion shows a dense infiltrate with macrophages and plasma cells. Focal collections of neutrophils and increased vessels are present near the ulcer base, while the periphery shows pseudoepitheliomatous hyperplasia. Demonstration of intracellular Donovon bodies is diagnostic. Staining with Giemsa or Warthin-starry method increases positive yield in identifying the organism.

Differential diagnosis

Lesions may resemble chancre or chancroid early in the course, but classical button induration and lymphadenopathy differentiate syphilis from donovanosis. Chancroid is recognized classically by

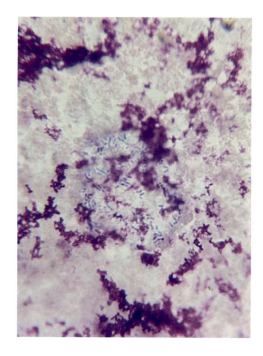

FIGURE 4.10 Tissue smear demonstrating intracellular donovan bodies. Giemsa stain 100×. (Photograph by Dr Rashmi Mahajan.)

multiple painful ulcers, with an undermined edge and necrotic slough associated with painful suppurative lymphadenopathy.

Bubo of LGV can be confused with pseudobubo of donovanosis.

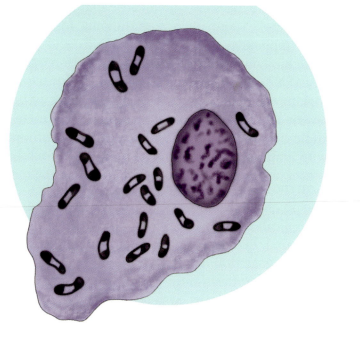

FIGURE 4.11 Diagrammatic representation of 'Safety-pin' appearance of Donovan bodies. (Photograph by Aashka Mehta.)

Herpes genitalis complicated with HIV can present with granuloma-like lesions (pseudo-granuloma herpeticum). The presence of multi-nucleate giant cells, absence of donovan bodies and response to acyclovir go in favor of herpetic infection.

Squamous cell carcinoma is another important differential to be ruled out with a biopsy.

Course and prognosis
If left untreated, the disease progresses relentlessly. Recurrence in already healed areas can occur. Persistent edema of the distal tissues can cause pseudoelephantiasis. Rectovaginal fistulae are an important complication. Females may suffer from stenosis of the urethra, vulva or anal orifice, particularly in the sclerotic type. Associated HIV infection may result in aggressive ulceration and a poor tendency for healing

Treatment
According to CDC guidelines 2021, recommended regimens include azithromycin l g orally once per week or 500 mg daily for >3 weeks and until all lesions have healed completely. Alternative regimens include doxycycline 100 mg orally twice daily for at least 3 weeks or erythromycin base 500 mg orally 4 times/day or trimethoprim-sulphamethoxazole double strength (160 mg/1800 mg) one tablet each twice daily, for at least 3 weeks and until all lesions have healed completely.

Pearl
The ulcerative form of granuloma inguinale closely mimics vulvar carcinoma, and a biopsy is essential to differentiate the two.

Recommended reading
1. Workowski KA, et al. MMWR Recomm Rep (2021). PMID: 34292926.
2. O'Farrell N. Int J STD AIDS (2001). PMID: 11394976.
3. Sand FL, et al. J Obstet Gynaecol (2017). PMID: 28397528.

Gonorrhea

Introduction
Gonorrhea (gonos-seed, rhoea-flow) is one of the most common STIs across the world.

Epidemiology
The incidence of gonorrhea has declined in recent years, with an increase in non-gonococcal urethritis cases. Countries in South East Asia have been showing declining numbers as per the WHO Bulletin 2021. This decline may be due to increased medical facilities, use of over-the-counter drugs, increased condom distribution and use and awareness about AIDS. There are increasing reports of resistance to antimicrobials for gonorrhea, complicating its treatment.

Pathophysiology
Neisseria gonorrhea is a gram-negative, non-motile, non-spore-forming diplococci, present intracellularly in neutrophils. Primary infection commonly occurs in the columnar epithelium, which may also occur in the stratified squamous epithelium of the vagina in prepubertal girls (gonococcal vulvovaginitis). Gonococci are able to invade the host and persist in the blood stream with Pili E and Opa. It is followed by endocytosis and pseudopod formation. Tissue damage occurs due to lipo oligo saccharide (LOS). The attracted neutrophils together with the serum and desquamated epithelium form the discharge.

Presenting complaints
More often, the disease in women may be asymptomatic. The classical symptoms include mucopurulent cervical discharge and burning micturition, frequency and urgency.

Clinical examination
The most prominent physical finding is the involvement of Skene's glands or Bartholin's glands or inflammation of the cervix. There may be peri-meatal erythema and edema, mucopurulent cervical discharge, cervical erythema, edema and friability. Gonococcal vulvovaginitis can occur in prepubertal girls because of thin vaginal epithelium with low glycogen, neutral pH and non-production of cervical mucus, lack of protective labial fat pads. It may be asymptomatic or may present with vaginal purulent discharge.

Ano-rectal gonorrhea may be primary or secondary to initial genito-urinary infection, presenting with anal pruritus, tenesmus, discharge and constipation. Pharyngeal infection due to urogenital sexual contact can present with fever, tonsillitis and cervical lymphadenopathy.

Systemic findings

Disseminated gonococcal infection may present as arthritis-dermatitis syndrome with high fever, joint pain, pustules, petechiae or ecchymosis.

Perihepatitis (Fitz-Hugh-Curtis syndrome) occurs because of the spread from the fallopian tube to the peritoneal cavity, along the paracolic gutter to reach subphrenic space. They present with right upper quadrant pain radiating to the shoulder, increasing deep inspiration.

Other complications include gonococcal arthritis, meningitis and endocarditis.

Laboratory examination

A gram stain of the discharge show gram-negative diplococci, within neutrophils. Culture in modified Thayer-Martin medium, serology and PCR are other tests available for diagnosis. The NAAT is the most sensitive.

Differential diagnosis

Nongonococcal urethritis (NGU), which is diagnosed when microscopy of urethral secretions indicates inflammation without gram-negative intracellular diplococci, is caused by *Chlamydia trachomatis*, *Mycoplasma genitalium*, *Trichomonas vaginalis*, *Ureaplasma*, HSV, Adeno and Epstein-Barr virus in few cases.

Course and prognosis

Local spread in women may lead to salpingitis, endometritis, Bartholin gland abscess, pelvic inflammatory disease (PID) and infertility.

Treatment

The CDC 2021 guidelines recommend ceftriaxone 500 mg IM in a single dose for persons weighing <150 kg (1 g for weight >150 kg). For disseminated gonococcal infection, cefotaxime 1 g IV every 8 hours or ceftizoxime 1 g every 8 hours is recommended. If chlamydial infection has not been excluded, treatment of chlamydia with doxycycline 100 mg orally 2 times/day for 7 days should be given.

Pearl

Women with suspected gonococcal urethritis should concomitantly receive treatment for chlamydia.

Recommended reading

1. Sharma M, et al. Bull World Health Organ (2021). PMID: 33953448.
2. Workowski KA, et al. MMWR Recomm Rep (2021). PMID: 34292926.
3. Dei M, et al. Best Pract Res Clin Obstet Gynaecol (2010). PMID: 19884044.
4. Sand FL, et al. J Obstet Gynaecol (2017). PMID: 28397528.

Chlamydia

Introduction

Chlamydia is one of the most common STIs in people worldwide. Serovars A, B, Ba and C are associated with trachoma, serovars D-K are associated with genital tract infections, and L1–L3 are associated with LGV.

Epidemiology

Chlamydia causes about half of the cases of mucopurulent cervicitis and 20%–40% of cases of PID. It accounts for 15%–40% of cases of NGU, which is diagnosed when microscopy of urethral secretions indicates inflammation without gram-negative intracellular diplococci. Vulvovaginal infection can occur in prepubertal girls because of sexual contact or through perinatal inoculation from infected cervical secretions during delivery

Pathophysiology

Chlamydia is an obligate intracellular bacterial pathogen. The infectious form is called as elementary body (EB) which is metabolically inert. It attaches to a susceptible host cell and finally condenses to form elementary bodies which are released after the lysis of the cell.

The incubation period is variable (1–3 weeks).

Presenting complaints

Women with chlamydial infection are usually asymptomatic; few may complain of a scanty mucopurulent discharge or post coital bleeding.

Clinical examination

Examination may reveal a urethral discharge, peri-meatal erythema or edema. The cervix may show cervicitis with cervical ectopy, presenting as an edematous, congested, cervix which bleeds easily.

Systemic findings

Perihepatitis (Fitz-Hugh-Curtis syndrome) occurs when organisms spread from the fallopian tube to the peritoneal cavity, along the paracolic gutter to reach subphrenic space. Right upper quadrant pain radiating to shoulder is seen.

Laboratory examination

Gram-stained endocervical or urethral smears, first void urine specimen, reveal an increased number of white blood cells without gram-negative diplococci. Smears can be cultured on McCoy, HeLa cells. Other tests include antigen detection, DNA amplification, serology or NAATs (most sensitive).

Differential diagnosis

Cervicitis and urethritis caused by chlamydia resemble gonococcal infection, but chlamydial infection has a long incubation period and presents with scanty and less purulent discharge. Post gonococcal urethritis usually develops after 2 weeks of adequate treatment of gonorrhea but not in chlamydia.

Other causes of urethral discharge include *Mycoplasma genitalium* (detected by NAAT) and *Trichomonas vaginalis* (characteristic green frothy discharge).

Course and prognosis

Chlamydia can cause purulent bartholinitis, salpingitis and endometritis with abnormal vaginal bleeding. Long-term sequelae include PID, tubal infertility, tubo-ovarian abscess and ectopic pregnancy.

Treatment

Treatment guidelines as per CDC 2021 include doxycycline 100 mg orally 2 times/day for 7 days or azithromycin 1 g orally in a single dose or levofloxacin 500 mg orally once daily for 7 days. The guidelines also include single-dose azithromycin 1 g orally in pregnant women.

Pearls

Patients treated for chlamydia should be instructed about sexual abstinence for 7 days after therapy and resolution of symptoms.

Any case of suspected gonococcal urethritis must be simultaneously treated for chlamydia.

Recommended reading

1. Workowski KA, et al. MMWR Recomm Rep (2021). PMID: 34292926.
2. Dei M, et al. Best Pract Res Clin Obstet Gynaecol (2010). PMID: 19884044.
3. Sand FL, et al. J Obstet Gynaecol (2017). PMID: 28397528.

Sexually transmitted infections in HIV

Syphilis

- Unusual clinical features of syphilis can be seen in HIV-coinfected patients. Atypical presentation with multiple chancres, rapid progression to the tertiary stage, syphilitic aortitis, serological non reactivity, relapse or failure of treatment may be seen.
- Neurological involvement can occur in the early stages of syphilis despite adequate treatment in HIV-coinfected patients.
- Malignant syphilis or lues maligna is an uncommon form of secondary syphilis, which usually occurs in HIV infection.

Chancroid

- Chancroid enhances the risk of HIV infection by disrupting the mucosal integrity, increasing the viral shedding and increasing the susceptibility to HIV infection.
- Presentation of chancroid in HIV-positive patients may be severe and atypical like extensive necrotizing lesions, multiple buboes and maggot formation.

Granuloma inguinale

- Patients diagnosed with granuloma inguinale should be suspected of HIV and tested for the same. HIV-positive patients with granuloma inguinale may have ulcers persisting for a longer duration; more tissue destruction and may require more intensive antibiotic therapy.
- HIV also increases the chances of squamous cell carcinoma in donovanosis.

Lymphogranuloma venereum

- The disease duration of LGV may be prolonged in HIV-positive patients. An atypical presentation of Parinaud's oculoglandular

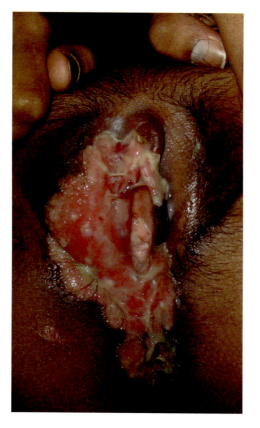

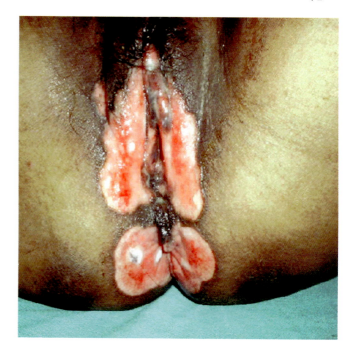

FIGURE 4.13 This patient of herpes genitalis may be misdiagnosed as Granuloma inguinale. (Photograph by Dr Janak Maniar.)

FIGURE 4.12 Extensive ulceration of herpes genitalis in a seropositive patient. (Photograph by Dr Nina Madnani.)

syndrome with unilateral follicular conjunctivitis and enlargement of preauricular lymph nodes with inguinal lymphadenopathy have been reported in a patient with HIV and LGV coinfection.

Gonorrhea

- Urethritis and cervicitis increase the risk of HIV shedding and the risk of transmission. Patients with HIV have more severe symptoms associated with PID.

Chlamydia

- Non-gonococcal urethritis and cervicitis also increase the transmission of HIV.

Herpes genitalis

- Lesions of Herpes become more aggressive and extensive with delayed healing.
- These require prolonged treatment and heal with scarring.
- Non-healing genital ulcer in a seropositive patient should always be investigated for herpes genitalis (Figures 4.12 and 4.13).

5

VULVOVAGINAL DISCHARGES

Pavithra Vani

Contents

Vulvovaginal discharge is a distressing symptom and a cause for 5–10 million outpatient department visits worldwide. The discharge can be asymptomatic in up to 50% of females, leading to morbidities including maternal and fetal complications.

Physiological discharge is transient, clear to whitish, and mostly odorless. Up to 4 ml is considered normal. The source of the discharge can be from the urethra, vulva, vagina, cervix, uterus or salpinx. This discharge is composed of mucoid endocervical secretions, sloughed epithelial cells, normal vaginal flora and vaginal transudate. It may be seen during menarche, in the reproductive years, premenstrual, postmenstrual, periovulatory, during sexual arousal, postcoital, during pregnancy, lactation and with the use of hygiene products (Figure 5.1).

The pH of the vagina varies considerably during a women's life. It is 7 in pemenarchal girls but acidic (4–4.5) in reproductive-aged women. It becomes 6 before and during menses and in postmenopausal women not on hormone replacement therapy (HRT).

Pathological causes of vaginal discharge can be infective or non-infective.

The common infective causes are sexually transmitted infections (STIs) like gonorrhea, trichomoniasis, chlamydia, herpes genitalis, syphilis, and reproductive tract infections (RTIs) like candidiasis, bacterial vaginosis (BV), Human papillomavirus (HPV) and mixed infections.

Non-infective causes of vaginal discharge include cytolytic vaginitis (CV), contact dermatitis, foreign

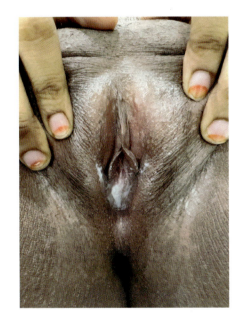

FIGURE 5.1 Normal vaginal discharge seen in this lady on the 14th day of her cycle. (Photograph by Dr Nina Madnani.)

body, inflammatory dermatoses like lichen planus, immune-mediated like pemphigus, pemphigoid, desquamative inflammatory vaginitis (DIV) and tumors.

Some predisposing factors include pathogenic organisms, altered vaginal flora due to pH changes, unprotected sex (alkaline semen favors the growth of certain bacteria), antibiotics, menstruation, pregnancy, intrauterine devices (IUD), harsh soaps, chemicals, irritant or allergic reactions, tumors.

It is important to distinguish physiological discharge from pathological to prevent unnecessary mental trauma, social stigma and interventions.

A thorough history, examination and relevant investigations not miss the diagnosis to prevent complications which can give rise to high morbidity and mortality.

Trichomonas vaginalis

Introduction
Vaginal trichomoniasis is the commonest non-viral STI worldwide. Humans are the only host for this protozoal infection caused by *Trichomonas vaginalis (T. vaginalis)*. This infection can co-exist with other STIs and may be suggestive of high-risk behavior. Up to 25% of infected individuals may be asymptomatic.

Epidemiology
Around 6–16% of vaginal discharge cases may be due to *T. vaginalis*. This infection is most prevalent in the third decade in sexually active women. It can be found in the female lower genital tract, male urethra and prostate. It can survive up to 24 hours in urine, semen and water by forming pseudocysts. Co-infection with BV or gonorrhea can be found in up to 40% women. *T. vaginalis* increases HIV transmission can occur.

Pathophysiology
Around 5–28 days post exposure, *T. vaginalis* adheres to and kills host cells via cadherin-like proteins. It also disrupts the vaginal ecosystem, causing inflammation by host immune system activation.

Presenting complaints
Women can complain of varied symptoms like itching, discharge, dysuria, dyspareunia, postcoital bleeding. The partner may have a history suggestive of urethritis, epididymitis or prostatitis.

Clinical examination
The vulva may be erythematous and edematous, with a profuse, thin, frothy, yellowish to greenish discharge. The ectocervix may show strawberry red patches with petechiae (strawberry cervix) (Figure 5.2).

Systemic findings
Women may have abdominal pain secondary to pelvic inflammatory disease (PID) as an outcome of the infection.

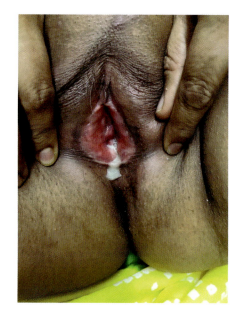

FIGURE 5.2   Inflamed vulva with yellowish-green frothy discharge. (Photograph by Dr Nina Madnani.)

Laboratory examination
Vaginal pH is more than 6. The whiff test is occasionally positive in *T. vaginalis*. In a wet mount (which is 50–70% sensitive), *T. vaginalis* is seen as an oval to pear-shaped motile organism with typical jerky or spring-like motility.

Culture (Diamond's modified medium) is positive in 3 days. Nucleic Acid Amplification Test (NAAT) has over 90% sensitivity and specificity and is used for definitive diagnosis. Rapid tests, oligonucleotide probe, OSOM Trichomonas Rapid Test and XenoStrip TM-TV275 are immuno-chromatographic assays that detect *T. vaginalis* antigens in vaginal swabs.

Cytology
Smears of the discharge show an inflammatory picture. Organisms are generally not seen as they lose character during fixing and staining.

Differential diagnosis
BV (grayish-white discharge with fishy odor), streptococcal vaginitis (can cause profuse discharge), candidiasis (curdy white, cottage-cheese like) and malignancy (blood stained and foul smelling).

Course and prognosis
Infection with *T. vaginalis* can be recurrent. If untreated, the infection can smolder and lead to

infertility due to tubal blockage, reduced sperm motility and other pregnancy complications.

Chronic infections can lead to psychiatric comorbidities.

Treatment

Metronidazole 500 mg twice daily for 7 days or 2 gm orally single dose, or tinidazole 2 gm single dose is usually curative. Treatment of the partner is essential. Test of cure with NAAT 2 weeks to within 3 months of completion of treatment may be done. Trichomoniasis must be treated during pregnancy, and metronidazole is the drug of choice.

Pearl

Early effective treatment can prevent infertility and pregnancy-related complications.

Recommended reading

1. Amrin SS, et al. Indian J Sex Transm Dis AIDS (2021). PMID: 34765936.
2. Mabaso N, et al. S Afr J Infect Dis (2021). PMID: 34485502.

Bacterial vaginosis

Introduction

BV is the commonest cause of vaginal infection in the reproductive age group which can lead to many complications. It may be asymptomatic in up to 50% of the affected individuals. It increases the risk of other STIs.

Epidemiology

More than 10 million cases per year have been reported in India. It is commonest in sexually active women between the ages of 15 and 45 years. It is caused by overgrowth of predominantly anaerobic organisms like *Gardnerella*, *Prevotella species*, *Mycoplasma hominis*, *Mobiluncus species*, etc. *Gardnerella* (previously called *Haemophilus*) is the most frequent of these. Aerobic infection due to *Staphylococci*, *Streptococci* and *E. coli* can also cause BV.

Pathophysiology

Reduction or lack of *lactobacilli* results in an altered vaginal ecosystem leading to the overgrowth of predominantly anaerobic organisms. Predisposing factors include having multiple sexual partners, smoking, douching etc.

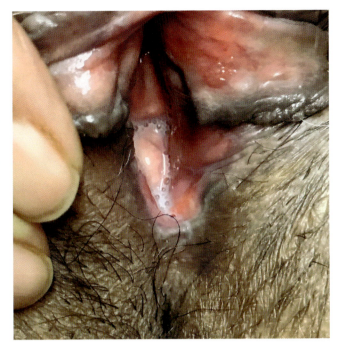

FIGURE 5.3 Whitish copious discharge with minimal vulvar inflammation. (Photograph by Dr Nina Madnani.)

Presenting complaints

Vaginal discharge with or without itching and burning, and/or occasional dysuria are the common presenting complaints (Figure 5.3).

Clinical examination

The woman has a grayish-white vaginal discharge with a fishy odor. The vaginal pH is more than 4.5. Vaginal walls appear normal on examination and vulva may show erythema.

Laboratory examination

A swab of the discharge mounted in normal saline shows clue cells (epithelial cells studded with coccobacilli), decreased or absent *lactobacilli* on wet preparation. A positive 'whiff' test – fishy odor present on the addition of an alkaline-like potassium hydroxide to the secretions. Various diagnostic criteria (Amsels Criteria, Nugents Scoring System and Hay Ison Criteria) have been described with varying sensitivity.

Differential diagnosis

The discharge of BV must be differentiated from that of trichomoniasis (greenish-yellow, frothy), candidiasis (curdy white, cottage-cheese like) and malignancy (purulent/blood stained).

Course and prognosis

Untreated, it may resolve within days or weeks but tends to be recurrent. PID, infertility, tubal pregnancy, preterm labor, loss of pregnancy and ascending infections like endometritis are some of the long-term complications. BV increases susceptibility to STIs.

Treatment

Metronidazole 500 mg twice a day for 1 week, or 2 gm single dose. Intravaginal clindamycin 2% cream was inserted twice daily for 7 days or metronidazole gel (0.75%) inserted twice daily for 5 days. Clindamycin 300 mg orally twice a day for 7 days/secnidazole 2 gm oral single dose has also been used. For recurrent BV, intravaginal metronidazole gel twice weekly for 4 months is recommended.

Pearl

BV is a strong risk factor for HIV infection.

Recommended reading

1. Chopra D, et al. Indian J Sex Transm Dis (2015). PMID: 26392656.
2. Bagnall P, et al. JAAPA (2017). PMID: 29135564.

Cytolytic vaginosis

Introduction

Also called lactobacillus overgrowth syndrome or Doderlein's cytolysis, CV is a lesser-known cause of vaginal discharge, frequently misdiagnosed because the symptoms mimic those of vulvovaginal candidiasis.

Epidemiology

Around 5–7% of cases of vaginal discharge unresponsive to antifungals are due to this condition, while 16% has been reported in a recent study from north India (Puri). CV is common in the 2nd to 4th decade of life. Diabetes can be a predisposing factor.

Pathophysiology

Overgrowth of *Lactobacilli alone* or in combination with other bacteria results in an increase in lactic acid and hydrogen peroxide, which irritates the vaginal epithelium resulting in cell dissolution.

This causes dysuria in the affected individuals. *Lactobacilli* are more abundant in women with high serum glucose levels. It has also been observed that symptoms will be more during the luteal phase, which is associated with increased colonization of *lactobacilli*.

Presenting complaints

Patients present with vulvar pruritus, soreness, a thick discharge, dyspareunia, urge incontinence and a cyclical worsening in the luteal phase of the menstrual cycle.

Clinical examination

The clinical picture mimics that of vulvovaginal candidiasis, with an inflamed, red vulva, edema and a thick whitish curdy discharge. The vaginal pH is 3.5–4.5.

Laboratory examination

Pap smear shows cytolysis of epithelial cells, naked nuclei, abundant *lactobacilli*, 'false clue cells' formed by *lactobacilli* covering the fragmented epithelial cells, which may be confused with the 'clue cells' of BV. Coccobacilli, pseudohyphae and spores are absent.

Differential diagnosis

This condition closely mimics VVC (growth on Sabouraud's dextrose agar confirmatory, good response to anti-fungals). The discharge in BV has a characteristic fishy odor, and vulvar inflammation is minimal, while in trichomoniasis, the patients have a greenish frothy discharge, and the diagnosis is confirmed by a wet mount.

Course

Maybe recurrent if underlying co-morbidities are not treated.

Treatment

Sodium bicarbonate douching (1–2 tsp in 4 cups warm water) or pessaries (baking soda filled in gelatin capsules and inserted into the vagina) and sitz baths are helpful to allay the symptoms.

Pearl

A suspected vulvovaginal candidiasis not responding to anti-fungal treatment should raise doubt about cytolytic vaginosis.

Recommended reading

1. Suresh A, et al. Indian J Sex Transm Dis AIDS (2009). PMID: 21938117.
2. Puri S. Ann Trop Pathol (2020). DOI: 10.4103/atp. atp_18_19.

Foreign body

Introduction

Vaginal discharge can be due to a foreign body in the vagina, cervix or uterus. Various culprit objects have been reported.

Epidemiology

Around 4% of pediatric patients attending gynecology outpatient clinics come due to foreign bodies in the vagina. The objects found are age related. In children, seeds, nuts, toys, tissue paper, pencils, hair pins, safety pins and household objects like batteries are common. In adults, reported objects include tampons, pessaries and other medical devices (like IUDs used for contraception), condoms, menstrual cups, sexual gratification objects and illicit substances like drugs. In children with foreign bodies, sexual abuse needs to be considered. Retained surgical gauze should be suspected in postpartum patients (Figure 5.4).

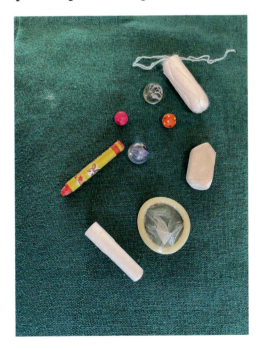

FIGURE 5.4 Common objects inserted into the vagina as foreign bodies – crayon, beads, marble, eraser, pen cap, tampon and condom. (Photograph by Dr Nina Madnani.)

Pathophysiology

Mucosal injury can become a nidus for infection.

Presenting complaints

Foreign bodies can present with a myriad of complaints such as foul-smelling vaginal discharge, which maybe persistent or recurrent especially in children. Vaginal bleeding, vulvar discomfort, pruritus and rashes may be other concerns. Often patients may present with dysuria, incontinence, hematuria, dyspareunia, abdominal and pelvic pain.

Clinical examination

Seropurulent to purulent vaginal discharge, occasionally blood stained, and foul smelling with or without vulvar inflammation may be seen at the introitus. A speculum examination shows vaginal inflammation and discharge which, after cleaning, may disclose the foreign body. Vaginoscopy can be very helpful in locating the object. Pelvic or abdominal tenderness may be present.

Systemic findings

Fever, tachycardia and hypotension can be early signs of sepsis.

Laboratory examination

Smear for Gram's stain and culture. Imaging of the pelvis with X-rays, ultrasonogram and magnetic resonance imaging (MRI) may be necessary, especially in the pediatric age group, where a vaginal examination is difficult.

Differential diagnosis

Some common causes of vaginal discharge must be ruled out, including:

- Infections such as trichomoniasis (frothy green discharge), candidiasis (curdy-white discharge with intense pruritus and soreness) and gonorrhoea (thick white pus and gram stain showing intracellular gram-negative diplococci).
- Sexual abuse (signs of injury at the introitus with a positive history of abuse).
- Malignancy (seen in elderly, accompanied with foul smelling, blood-tinged discharge).

Course and prognosis

Retention of the foreign object for prolonged periods can lead to vaginolith, urethrovaginal or rectovaginal fistula or even septicemia/toxemia. Repeated episodes in an individual may indicate psychological disturbance or sexual abuse.

Treatment

Removal of the causative object is curative. Systemic antibiotics may be necessary for impending toxemia. Psychological evaluation for repeated episodes in an individual or in sexual abuse is required.

Pearl

Recurrent, purulent vaginal discharge needs a high index of suspicion of a foreign body.

Recommended reading

1. Saidman JM, et al. J Ultrasound (2021). PMID: 34145533.
2. Ma W, et al. Pediatr Surg Int (2022). PMID: 35129659.
3. Kumari P, et al. J Evolution Med Dent Sci (2020). DOI: 10.14260/jemds/2020/540.

6

INFLAMMATORY DISORDERS OF THE VULVA

Nina Madnani

Contents

Intertrigo

Introduction

Intertrigo, an inflammatory condition of body folds or closely opposing surfaces, is a common condition which is frequently seen in women in hot and humid climates or in those with bowel incontinence.

Epidemiology

The incidence of intertrigo is difficult to quantify, as no studies are available. It is common in obese and overweight people with deep body folds, diabetics, and those on immunosuppressive medications. Professional runners/athletes often suffer from intertrigo.

Pathophysiology

Excessive sweating keep the folds macerated, and easily traumatized with friction. Tight thick trousers aggravate the condition. Secondary fungal and bacterial infections complicate the condition.

Presenting complaints

Patients complain of severe burning, itching soreness in the body folds, especially the groins. The pruritis and burning often disturb sleep and reduce their quality of life (QoL). Common activities like walking, cycling, and exercising become painful.

Clinical examination

Few or all body folds can be involved including inframammary and under a pendulous abdominal fold. The areas show well-marginated erythema, with maceration and a musty odor when complicated by superadded bacterial/fungal infection. The area may be studded with papules/papulopustules, excoriations, and erosions (Figure 6.1).

Dermoscopy

The findings would be those of eczematous dermatitis with a patchy distribution of dotted vessels and yellow sero-crusts.

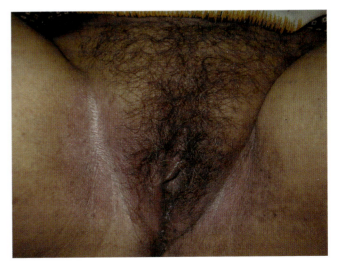

FIGURE 6.1 Obese women are prone to intertrigo due to deep folds, friction, and maceration. (Photograph by Dr Nisha Chaturvedi.)

DOI: 10.1201/9781003284116-6

Lab examination

Smears for bacterial and fungal culture may be requested only if a secondary infection is suspected. A skin biopsy may be helpful to differentiate from other conditions like psoriasis, candidiasis, or a tinea cruris.

Histopathology

A spongiotic process is seen. A periodic acid-Schiff (PAS) stain to rule out candida.

Differential diagnosis

Candidiasis, psoriasis, and seborrheic dermatitis are the closest differentials. Hailey-Hailey disease and extramammary Paget disease are:

- Intertriginous candidiasis in addition to the bright pink well-defined lesions would have satellite papulo -pustules and fissuring.
- Psoriatic lesions are well demarcated, bright pink with mild scaling. Other sites like scalp, extensor aspects, nails, and joints should also be examined. The classic location is the intergluteal fold.
- Seborrheic dermatitis lesions have yellowish scale crusts. Other sites such as eyebrows, retro-auricular, pre-sternal area, and the upper back are sites commonly affected.

Course and prognosis

This condition waxes and wanes depending on the weather condition and weight of the individual.

Treatment

Air drying the area is extremely important. Cotton underpants, akin to boxer pants, are recommended to prevent skin-to-skin rubbing. A mild anti-bacterial-steroid combination is useful in reducing inflammation. Diaper creams are also helpful. Systemic antihistamines are required to allay the itch. A diaper rash cream/zinc-oxide cream soothes and prevents friction. Weight loss and loose cotton clothing need to be encouraged for long-term remission.

Pearl

Suspect intertrigo when the intensity of the discomfort reported by the patient does not match the clinical findings.

Recommended reading

1. Hagerman GF, et al. Clin Colon Rectal Surg. 2019. PMID: 31507350.
2. Kottner J, et al. Int J Nurs Stud. 2020. PMID: 32105975.

Seborrheic dermatitis

Introduction

Although seborrheic dermatitis commonly involves the scalp, medial eyebrows, glabella, nasolabial, V of the chest and back, and other intertriginous folds, it can also involve the vulva and the inguinal folds. This area is often missed by the examining physician as a result of which women may suffer for years before they seek treatment for this distressing condition.

Epidemiology

Exact statistics of the incidence is not known, but it is more common in women between 30 and 60 years of age.

Pathogenesis

Stress, obesity, sweating, alcohol, fatigue, Parkinson's, and immunosuppression are triggers. Malassezia furfur colonization is considered an important factor for inflammation.

Presenting complaints

A musty odor is a common complaint. Itching, burning, inability to wear undergarments, and difficulty in walking and exercising make the woman's QoL poor. Sexual intimacy is compromised.

Clinical examination

The entire vulva up to the perianal region, the inguinal folds, and often extending onto the medial thighs, shows a bright pink or dusky pink erythema with mild scaling. Satellite papules may be seen. Other sites like the scalp, medial eyebrows, and naso labial folds may be involved and can often give supportive evidence for the clinical diagnosis. Mild cases may show subtle erythema in the inguinal folds. Fissures can be seen in the interlabial folds, sulci, natal cleft, and posterior fourchette (Figures 6.2 and 6.3).

Lab investigations

A KOH mount may show Malassezia furfur. A patch test may be required to rule out contact dermatitis.

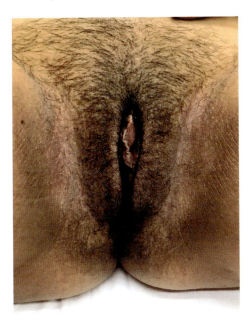

FIGURE 6.2 Unlike seborrheic dermatitis of the scalp, the vulva shows minimal seborrhea with fine scaling. (Photograph by Dr Nina Madnani.)

Histopathology
As this is an eczematous process, hyperkeratosis, irregular acanthosis, mild spongiosis, and a perivascular lymphocytic infiltration are the features seen.

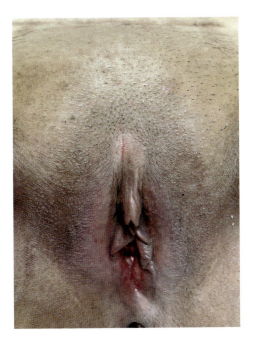

FIGURE 6.3 Interlabial fissures may be a component of seborrheic dermatitis, as seen in this image. (Photograph by Dr Nisha Chaturvedi.)

Dermoscopy
Mild yellowish scaling irregularly arranged dotted vessels on a background of erythema.

Differential diagnosis
This condition is often difficult to distinguish from other eczematous processes like atopic dermatitis, contact dermatitis both allergic and irritant, candidiasis, and inverse psoriasis.

Management
Weight loss if obese is extremely important to reduce sweating, and friction in the folds. Mid-potency corticosteroids several times a week and then substituted with tacrolimus ointment (0.03/0.1%) or pimecrolimus cream are required.

Course and prognosis
The condition has a tendency to relapse during periods of stress, or weather changes where sweating is excessive.

Pearl
In darker skin types, the erythema may not be so evident, so examination of other seborrheic sites is important.

Recommended reading
1. Sand FL, et al. J Obstet Gynaecol (2018). PMID: 28780897.
2. Pichardo-Geisinger R. Obstet Gynecol Clin North Am (2017). PMID: 28778637.

Eczemas/dermatitis: Atopic/contact (Irritant/Allergic)

Introduction
Eczemas are the commonest cause of the vulvar itch, and are a morphological description of an "umbrella" term, encompassing atopic dermatitis and allergic or irritant contact dermatitis among others. Clinically, they may be difficult to differentiate in many patients, and a biopsy or patch test may be required for the diagnosis. Most often, these cases are missed, and the women are repeatedly misdiagnosed as having a fungal infection and administered systemic fluconazole with no relief.

Epidemiology

Approximately 0.5–10% of women suffer from vulvar eczema. The incidence of atopic dermatitis has been steadily increasing, especially in urban populations. With the availability of a plethora of vulvar care products, menstrual products, clothes, hair-removal creams, etc, the incidence of allergic contact dermatitis is steadily rising, while harsh cleanser usage in this sensitive area can lead to an irritant contact dermatitis.

Pathophysiology

Atopic dermatitis is a chronic inflammatory disorder resulting from a genetically programmed defective skin barrier that allows high levels of trans epidermal water loss. This is especially evident on the vulvar skin, which by virtue of its anatomical location is subjected to sweating, warmth, maceration, menstrual products, and friction from clothing, besides various detergents used to keep the area "clean" by obsessive individuals.

Allergic contact dermatitis is a delayed type of hypersensitivity reaction seen in individuals who have been previously sensitized to the antigen/allergen, and does not affect the entire population. Irritant contact dermatitis results from contact with a toxic substance/chemical and can affect every individual by triggering off innate immunity. The irritant directly damages the epidermal cells.

Presenting complaints

Pruritis, pain, burning, and dyspareunia are the commonest complaints of all 3. Intractable itching, more at night, is a common complaint. Soiling of the underpants either with blood or serum in very acute or severe cases can occur.

Clinical findings

The areas involved include not only the labia majora but also the modified mucous membranes and the perianal area. Extragenital sites (nape of the neck, flexures, shins, etc) are often concurrently involved and need to be looked out for.

The appearance will vary depending on whether the dermatitis is acute, subacute, or chronic.

In the acute stage, the labia will show edema, erythema, and some areas of vesiculation and oozing. Erythema may be difficult to discern in darker skin types. Erosions and excoriations may be evident (Figures 6.4–6.7).

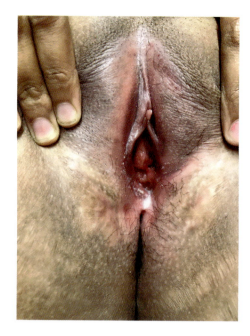

FIGURE 6.4 Acute contact dermatitis following the use of depilatory cream. (Photograph by Dr Nina Madnani.)

In the subacute stage, the edema may be absent or subtle, erythema less intense, with evidence of early lichenification.

Chronic eczema will show evidence of accentuation of skin markings (lichenification), thickening, and dyspigmentation in darker skins.

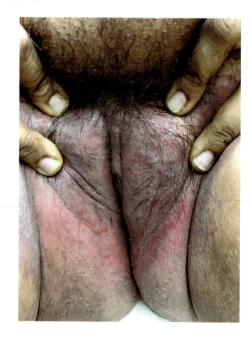

FIGURE 6.5 This lady scrubbed herself with Dettol liquid. Notice the bright erythema and superficial erosion due to the irritant effect. (Photograph by Dr Nina Madnani.)

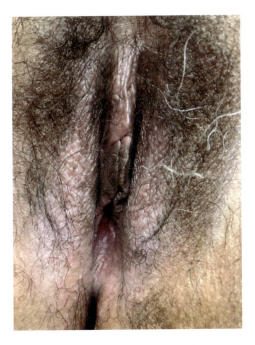

FIGURE 6.6 Allergic contact dermatitis to a popular synthetic sanitary napkin presenting as subacute eczematization. (Photograph by Dr Nina Madnani.)

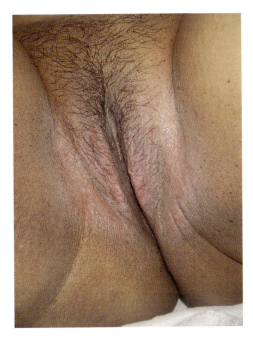

FIGURE 6.7 Synthetic sanitary pads with "wings" can give an allergic contact dermatitis in the genito crural folds as seen in this lady. She was misdiagnosed with vulvar psoriasis. (Photograph by Dr Nisha Chaturvedi.)

Irritant contact dermatitis will be more inflamed and show deep erosions. Prominent edema of the vulva will be apparent.

Lab investigations

Patch testing may be useful in a c/o vulvar dermatitis which fails to give the expected response to management. In such cases, it may be carried out with standard series and sometimes with the actual product suspected. It requires great experience to read the results.

Histopathology

A biopsy is useful only to differentiate dermatitis from other differentials like psoriasis or candidiasis, which look clinically similar.

An acute stage shows a spongiotic process, whereas a chronic stage will show acanthosis, irregular and thickened epidermal rete ridges, prominent granular layer, and fibrosis in the papillary dermis.

Differential diagnosis

Psoriasis, seborrheic dermatitis, candidiasis, HSIL (high-grade squamous intraepithelial lesion), and EMPD (extramammary Paget's disease) need to be differentiated from the eczemas (Figure 6.8).

Management

It is essential to break the itch-scratch cycle, repair the barrier function, and reduce inflammation.

Counseling and education on vulvar cleansing only with water or non-soap cleansers, avoidance of wet wipes, perfumed deodorants, anti-perspirants, synthetic underpants, harsh detergents, and medicated non-prescription creams are important to allow the skin barrier repair process.

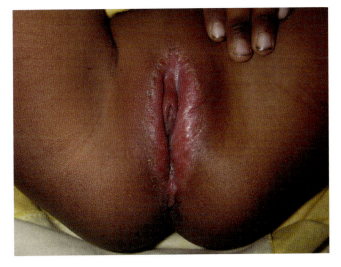

FIGURE 6.8 Psoriasis in a child can easily be mistaken as an irritant contact dermatitis. Notice the well-defined lesion with silvery scales at the periphery. (Photograph by Dr Nisha Chaturvedi.)

Keeping the area dry, topical emollient creams and mid-potency corticosteroids help to reduce inflammation. Non-steroidal applications of tacrolimus/pimecrolimus can be phased in.

Antihistamines, sedating at night to break the itch cycle, are useful.

Oral corticosteroids in non-responders for a short period of a few weeks may assist in bringing the inflammation and itch under control

Prognosis

Eczemas in this region tend to be more persistent by virtue of the environmental conditions and triggering factors. Hence, relapses are common.

Pearl

These chronic conditions need counseling and a lot of hand-holding to bring the disease under control.

Recommended reading

1. Woelber L, et al. Dtsch Arztebl Int (2020). PMID: 32181734.
2. Pichardo-Geisinger R. Obstet Gynecol Clin North Am (2017). PMID: 28778637.

Lichen simplex/lichen simplex chronicus

Introduction

This is a pruritic, chronic endogenous eczematous condition, perpetuated with the "itch-scratch cycle" and lasting for several months or years. The itch described by the woman is colloquially called "meethee" or "sweet" itch, more at night.

Epidemiology

No data exists specifically for lichen simplex chronicus (LSC) but is seen across all races and skin colors. Adult women between 30 and 50 generally suffer from this condition. An atopic diathesis may be present in some of the patients.

Pathophysiology

This endogenous eczema often gets triggered off by synthetic clothing, sweating, or psychological stress. Anogenital pruritis is a very common "stress-busting" site. The action of itching causes injury to the epidermis and stimulates nerve impulses which heighten the itch impulse. Also, repeated scratching leads to thickening (lichenification) and barrier dysfunction. This cycle of

itch-scratch is self-perpetuating. LSC may be complicated by a contact dermatitis or a super-added bacterial/candidal infection.

Presenting complaints

Intractable itching, especially at night, is the hallmark of LSC. Once the patient itches the area, she is unable to stop as it gives her both pain and pleasure. Burning is another symptom. Often, the vulvar itch extends to the perianal area.

Clinical examination

The areas involved may be erythematous in lighter skin types, deeply pigmented or grayish-white in darker skin types, with thickening and lichenification. Both the keratinized and non-keratinized skin are involved, with the labia majora taking the brunt. Extension to the perianal skin may be seen. Excoriations and erosions may be evident (Figures 6.9–6.12).

Lab investigations

A swab should be taken when a superadded bacterial/fungal infection is suspected.

Dermoscopy

In this chronic eczematous condition, the findings include uniform dotted vessels with a white halo (Figure 6.13).

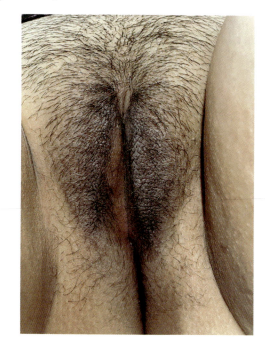

FIGURE 6.9 Early lesion showing lichenification on the extensor aspect of labia majora. (Photograph by Dr Nina Madnani.)

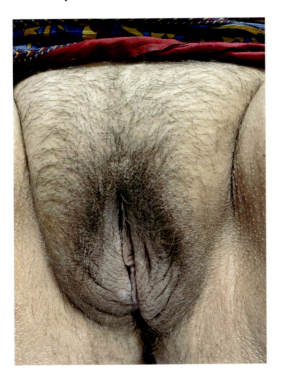

FIGURE 6.10   Another patient with lichenification and vulvar laxity (saggy look).

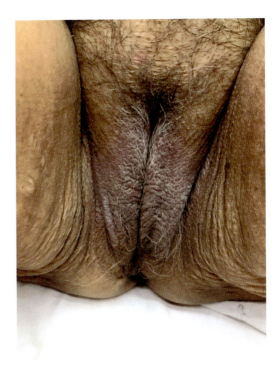

FIGURE 6.12   Both labia majorae are lichenified secondary to chronic itching. Photograph by Dr Nina Madnani.

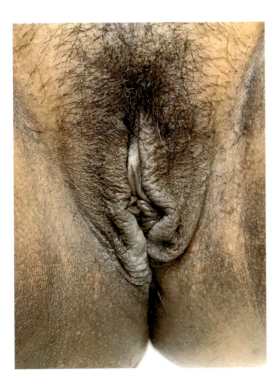

FIGURE 6.11   Chronic itching and lichenification give the appearance of vulvar laxity (saggy look). Photograph by Dr Nina Madnani.

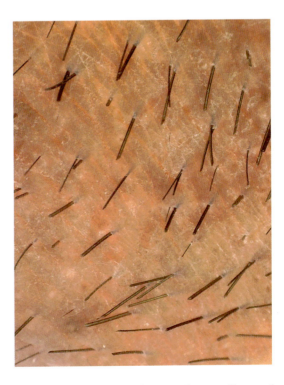

FIGURE 6.13   Irregular scales, yellow clods, and irregularly distributed dotted vessels. Dinolite Digital Microscope, WF-20, polarized, 10×. (Photograph by Dr Nina Madnani.)

Histopathology

Epidermis shows hyperkeratosis, acanthosis, psoriasiform hyperplasia, and a chronic inflammatory infiltrate in the dermis. Often, vulvar LSC does not show vertically oriented collagen bundles, as seen in biopsy specimens from extragenital sites.

Differential diagnosis

Although the appearance of LSC is so classical, a close differential would be an allergic/irritant contact dermatitis, psoriasis, lichen planus, and candidiasis.

Management

It is imperative to break the "itch-scratch" cycle with sedative antihistamines or anxiolytics. Repair of the barrier function with emollients, reduction of the inflammation, and lichenification often may require short bursts of mid to high-potency corticosteroids. Intra-lesional triamcinolone acetonide 5 mg/ml may be injected into unresponsive areas. Calcineurin inhibitors like tacrolimus and pimecrolimus are other options but may cause stinging in some patients.

Prognosis

This condition may smolder for years and requires counseling to improve compliance. Many may improve, but often relapse once again. The women become demotivated, and their self-esteem and self-worth get impaired. Sexual intimacy is impaired.

Pearls

The clues to diagnosing LSC are lichenification, a leathery look, and a grayish-moist appearance.

Always check the perianal area.

Nails may be glossy due to chronic itching.

Recommended reading

1. Verma SB. Indian Dermatol Online J (2021). PMID: 34430467.
2. Virgili A, et al. J Reprod Med (2001). PMID: 11354834.

Psoriasis

Introduction

Psoriasis is a common, chronic, autoimmune inflammatory disorder, which is considered "difficult" when it involves the genitals. "Inverse" psoriasis is the term given for the disease occurring in folds and not on the normal extensor areas. Women with psoriasis do not disclose their genital involvement and need to be specifically asked. Although genital psoriasis theoretically involves a small percentage of the body surface, it has a huge negative impact on the patient's daily routine activities, her QoL, and sexual intimacy.

Epidemiology

Around 29–46% of women with psoriasis have "inverse" psoriasis and 80% of women with "inverse" psoriasis have genital involvement. Children and infants may have diaper psoriasis, which may be mistaken as diaper dermatitis. The age of women with genital psoriasis varies between 20 and 40 years, but it is also seen in children.

Pathophysiology

The Koebner's phenomena of the constant rubbing of the vulvar area and folds due to clothing, friction, and in day-to-day activities suggest that its pathophysiology is similar to that of plaque psoriasis. Stress, obesity, smoking, and alcohol are the other triggering factors. Epidermal hyperplasia is the result of an inflammatory process driven by cytokines like tumor necrosis factor (TNF)-alfa, interleukin (IL)-17A, and IL-23.

Presenting complaints

Soreness, intractable itching, burning and dyspareunia, and inability to tolerate the wearing of underpants are the common complaints. Daily activities like walking, cycling, exercising become painful and difficult. The itching is often severe enough to cause sleepless nights.

Clinical examination

Typical erythematous scaly plaques are common on the mons pubis. The genitocrural folds show well-demarcated plaques, bright pink or pigmented crusted plaques with maceration. Scaling may be absent. Macerated areas may emanate a musty smell. The Auspitz sign, which is characteristic of psoriasis, may not be elicitable in inverse psoriasis (Figures 6.14 and 6.15).

Other body areas including the nails, scalp, and joints need to be examined for evidence of psoriasis, and if present, makes diagnosis simpler (Figure 6.16).

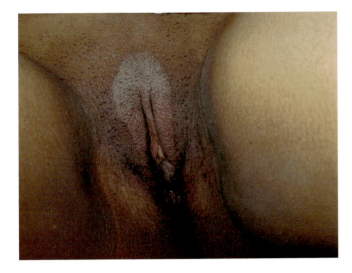

FIGURE 6.14 Grayish pink, well-demarcated plaque with fine scaling. (Photograph by Dr Nina Madnani.)

Lab examination

Skin biopsy is the key to confirming psoriasis as well as differentiating it from other conditions. Patients with genital psoriasis are more prone to have a metabolic disease, and hence need to be worked up with lipid profile, liver function tests, blood sugars, Vit D3 levels, and evaluation of the cardiac status.

Dermoscopy

Vulvar psoriasis typically shows regular dotted vessels on a pinkish background, with regularly arranged scales, which may be fewer in macerated areas (Figure 6.17).

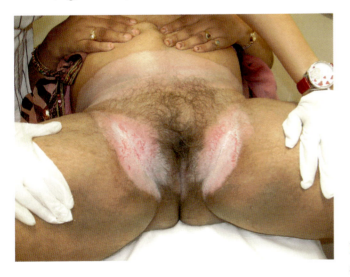

FIGURE 6.15 Erythematous plaques on vulva and body folds with fine silvery white scaling. (Photograph by Dr Nina Madnani.)

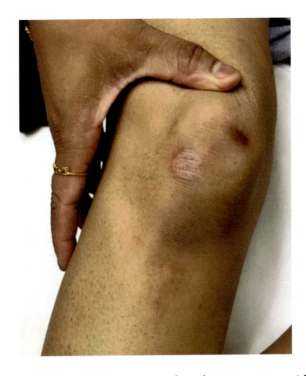

FIGURE 6.16 Psoriasis elsewhere may provide a clue to making a diagnosis of vulvar psoriasis. (Photograph by Dr Nina Madnani.)

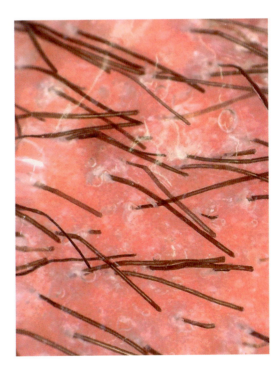

FIGURE 6.17 Dermoscopy shows regularly arranged scales and dotted vessels on a pinkish background. Dinolite Digital Microscope, WF-20, polarized, 10×. (Photograph by Dr Nina Madnani.)

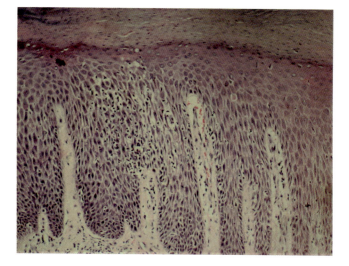

FIGURE 6.18 Psoriasiform epidermal hyperplasia, diminished granular layer, and confluent parakeratosis, supra-papillary thinning, dilated capillaries in the dermal papilla, and epidermal lymphocytes (exocytosis). (Photograph by Dr Rajiv Joshi.)

Histopathology

The epidermis may not show hyperkeratosis normally seen in a psoriatic plaque but shows peg-shaped elongated rete ridges with supra-papillary thinning, dilated blood vessels with extravasation of erythrocytes. A sparse perivascular lymphocytic infiltrate is seen. Some areas may show mild spongiosis (Figure 6.18).

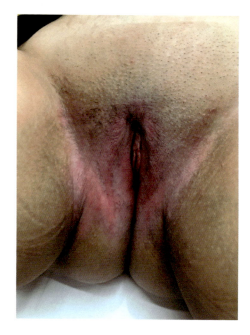

FIGURE 6.19 Flexural erythema with minimal scaling can mimic seborrheic dermatitis sans yellow crust. (Photograph by Dr Nina Madnani.)

Differential diagnosis

Inflammatory and infective conditions like Intertrigo, seborrheic dermatitis, incontinence dermatitis, extramammary Paget disease, lichen sclerosus, lichen planus, fungal infections, and plasma-cell vulvitis need to be differentiated from inverse/genital psoriasis (Figures 6.19 and 6.20).

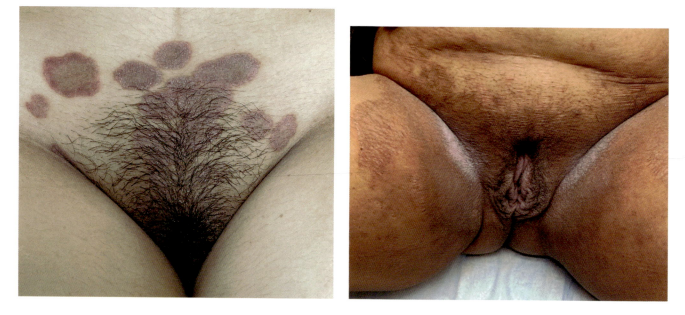

FIGURE 6.20 (a) This patient with plaque-type psoriasis (biopsy proven) can be easily mistaken for tinea infection. (b) This lady with inverse psoriasis has a concomitant dermatophyte infection. (Photograph by Dr Nina Madnani.)

Treatment

Weight loss and lifestyle changes are important for long-term relief. Tight-fitting trousers and underpants should be avoided to prevent koebnerization. Topical mid-potency corticosteroids phased into topical tacrolimus; vitamin D analogues, together with emollients, can be used as first-line therapy. Non-responders may need systemic medication from the following: cyclosporin, methotrexate, apremilast, TNF-alfa inhibitors like adalimumab, infliximab, etanercept, IL-17 antagonists like secukinumab, IL-23 inhibitors, in addition to newer biologics in the pipeline (Figure 6.21).

Course and prognosis

Inverse psoriasis is a chronic disabling condition, especially in the obese and diabetics. Due to the constant friction and maceration, koebnerization can keep the disease smoldering for years. The intense pruritus can severely affect the QoL. Biologics have given new hope in the management of this difficult condition. Botulinum toxin A has been tried to reduce hyperhidrosis in obese women (Figure 6.22).

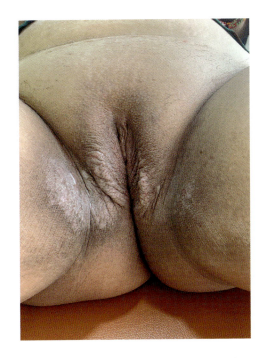

FIGURE 6.22 Lichenification, a secondary event on an itchy psoriatic plaque. (Photograph by Dr Nisha Chaturvedi.)

Pearls

A well-defined pinkish plaque in the intergluteal cleft is strongly suggestive of psoriasis (Figure 6.23).

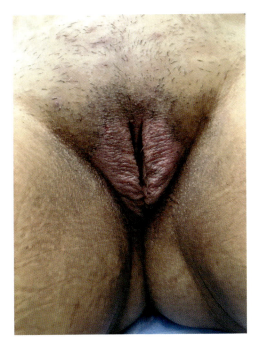

FIGURE 6.21 Well-demarcated thickened pinkish-gray plaques on both labia, indicating rubbed psoriasis. (Photograph by Dr Nina Madnani.)

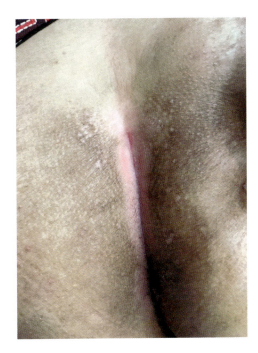

FIGURE 6.23 Intergluteal cleft involvement is sometimes the only site involved in obese women. (Photograph by Dr Nina Madnani.)

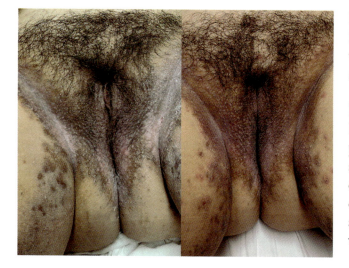

FIGURE 6.24 Psoriasis healing with post-inflammatory hyperpigmentation. (Photograph by Dr Nina Madnani.)

In patients with the skin of color, psoriasis can heal with deep hyperpigmentation (Figure 6.24).

Recommended reading

1. Micali G, et al. Clin Cosmet Investig Dermatol (2019). PMID: 32099435.
2. Hagerman GF, et al. Clin Colon Rectal Surg (2019). PMID: 31507350.
3. Hong JJ, et al. Dermatol Ther (Heidelb) (2021). PMID: 33914293.
4. Beck KM, et al. Dermatol Ther (Heidelb) (2018). PMID: 30145740.

Vulvar lichen planus

Introduction

Lichen planus (LP) is an autoimmune inflammatory condition that can involve the skin, scalp, nails, and mucosa in patients of all age groups from infancy to menopause. Vulvar Lichen Planus (VLP) is commoner in women between 30 and 50 years of age. The erosive mucosal form is relentless, ultimately leading to scarring.

Epidemiology

The exact incidence of vulvar LP is not known, but some studies show an incidence of 3.7%, of which 17.6% are the erosive type. A majority of women with oral LP can have VLP and vice versa. The association of autoimmune disease such as thyroid, coeliac disease, alopecia areata, and erosive LP is well known.

Pathophysiology

LP is considered to be a T-cell-mediated disease, with resultant damage to the basement membrane and pigmentary incontinence.

Presenting complaints

Pruritis and pain are the two commonest complaints. Women with VLP may seek treatment several months to years after the onset of the disease. The erosive ones generally have severe dysuria and dyspareunia, with vaginal discharge and post-coital bleeding, and may reach us late, wherein vaginal scarring has already set in.

Clinical examination

Every patient with VLP needs to be examined for extragenital lesions on the skin, scalp, nails, and mucous membranes. VLP has 3 variants: Classical, hypertrophic, and erosive form. The classical form has the typical violaceous flat-topped polygonal papules in groups. The hypertrophic variety has violaceous hyperkeratotic papules and plaques, while the erosive variety has a bright red glazed appearance at the introitus and vagina. The tissue may be hemorrhagic or friable. Plurimucosal LP or vulvo-vaginal-gingival (VVG) syndrome described by Pellise, involves the buccal mucosa, the vulva, and vagina. Severe cases may affect the pharynx and/or the anal mucosa. A lacy pattern typical of LP may be seen in the vulva and buccal mucosa. Neglected patients may have the entire vulva scarred with only a minute opening suggestive of the vagina. The incidence of oral LP in women with erosive vulvo-vaginal LP varies between 40 and 100% (Figures 6.25–6.30).

Rarely, lichen planus pigmentosus can involve the vulva in extensive disease leaving behind post-inflammatory hyperpigmentation.

Dermoscopy

Classic lichen planus will show Wickham's stria which are white lines crisscrossing with peripheral dotted vessels (Figure 6.31).

Hypertrophic LP will, in addition, show comedo-like openings.

Erosive LP may show Wickham's striae at the periphery, but mostly a dark pink background with erosions and dotted vessels

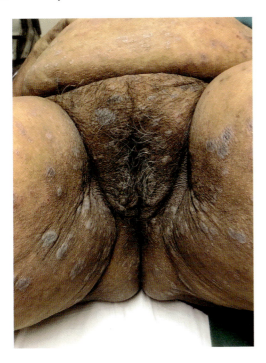

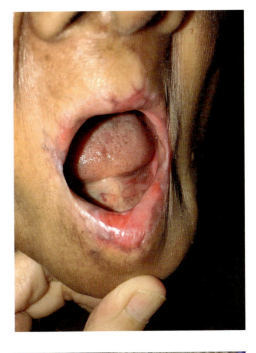

FIGURE 6.25 Grayish flat-topped papules and plaques, extending over the vulva, genitocrural folds, and upper inner thighs. (Photograph by Dr Nina Madnani.)

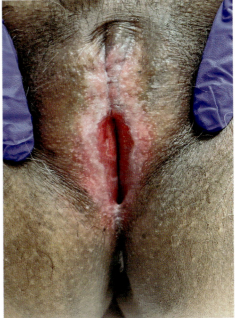

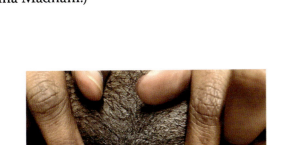

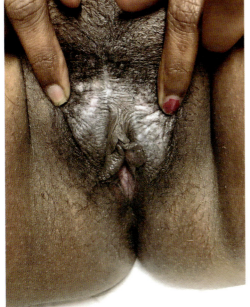

FIGURE 6.26 Differential here is Lichen simplex chronicus. The presence of flat-topped papules clinches the diagnosis of lichen planus. (Photograph by Dr Nina Madnani.)

FIGURE 6.27 **(a and b)** Chronic inflammation in VVG syndrome results in severe scarring in the oral cavity with loss of teeth and destruction of the vulva with a small residual opening. (Photographs by Dr Nina Madnani.)

Histopathology

Classical VLP shows typical features of an interface dermatitis, with a lichenoid infiltrate mainly of lymphocytes, hugging the epidermis. Basal cell degeneration is seen. The hypertrophic variety will have a thicker acanthotic epidermis with

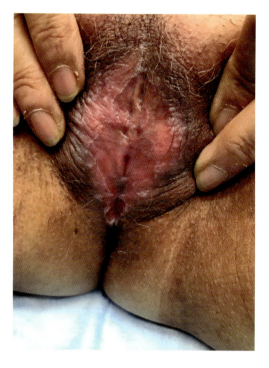

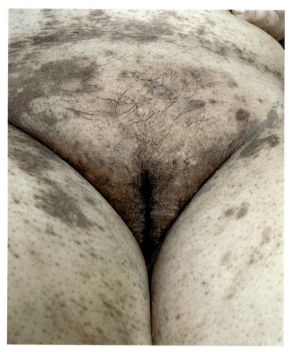

FIGURE 6.28 Notice the lacy pattern and violaceous papules at the border. (Photograph by Dr Nina Madnani.)

FIGURE 6.30 This lady had extensive lichen planus pigmentosus with active follicular LP. (Photograph by Dr Nina Madnani.)

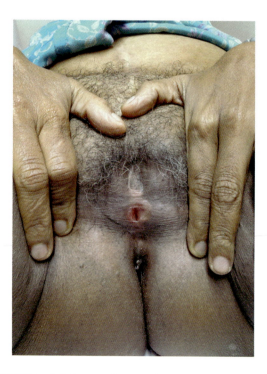

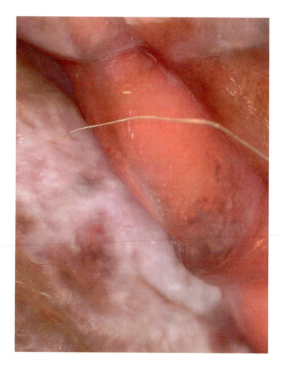

FIGURE 6.29 Lichen planus is an important differential to consider in a scarred vulva. (Photograph by Dr Nina Madnani.)

FIGURE 6.31 Criss-crossing of white lines of Wickham's striae with peripheral dotted vessels. Dinolite Digital Microscope, WF-20, polarized, 10×. (Photograph by Dr Nina Madnani.)

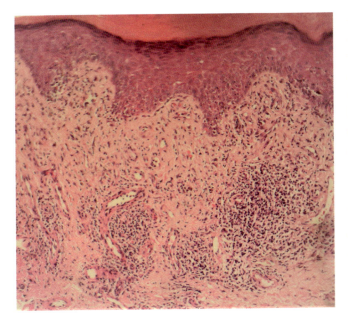

FIGURE 6.32 Lichen Planus 1: H & E, 100×, epidermal acanthosis with wedge-shaped hypergranulosis, perivascular, and interstitial lymphocytic infiltrate. (Photograph by Dr Rajiv Joshi.)

similar interface changes. The erosive variety does not have any classical histopathology, and biopsy is recommended only to rule out a malignancy (Figure 6.32).

Differential diagnosis

The erosive form needs to be distinguished from other conditions like pemphigus vulgaris, mucosal pemphigoid, Steven Johnson syndrome, graft versus host disease (GVHD), and desquamative inflammatory vaginitis. GVHD is seen in the bone marrow and stem cell transplant patients. Mucosal erosions and lichen planus can occur in both acute and chronic forms.

Management

The classical and hypertrophic varieties are managed similarly to LP elsewhere on the body.

The mucosal variety is a therapeutic nightmare, which requires topical treatment with super-potent clobetasol propionate 0.05% twice a day initially and then tapered off as required or replaced by a lower potency corticosteroid ointment. Topical calcineurin inhibitors tacrolimus and pimecrolimus are steroid sparing, but some patients are intolerant to them. Vaginal hydrocortisone creams inserted daily may prevent adhesions and scarring. Surgery is required to break

adhesions and needs to be followed with dilators and topical corticosteroids (within 24 hours of surgery), as relapse is the norm. Systemic corticosteroid in a dose of 0.5 mg/kg per day or cyclosporine 5–6 mg/kg in divided doses gives fast results but cannot be given long term. Mycophenolate mofetil 500 mg 2–3 times daily has a slower onset. Methotrexate has shown mixed results. Hydroxychloroquine is not so effective for vulvar LP. Mycophenolate mofetil 500 mg twice or thrice a day is required for unresponsive active disease.

Course and prognosis

Classic cases after healing leave behind post-inflammatory hyperpigmentation. Erosive forms progress relentlessly and require active intervention to slow down the scarring. Dysesthesia is a common complication for such patients. Around 1–3% of erosive LP may develop cancers and require constant monitoring.

The classical and hypertrophic varieties respond well, although squamous cell carcinomas may be an outcome in the hypertrophic variety.

Pearl

Vulvar erosion with scarring, think of lichen planus.

When suspecting vulvar lichen planus, check for LP elsewhere.

Recommended reading

1. Fruchter R, et al. Int J Womens Dermatol (2017). PMID: 28492056.
2. Micheletti L, et al. Br J Dermatol (2000). PMID: 11122067.
3. Santegoets LA, et al. J Low Genit Tract Dis (2010). PMID: 20885160.
4. Simpson RC, et al. Br J Dermatol (2012). PMID: 22384934.
5. Dash S, et al. Clin Exp Dermatol (2021). PMID: 33484573.

Lichen sclerosus

Introduction

In 1976, ISSVD recommended the abolition of the term "lichen sclerosus et atrophicus" (LSA), replacing it with Lichen sclerosus (LS). This condition is often missed, and there is a delay of several years before the diagnosis is made.

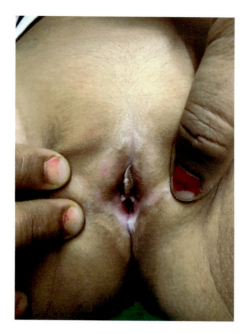

FIGURE 6.33 Pre-adolescent with early lichen sclerosus. (Photograph by Dr Nina Madnani.)

Epidemiology

The exact prevalence is not known as the disease may be asymptomatic initially, but an incidence of 1 in 30 older women and 1 in 900 prepubertal girls has been reported. The disease has a biphasic onset: pre-pubertal and post-menopausal, but it can affect any age (Figure 6.33).

Pathophysiology

Although the exact etiology is not known, LS is considered to be an autoimmune disease associated with other autoimmune conditions like thyroid disease, psoriasis, type 1 diabetes, systemic lupus erythematosus, systemic sclerosis, pernicious anemia among others. A genetic predisposition, immune dysregulation, inflammation, abnormal collagen metabolism, and triggers like friction due to tight clothing and urinary incontinence have been hypothesised.

Presenting complaints

The women may come with one or more of the following: vulvar or anal itching, which is intractable at night, irritation and/soreness, urethral and vaginal discharge, painful skin fissuring, dysuria, dyspareunia, urinary and fecal incontinence, or may be asymptomatic.

Constipation is a common complaint in children with LS.

Clinical examination

LS can involve the vulva up to the perianal region, giving a classical "figure-of-eight" distribution. It involves the clitoris, clitoral hood, labia minora, vestibule, and perianal area but very rarely the vagina. Early disease may just show evidence of pallor, but as the disease progresses, pale, ivory-colored lesions of partially atrophic skin give the typical crinkling or cellophane paper-type appearance. Purpura/ecchymosis due to localized hemorrhage of the skin, ulcerations/erosions/fissuring, and rarely blisters may be evident. Darker skin types, especially Fitz. Types 5 and 6 may show depigmentation akin to vitiligo. The vulvar components start "disappearing", and missing vulvar parts is the hallmark of LS. As the disease progresses, hyperkeratotic areas and sclerosis indicating varying degrees of scarring are seen (Figures 6.34–6.38).

Extragenital lesions may be seen on the neck, trunk, upper extremities, and thighs.

Lab examination

LS can be diagnosed easily by careful history taking and clinical examination. The "missing" parts are pathognomonic. Biopsy in children is generally

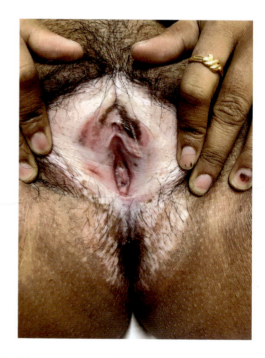

FIGURE 6.34 Vulvar LS extending to the perianal area in a classic figure of 8 patterns. (Photograph by Dr Nina Madnani.)

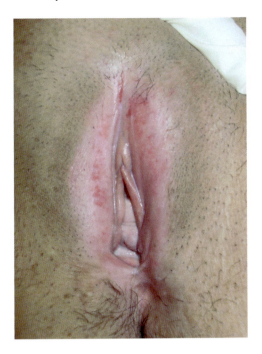

FIGURE 6.35 Petechiae are a prominent finding in early disease. (Photograph by Dr Nina Madnani.)

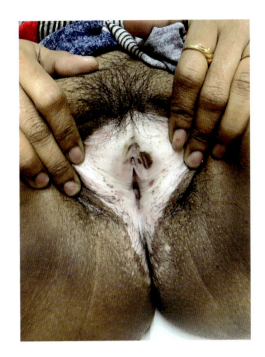

FIGURE 6.37 Mimics vitiligo in the skin of color. (Photograph by Dr Nina Madnani.)

not recommended. Biopsy in adults is done in unusual presentations or to sample non-responsive suspicious areas to exclude vulvar intraepithelial neoplasia (VIN). Work-up for the associated auto-immune diseases is essential (Figure 6.39).

Dermoscopy

White structureless area, hairpin vessels, comma vessels, and linear branching vessels are seen, and at places, superficial erosions if the area has been scratched. Comedo-like openings are absent in genital LS (Figure 6.40).

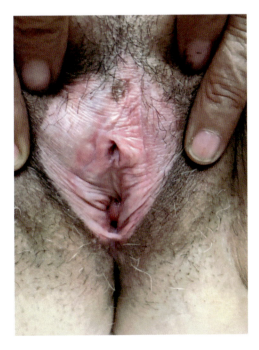

FIGURE 6.36 Agglutination of labia, clitoris, and clitoral hood, cigarette paper wrinkling. (Photograph by Dr Nina Madnani.)

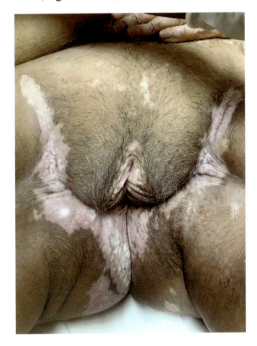

FIGURE 6.38 Extensive LS extending into the genito-crural folds with areas of hyperkeratosis. (Photograph by Dr Nina Madnani.)

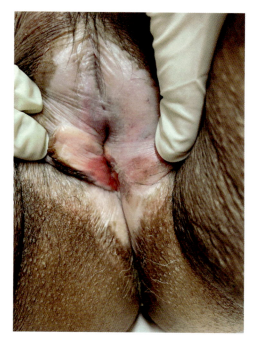

FIGURE 6.39 Hyperkeratosis or erosions not responsive to topical therapy warrant biopsy to rule out malignancy. (Photograph by Dr Nina Madnani.)

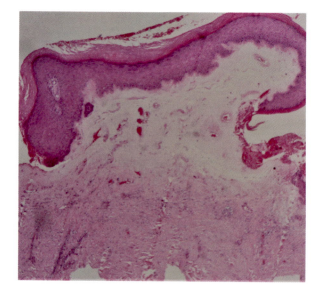

FIGURE 6.41 Lichen sclerosis 2: H & E, 100×, pale sclerotic upper dermis, interstitially scattered lymphocytic infiltrate beneath the sclerosis. (Photograph by Dr Rajiv Joshi.)

Histopathology

Biopsy from a white sclerotic area has three zones, viz, an atrophic epidermis, hyalinized mid zone, and a lichenoid infiltrate (Figure 6.41).

Differential diagnosis

LS is commonly mistaken as vitiligo, or candidiasis. Vitiliginous patches are stark white, well demarcated, and not associated with induration or sclerosis of the vulvar parts. Often early LS may resemble vitiligo, but a biopsy is confirmatory. Other differentials include psoriasis, lichen planus, or a VIN.

Management

LS is a chronic disease and requires lifelong follow-up. Extensive studies have evidence supporting the use of super-potent topical corticosteroid clobetasol propionate 0.5% as single therapy. Application is recommended twice a day for 2 weeks, then once a week till itch is relieved, and then can be replaced with lower potency topical corticosteroid as need based. Topical calcineurin inhibitors like tacrolimus and pimecrolimus serve as steroid spares, but in the authors' experience, many are intolerant to the severe stinging which occurs with the applications. Antihistamines (sedative at night) are required in the first few weeks. Follow-up is recommended 3 monthly, six monthly and then yearly for life.

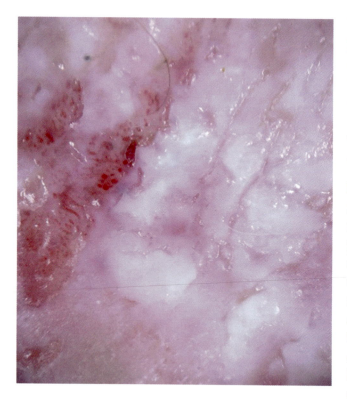

FIGURE 6.40 Dermoscopy showing white structureless area, red erosions, and polymorphous vessels on a pinkish background. (Photograph by Dr Nina Madnani.)

Topical testosterone has no role and has been abandoned. Fractional lasers and platelet-rich plasma (PRP) local injections as a recommended therapy require larger studies before they can be recommended in the therapeutic ladder.

Course and prognosis
Response to topical clobetasol propionate is excellent, relieving the itch in a few weeks. In total, 3–5% of untreated women with vulvar LS may develop a malignancy, and this serves to emphasize the need for regular follow-up (Figures 6.42 and 6.43).

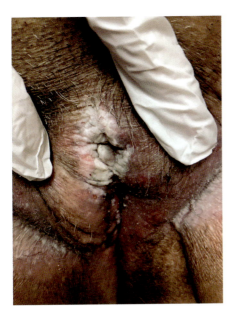

FIGURE 6.42 This 76-year-old lady comes with a recurrence of her squamous cell carcinoma (SCC). Note the underlying LS lesion. (Photograph by Dr Nina Madnani.)

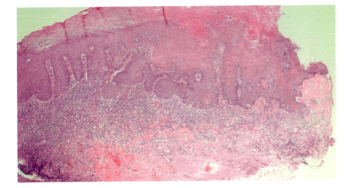

FIGURE 6.43 H & E, 100×, irregular epidermal hyperplasia with lichenoid lymphocytic infiltrate, atypia of lower epidermis, and sclerosis of the upper dermis at one end of the sections. (Photograph by Dr Rajiv Joshi.)

Pearl
Vitiligoid LS has been reported in darker skins, wherein the lesions look typically like vitiligo, but the histopathology is of LS. Sparing of clitoris and clitoral hood is a clue to vitiligoid LS. Biopsy is important in such cases (Figures 6.44 and 6.45).

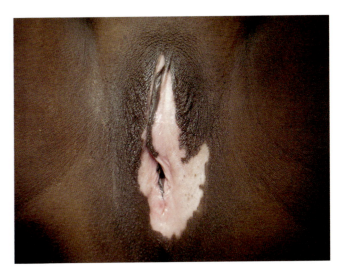

FIGURE 6.44 This was mistaken for vitiligo, but biopsy proved it as lichen sclerosus. (Photograph by Dr Nisha Chaturvedi.)

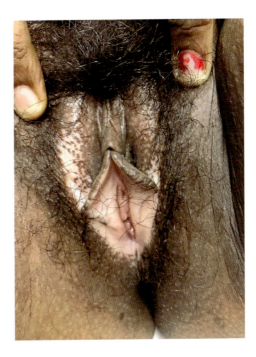

FIGURE 6.45 Vitiligoid Lichen sclerosus responds with perifollicular re-pigmentation. (Photograph by Dr Nina Madnani.)

Recommended reading

1. Corazza M, et al. Biomedicines (2021). PMID: 34440154.
2. Cooper SM, et al. Arch Dermatol (2008). PMID: 19015417.
3. Singh N, et al. Obstet Gynecol Int (2020). PMID: 32373174.
4. Bleeker MC, et al. Cancer Epidemiol Biomarkers Prev (2016). PMID: 27257093.

Plasma cell vulvitis

Introduction

This is an uncommon condition, also known as Zoon vulvitis, seen on the vulva and oral mucosa. It was first reported in 1954 by Garnier.

Epidemiology

Plasma cell vulvitis is a disease affecting adults between the second and seventh decade of life. The exact incidence is not known as there are very few published cases.

Pathophysiology

It appears to be a non-specific reactive response to trauma or infections, although an autoimmune or a hormonal etiology has been considered. The exact etiology is still not clear.

Presenting complaints

The chief complaint is itching, followed by burning and dyspareunia. Patients often complain of dysuria.

Clinical examination

Zoon vulvitis lesions are usually bilaterally symmetrical, bright orange-red, and may have a velvety surface or sometimes erosions. The entire mucosal surface of the vulva can be affected (Figure 6.46).

Lab investigations

Swabs must be taken to rule out an infective etiology.

Histopathology

This is diagnostic. The dermis shows a lichenoid infiltrate with sheets of plasma cells in the upper and mid dermis. Vascular dilatation with extravasation of red blood cells is seen.

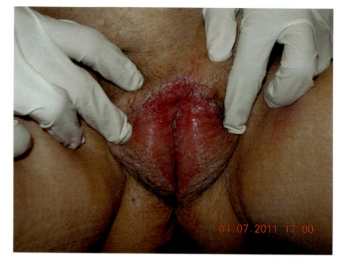

FIGURE 6.46 Glazed well-demarcated erythema involving the labia. (Photograph by Dr Nina Madnani.)

Differential diagnosis

Erosive LP, irritant contact dermatitis, and pemphigus are some conditions to be differentiated.

Erosive LP shows bright red, painful erosions in the vestibule with scarring and narrowing of the introitus. A Lacy pattern may be seen at the periphery of the erosions. The gingiva may show erosions.

A patient with irritant contact dermatitis will give a history of using strong detergents or chemicals on the vulva, which may show well-demarcated erythema and edema of the labia and vestibule.

Pemphigus vulgaris can involve the labia minora and lower vagina with evanescent blisters that rupture to give erosions. Oral mucosa and other body sites may also be involved. A Tzanck smear is useful as an early diagnostic tool. It shows acantholytic cells.

Course and prognosis

Patient's QoL is seriously impaired with this disease as it is often refractory to treatment and has a tendency to continue for weeks to months.

Management

Topical corticosteroids (super-potent and mid-potent) alone or in combination with fusidic acid have been used, initially twice a day application and then tapered off as per response. Topical tacrolimus 0.1% may be used as a steroid-sparing agent.

Systemic agents including antibiotics like doxycycline, minocycline, cyclosporine, and acitretin are some of the other agents used. This condition is often unresponsive to treatment, and cryotherapy or CO_2 laser ablation may need to be considered in refractory cases.

Pearls

This is an uncommon condition often missed or misdiagnosed.

A red vulva not responding to therapy needs a biopsy to rule out plasma cell vulvitis.

Recommended reading

1. Sattler S, et al. Int J Womens Dermatol (2021). PMID: 35028377.
2. Virgili A, et al. Dermatology (2015). PMID: 25633048.

7

PRE-MALIGNANT VULVAR DERMATOSES

Nina Madnani

Contents

Vulvar intraepithelial neoplasia

Introduction

The classification of vulvar squamous intraepithelial lesions, or SILs (formerly known as vulvar intraepithelial neoplasia [VIN]) has undergone various modifications from 2005, and the latest classification by the International Society for the study of vulvar disease (ISSVD) in 2015 is now widely accepted.

It is categorized into the low-grade squamous intraepithelial lesion (LSIL) of the vulva (HPV effect/flat LSIL/flat condyloma), high-grade squamous intraepithelial lesion (HSIL) of the vulva (vulvar HSIL, VIN usual type) and dVIN (differentiated vulvar intraepithelial neoplasia) secondary to lichen sclerosus (LS) and lichen planus (LP). Entity previously described as Bowenoid papulosis is now included in HSIL.

Epidemiology

The incidence of HSIL has been increasing in recent years and is seen to be higher in a younger age group between 20 and 35 years of age. dVIN is reported in post-menopausal women, occurring on a pre-existing chronic inflammatory disease. It is unifocal and unicentric, and when untreated, can rapidly progress to a squamous cell carcinoma (SCC). dVIN forms < 5% of all VINs. uVIN (VIN usual type) is often multicentric and self-resolving. It is sexually transmitted and may have a slow progression to cancer.

Pathophysiology

Seventy-five percent of HSILs are found to be due to HPV 16, 18. Other risk factors include a low age of sexual activity, multiple lifetime sexual partners, pregnancy, immunosuppression, HIV, chronic hepatitis, transplant recipients and autoimmune connective tissue diseases.

The dVIN is HPV negative and usually on a background of LS or LP. Smoking is a risk factor, as is chronic vulvar irritation/inflammation and oxidative stress.

Presenting complaints

The lesion may be asymptomatic and be picked up at a routine check-up, or present as a chronic itch non-responsive to routine treatment. Some patients may complain of pain, dysuria, dyspareunia and a change in texture or color of the vulva. Thirty percent of LSIL patients may be asymptomatic.

Clinical examination

Careful and thorough examination of the vulva, perineum and perianal area is required. Pigmentated lesions are a common component of LSIL and HSIL in the skin of color. LSIL lesions may start as erythematous/pale/pigmented grouped papules, while HSIL presents as a well-demarcated pigmented raised patch or as warty growths. dVIN lesions present as erythema, induration, a nodule or an ulcer on a background of LS or LP. Lesions of dVIN may be so subtle that they are often missed (Figures 7.1–7.5).

Vulvoscopy can assist where lesions are inconspicuous.

Lab examination

Skin biopsy of a suspicious lesion is the single most important test. Persistent areas of thickening, induration and erosion/ulceration should be biopsied.

DOI: 10.1201/9781003284116-7

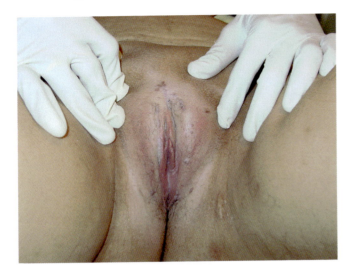

FIGURE 7.1 Multiple, flat-topped, pale, gray papules (LSIL). (Photograph by Dr Nina Madnani.)

Pap smears to rule out cervical intraepithelial neoplasia (CIN) and anal intraepithelial neoplasia (AIN) are essential. Further testing will depend on histopathological findings, to evaluate invasiveness.

Histopathology
Histopathological changes with uVIN are overt, while those with dVIN are subtle and difficult to diagnose. The uVIN changes may be warty or

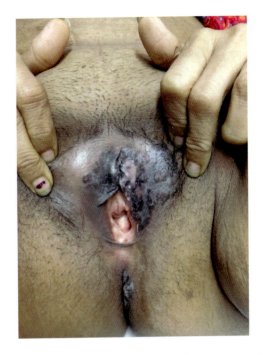

FIGURE 7.2 Extensive involvement of the labia, clitoris, perianal area with pigmented grayish plaques showing papules at the periphery. (Photograph by Dr Nina Madnani.)

basaloid. Warty-type uVIN shows hyperkeratosis with papillomatosis, acanthosis, with dyskeratotic cells, koilocytes and multinucleated cells showing

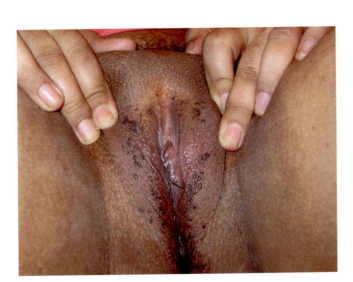

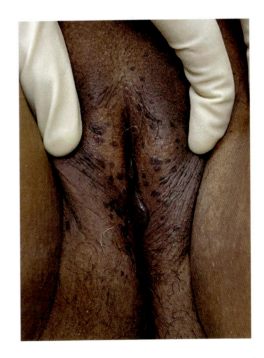

FIGURE 7.3 (a and b) Discreet to grouped, shiny pigmented papules over the vulva. Verruca plana are a close differential. (a – Photograph by Dr Nina Madnani. b – Photograph by Dr Dhanashree Bhide.)

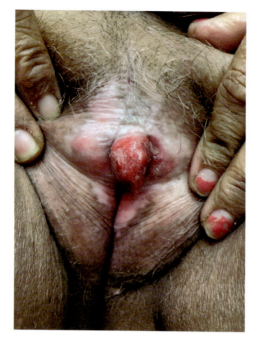

FIGURE 7.4 Sixty-eight years old lady with long-standing LS presented with a fleshy nodule. (Photograph by Dr Nina Madnani.)

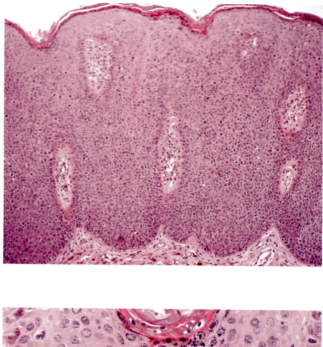

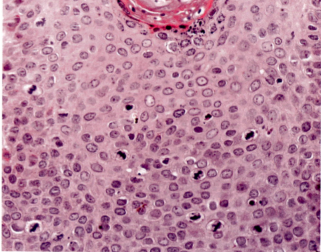

FIGURE 7.6 (**a**) H & E, 200× broad psoriasiform epidermal hyperplasia, surface-confluent parakeratotic scale, and loss of polarity of keratinocytes. (**b**) H & E, 400& E, numerous atypical mitotic figures and few dyskeratotic cells. (Photograph by Dr Rajiv Joshi.)

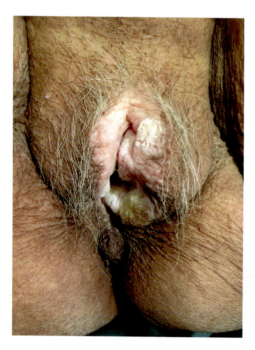

FIGURE 7.5 Notice the verrucus change on an existing LS. (Photograph by Dr Nina Madnani.)

mitotic changes and nuclear hyperchromasia. Appendages are rarely involved. The basaloid-type uVIN shows the entire epidermis replaced with basaloid cells (Figure 7.6a and b).

dVIN lesions have subtle changes. The epidermis shows anastomoses of the rete pegs, hypereosinophilia of the cells with prominent nucleoli and intercellular bridges. Skin appendages may be involved.

Differential diagnosis
Seborrheic warts, vulvar verrucae, eczemas, psoriasis and condyloma lata are the common conditions misdiagnosed.

Seborrhoeic warts are usually multiple, flat and warty, occur on keratinized surfaces and show classical features on dermoscopy.

Verrucae may be few, but are generally multiple, some forming large cauliflower-like masses.

Vulvar eczema involves larger areas of hair-bearing surfaces, while VIN lesions are more well demarcated.

Vulvar psoriasis may lack silvery scales when on non-hair-bearing parts.

Condyloma lata, secondary syphilitic lesions, are usually multiple, flat, whitish and well defined on non-hair-bearing parts.

Course and prognosis

uVIN: Typically, 1.2% of HSIL may undergo spontaneous regression, while less than 5% of untreated cases may progress to a vulvar squamous cell carcinoma (Figure 7.7).

dVIN: These lesions have a higher tendency to progress to a vulvar SCC in a shorter time. Forty percent of vulvar SCC had a dVIN adjacent (Figure 7.8).

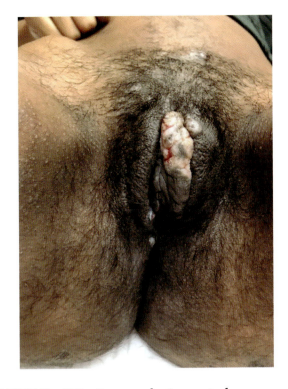

FIGURE 7.8 Large depigmented verrucous plaque involving clitoris, left labia minora in a patient with chronic lichen planus. Please note LP lesions on the pubis. (Photograph by Dr Nina Madnani.)

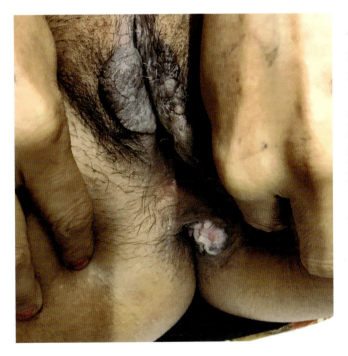

FIGURE 7.7 Large, greyish, irregular plaques showing asymmetric hyperpigmentation on the labia. Note the SCC arising in the perianal region. (Photograph by Dr Nina Madnani.)

Treatment

Guidelines of care have not evolved for VIN as the numbers are few.

Surgical excision is the gold standard with a clear margin of 5 mm. Often the surgery is mutilating, increasing morbidity. Multifocal lesions may require a vulvectomy. Moh's microsurgery has the best outcome. Relapse rates are generally high after excision. Topical 5% imiquimod has shown gratifying results in patients with HSIL, but larger studies are required for validation.

HPV vaccines are recommended by World Health Organization (WHO) to girls aged 9–15 (2 doses), and 15–26 (3 doses) in the prevention of HPV-related cervical cancer; those between 26 and 45 recommended if the physician feels the patients would benefit from the same.

Pearls

Pigmented HSIL lesions may often be missed in darker skin types. dVIN lesions need to be aggressively managed and followed up for life (Figure 7.9).

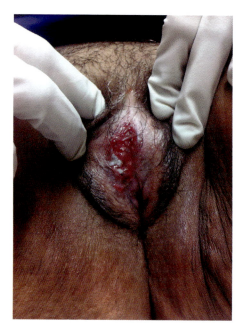

FIGURE 7.9 Bright pink, glazed erosion on a pre-existing LS should be biopsied. (Photograph by Dr Nina Madnani.)

Recommended reading

1. Bornstein J, et al. Obstet Gynecol (2016). PMID: 26942352.
2. Heller DS, et al. J Low Genit Tract Dis (2021). PMID: 33105449.
3. Wohlmuth C, et al. J Dtsch Dermatol Ges (2019). PMID: 31829526.
4. Faber MT, et al. Int J Cancer (2017). PMID: 28577297.
5. Hoang LN, et al. Pathology (2016). PMID: 27113549.

Bowen's disease

Introduction
Bowen's disease is a cutaneous SCC in situ, associated with the HPV virus. Approximately, 3–5% convert to an SCC.

Epidemiology
As it is a rare condition, and often missed, the exact incidence is not known.

Pathophysiology
Although the exact cause is not known, its association with HPV, especially HPV16, is conjectured.

Presenting complaints
Itch is the main complaint in the majority of the patients, but with chronic pruritis, patients may complain of a stinging sensation.

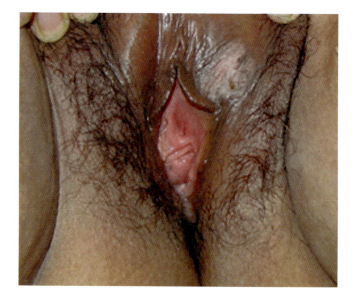

FIGURE 7.10 Well-demarcated scaly plaque with erosions on the left labia minora encroaching on the inner surface of the labia majora. (Photograph by Dr Nina Madnani.)

Clinical examination
The lesion may be a single well-defined erythematous/pigmented patch usually less than 3 cm in diameter with a surface crust or occasionally fissuring, and commonly mistaken as an eczematous patch. Occasionally, the patch may get eroded or ulcerated. The areas involved are the glabrous skin including the prepuce, clitoris and the labia minora (Figures 7.10 and 7.11).

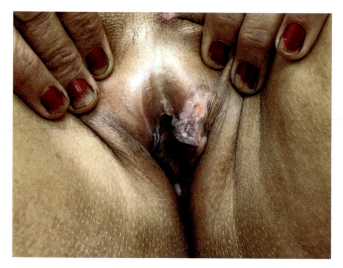

FIGURE 7.11 Plaque with dyspigmentation and ulceration resembling an SCC. (Photograph by Dr Yogesh Bhingradia.)

Dermoscopy

Scaly surfaces with dotted and glomerular vessels, gray/brown homogenous pigment and brown globules are features seen.

Lab examination

Skin biopsy is the most important test to be done.

Histopathology

The epidermis shows acanthosis with full-thickness dysplasia of the keratinocytes giving a "wind-blown" appearance. The dermis shows solar elastosis with a chronic inflammatory infiltrate (Figure 7.12).

Differential diagnosis

The closest differentials include eczematous dermatitis, psoriaisis, extramammary Paget disease (EMPD) and a fixed drug eruption.

A patient with eczematous dermatitis may have a history of atopy, or a contact allergen or irritant. The lesions will be more lichenified if chronic, or erythematous/oozing if acute.

Extramammary Pagets disease is usually seen in older women and can involve more extensive areas

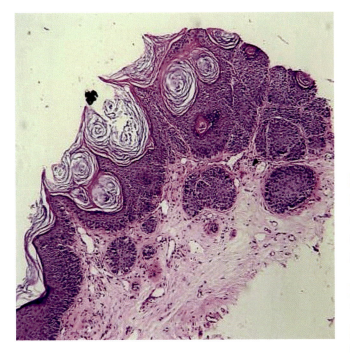

FIGURE 7.12 H & E 10× full thickness epidermal dysplasia with complete disorganization loss of maturation and lack of polarity of cells. (Photograph by Ankit Bharti.)

including the entire vulva, perineum and perianal region. Pruritis is very severe. Biopsy sows the typical pale Paget cells with vesicular nuclei.

Psoriatic lesions if in the folds will be pinkish and lack the typical silvery scales.

A fixed drug eruption is triggered by a drug, and occurs at the same place as earlier, often well-demarcated, pigmented, vesicular or crusted.

Course and prognosis

Prognosis is usually good, although between 3 and 12% may progress to a SCC.

Treatment

Surgical excision with a wide margin, and occasionally a vulvectomy when the need arises.

Non-surgical options include imiquimod, 5-fluorouracil, cidofovir and photodynamic therapy.

Pearl

Suspect Bowen's disease in a well-demarcated pigmented plaque less than 3 cm in diameter.

Recommended reading

1. Bath-Hextall FJ, et al. Cochrane Database Syst Rev (2013). PMID: 23794286.
2. Morton CA, et al. Br J Dermatol (2014). PMID: 24313974.
3. Scalvenzi M, et al. Open Access Maced J Med Sci (2019). PMID: 30894936.
4. Kang HK, et al. Ann Dermatol (2014). PMID: 24882981.
5. Thuijs NB, et al. Int J Cancer (2021). PMID: 32638382.

Extramammary Paget disease (EMPD)

Introduction

EMPD is a rare neoplasia arising from the apocrine glands of the axillae or anogenital region, often mistaken as an eczematous rash resulting in a delay in diagnosis.

Epidemiology

The exact incidence is unknown as cases go unreported. Women between 60 and 80 years are affected.

Although reported to be a disease seen more often in Caucasians, the author and colleagues from India have seen several cases sporadically over the years (unpublished) in the Indian population.

Pathophysiology

The malignancy may arise from the epidermis (primary EMPD), or as an extension from the ano-rectal, or the genito-urinary system (secondary EMPD).

Presenting complaints

Intractable itching is the commonest complaint in a majority of patients. Pain, oozing, hematuria, dysuria or rectal bleeding may be the primary complaint. An asymptomatic white patch may be an early complaint in some.

Clinical examination

The area of involvement may vary between a centimeter in diameter to extensive involvement of the vulva, perineum and perianal area, often encroaching onto the groins, upper thighs and buttocks. The lesions have a well-defined margin and may be erythematous, pigmented or depigmented. There may be oozing, crusting or ulceration, resembling a typical patch of eczema. Both mucosal and hair-bearing surfaces may be involved. A typical "strawberry and cream" appearance has alluded to the ulcerated areas with whitish crusts. In contrast, in the skin of color, this may appear as a dusky bluish-gray. Advanced cases can be extensively scarred with loss of normal anatomical parts. Induration and nodularity are red flags heralding deeper involvement. Inguinal nodes may be palpable in the invasive variety. EMPD in the skin of color tends to show areas of hyperpigmentation and depigmentation/hypopigmentation in the same lesion (Figures 7.13–7.17).

Dermoscopy

Although classical features have not been described, structureless white areas, structureless gray areas, glomerular vessels, dotted vessels, and milky areas are seen (Figure 7.18).

Lab examination

Around 10–30% of EMPD are associated with an internal malignancy. Skin biopsy with immuno-histochemistry is the diagnosis clincher. Other investigations required ruling out the site of origin or metastasis are X-ray chest, mammogram, ultrasound abdomen and pelvis, colonoscopy, cystoscopy, colposcopy and Papanicolaou (PAP) smear.

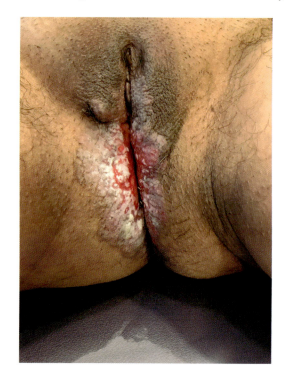

FIGURE 7.13 Eczematous-eroded palques involving labia majora and extending onto the perianal region. (Photograph by Dr Nina Madnani.)

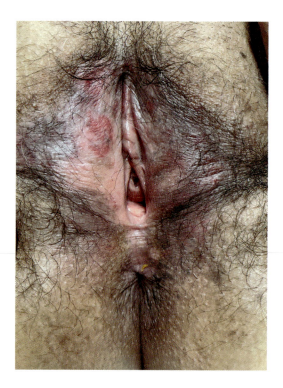

FIGURE 7.14 Lichenoid appearance with depigmented plaques in a case of EMPD. (Photograph by Dr Nina Madnani.)

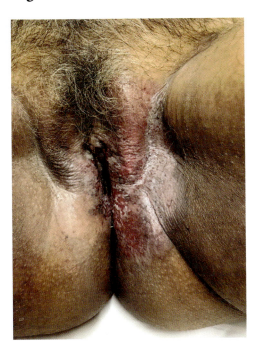

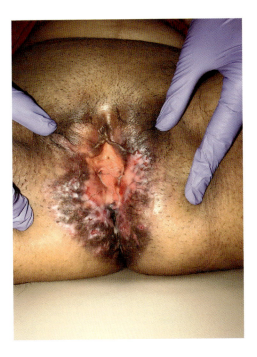

FIGURE 7.15 EMPD can often mimic eczematous dermatitis. (Photograph by Dr Nina Madnani.)

Histopathology

The Paget cells are typically large cells with pale cytoplasm and vesicular nuclei and involve the entire thickness of the epidermis. Near the basal

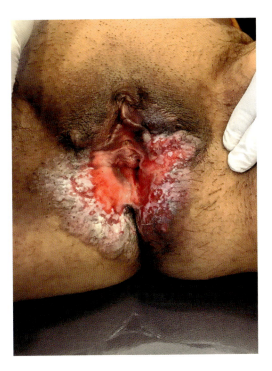

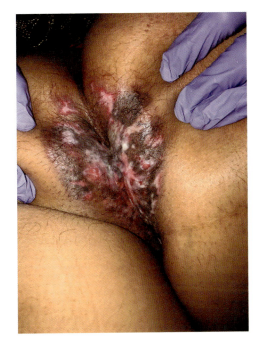

FIGURE 7.17 **(a and b)** This lady with extensive EMPD extending to the perianal region has both hyperpigmentation and depigmentation. (Photograph by Dr Nina Madnani.)

FIGURE 7.16 Ulceration with whitish crusts giving a 'Strawberry Cream' appearance. (Photograph by Dr Nina Madnani.)

layer, they are distributed singly but higher up are found in groups (Figure 7.19a and b).

These cells are positive for cytokeratin (CK)7, periodic acid-Schiff (PAS), gross cystic disease fluid protein (GCDFP)-15, carcinoembryonic antigen (CEA) and negative for S-100 stain.

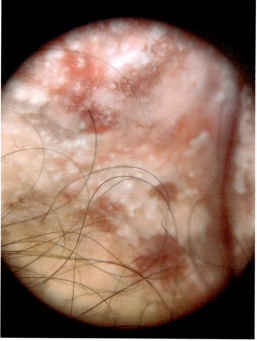

FIGURE 7.18 Dermoscopy shows milky red areas, white clouds, branching white lines, bluish-gray area and polymorphous blood vessels. Magnum Plus, polarized, 10×. (Photograph by Dr Dhanashree Bhide.)

If originating from an internal carcinoma, then the cells are negative for CK7, CEA, GCDFP-15 and positive for CK-20. A primary intraepidermal tumor will be CK7, GCDFP-15 positive and CK-20 negative. If of urothelial origin, it will show positivity with uroplakin-III.

Differential diagnosis

Eczematous dermatitis, psoriasis, erosive LP, Bowen's disease, LS, vitiligo, candidiasis, intertrigo, VIN, and superficial spreading melanoma (SSM) are the common differentials to be kept in mind.

The biopsy shows typical Paget cells, and immunohistochemistry eliminates other diagnoses. SSM is CK negative, PAS negative, CEA negative and S-100 positive.

Course and prognosis

EMPD can linger on indolently for years, but the invasive form, once it breaches the dermis, spreads rapidly. Long-term follow-up of the patients of EMPD is required to watch for invasiveness or

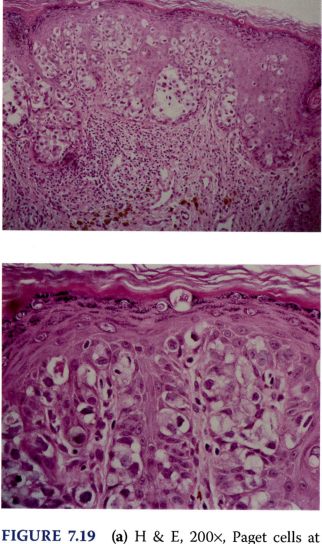

FIGURE 7.19 **(a)** H & E, 200×, Paget cells at all levels of the epidermis including stratum corneum, arranged as single cells as well as collections and even showing acinar structures within the epidermis. **(b)** H & E, 400×, high power of Paget cells. (Photograph by Dr Rajiv Joshi.)

relapse after treatment/surgery. Relapse after surgery varies between 40 and 45%, due to the multifocal nature.

Treatment

Surgical excision with a clear margin of 1–2 cm is the gold standard. Moh's microsurgery gives the best results. Radiotherapy is also useful. Systemic and topical chemotherapy are for cases unsuitable for excision or radiotherapy.

Topical imiquimod 4–5 times a week has shown promising results, but needs larger studies to recommend as a protocol, and can be used initially where surgery is not feasible or to decrease the lesion extent in primary EMPD.

Pearls

EMPD should be suspected in non-responsive vulvar eczema.

In darker skin types, a depigmented itchy patch raises the suspicion.

Recommended reading

1. St Claire K, et al. Dermatol Online J (2019). PMID: 31046904.
2. Nasioudis D, et al. Gynecol Oncol (2020). PMID: 31780234.
3. Ishizuki S, et al. Curr Oncol (2021). PMID: 34436026.
4. Anjana JS, et al. Indian J Surg Oncol (2021). PMID: 34658580.

8

MALIGNANT DERMATOSES

Kavitha Athotha

Contents

Squamous cell carcinoma

Introduction

Squamous cell carcinoma (SCC) accounts for 90% of vulvar carcinomas with vulvar intraepithelial neoplasia (VIN) being an important precursor. The increased incidence of SCC in younger women is supposed to be due to increasing oncogenic human papilloma virus (HPV) infections.

Epidemiology

In the Cancer registry in India, 2015 showed a rate of 0.2–0.5 per 1,00,000 women per year. Around 60% of vulvar SCC are seen in post-menopausal women.

Pathophysiology

SCC of the vulva develops by two different mechanisms. One is HPV-dependent pathway and is caused by HPV 16, 18 and 33, predominantly resulting in high-grade squamous intraepithelial neoplasia (HSIL), which may lead to SCC. This is commonly seen in younger women. The second type occurs more commonly in the elderly on a background of lichen sclerosus (LS) and differentiated vulvar intraepithelial neoplasia (dVIN) progressing to SCC. This is HPV negative.

Risk factors include elderly age group, multiple sexual partners, poor socio-economic status, cigarette smoking, HPV infections, human immunodeficiency virus infection, LS and VIN.

Presenting complaints

Can be asymptomatic or present with pruritus, burning sensation or pain, dysuria and dyspareunia or a lump or growth. Vulvar bleeding is more common in invasive disease.

Clinical examination

Labia majora, clitoris, perineal body and fourchette are the common sites but can involve any area. Lesions can be pigmented, white, skin colored or erythematous. They can present as a unifocal plaque, ulcer or an ill-defined mass. All vulvar, perianal skin surfaces, cervix and vagina should be evaluated (Figures 8.1–8.3).

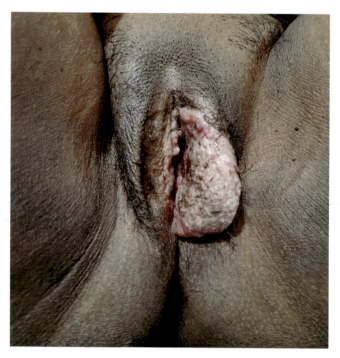

FIGURE 8.1 SCC can present as a warty outgrowth as seen in this patient. (Photography by Dr Kavitha Athota.)

DOI: 10.1201/9781003284116-8

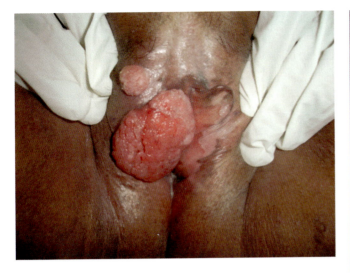

FIGURE 8.2 Bright pink verrucous exophytic growth on a lesion of LS. (Photograph by Dr Janak Maniar.)

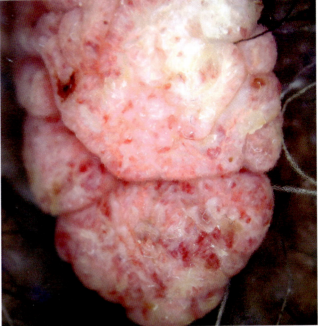

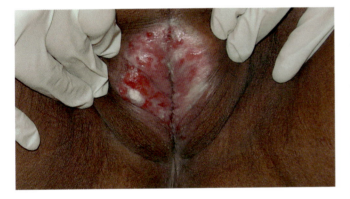

FIGURE 8.3 This lady with untreated lichen sclerosus presented with velvety red papules, plaques and erosions, which on biopsy was squamous cell carcinoma. (Photograph by Dr Nina Madnani.)

Systemic findings

Vulvar SCC metastasizes by direct spread, lymphatic and hematogenous routes. Direct extension to adjacent structures like vagina, urethra and anus can be seen. Lymphatic spread to ipsilateral inguinal lymph nodes is common in lesions that are unilateral and in lesions that are 2 mm or more.

Dermoscopy

dVIN, microinvasive SCC and invasive SCC are closely related entities to be differentiated on dermoscopy. The dermoscopic picture of a superficially invasive SCC (previously known as microinvasive SCC) shows a whitish background

FIGURE 8.4 Dermoscopy shows keratin crusts, perivascular whitish halos, white structureless areas, polymorphous vessels. Dinolite Digital Microscope, WF-20, polarized, 10×. (Photograph by Dr Nina Madnani.)

with polymorphous vessels like curvy, dotted, linear, irregular or hair-pin shaped. Invasive vulvar SCC is commonly identified by highly polymorphous vessels with curvy and linear-irregular vessels distributed centrally and hairpin vessels at the periphery. These features are to be differentiated from dVIN in which red color and curvy, short serpentine vessels predominate (Figure 8.4).

Histopathology

Biopsy is the gold standard in the diagnosis of SCC. Multiple biopsies of lesions of distinct morphologies increase the chance of detecting SCC. Three main types are identified viz keratinizing, basaloid and warty.

Keratinizing SCC or well-differentiated type: This pattern is the most frequent histologic type encountered. This is characterized by keratin pearls and by well or moderately differentiated cells with an absence of koilocytosis (Figure 8.5).

Basaloid type is composed of smaller cells with an increased nuclear-to-cytoplasmic ratio, and they do not form keratin. Squamous differentiation is seen towards the center of cell nests.

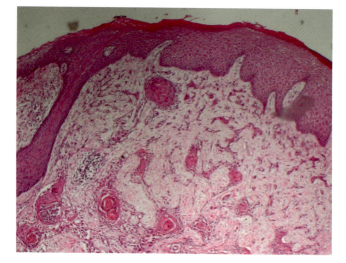

FIGURE 8.5   Biopsy showing well-differentiated SCC. Epidermal proliferation showing thickened and branching and coalescing rete ridges. Keratinocytes showing individual cell keratinization and formation of horn pearls. (Photograph by Dr Kavitha Athota.)

Warty carcinomas have koilocytosis, dyskeratosis, multinucleation, nuclear pleomorphism, hyperchromasia and abnormal mitotic figures.

Laboratory investigations

Colposcopy of the vulva may be needed to identify subclinical lesions which are not visualized on clinical examination. Imaging studies like X-ray chest, computerized tomography (CT), magnetic resonance imaging (MRI) and positron emission tomography (PET) are done to know the extent and spread of the disease. Cystoscopy and proctoscopy help in advanced cases to note the spread into the bladder and rectum, respectively.

Differential diagnosis

Inflammatory and benign lesions like LS, lichen planus (LP), VIN, Paget's disease of the vulva, condyloma acuminata, seborrheic keratoses, angiokeratoma, epidermal inclusion cysts, hidradenomas and pigmented lesions like melanocytic naevi and melanomas are to be differentiated.

Lichen scleroses have ivory white, atrophic, ecchymotis lesions with a very characteristic crinkled texture.

Hypertrophic LP presents as thickened hyperkeratotic plaques and can involve vaginal or oral mucosa also.

VIN lesions can be unifocal or multifocal, raised or verrucous but have no pathognomonic clinical features, so a biopsy is mandatory in all suspicious lesions.

Seborrheic keratoses are flat-topped, sharply demarcated, usually solitary plaques with a stuck-on appearance.

Course and prognosis

Although HPV-positive tumors are comparatively less aggressive, the ones originating from LP/LS tend to progress more rapidly. The prognosis depends on the stage of the disease and lymph node status. Well-differentiated tumors with negative lymph nodes have a good survival rate. Local and distant recurrences occur in 12–37% of patients with vulvar SCC. Most recurrences occur within 2 years after initial treatment (Figure 8.6).

Treatment

Primary treatment modality is surgery which is stage-dependent. Mohs micrographic surgery (MMS) is indicated for SCC not involving lymph nodes. Chemotherapy: Drugs like cisplatin, carboplatin, vinorelbine, paclitaxel and erlotinib are options used. Treatment for local recurrences is wide local excision (WLE), for groin recurrences, surgery with or without chemo-radiation and palliative treatment for distant recurrences.

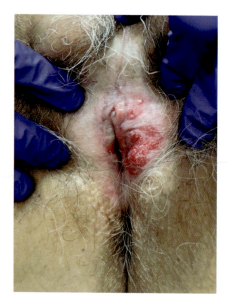

FIGURE 8.6   Biopsy-proven, well-differentiated squamous cell carcinoma arising from a long-standing, untreated case of LS. (Photograph by Dr Nina Madnani.)

Pearls
HPV vaccination is an important tool for the prevention of HPV-related SCC of the vulva in women.

Chronic inflammatory diseases like LS and LP should be treated aggressively in the elderly to prevent dVIN.

Recommended reading
1. Koh WJ, et al. J Natl Compr Canc Netw (2017). PMID: 28040721.
2. Tan A, et al. J Am Acad Dermatol (2019). PMID: 31349045.
3. Vaccari S, et al. Clin Exp Dermatol (2018). PMID: 29315730.

Verrucous carcinoma

Introduction
Verrucous carcinoma (VC) of the vulva is a slow-growing, locally invasive tumor. It was first described as a subtype of SCC by Ackerman in 1948. It constitutes less than 1% of vulvar cancers.

Epidemiology
VC is common in post-menopausal women. The etiology of VC is unknown, but an association with LS and lichen simplex chronicus is reported.

Pathophysiology
Role of HPV is reported in a few studies, but its role is controversial. Few studies state that VC is a discrete clinicopathological entity.

Presenting complaints
Pruritus and pain are the common presenting symptoms. Some complaint of a lump or growth on the vulva.

Clinical examination
VC commonly presents as a cauliflower growth, though ulceration and bleeding are the other manifestations. The most affected sites are labia majora, labia minora and posterior commissure. If left untreated, it may attain a voluminous size. VC has no lymph node spread and no metastases (Figures 8.7 and 8.8).

Histopathology
Histology reveals mild cellular atypia and very few mitotic figures compared to SCC. VC is characterized by a "pushing border" with a well-defined

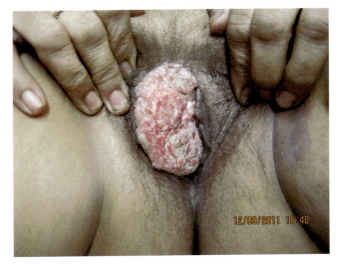

FIGURE 8.7 Sixty-five-year-old female came with a large, foul smelling, warty mass, obliterating her vulva. (Photograph by Dr Nina Madnani.)

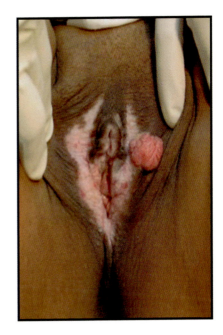

FIGURE 8.8 This lady had been mistakenly diagnosed as condyloma instead of verrucous carcinoma. (Photograph by Dr Nina Madnani.)

tumor-dermal interface without apparent infiltration. Acanthosis, parakeratosis, orthokeratosis, organized keratinocytes and characteristic bulbous rete ridges named as "baggy trousers" are the features of histopathology.

Differential diagnosis
Giant condyloma acuminatum (GCA, Buschke-Lowenstein tumor) presents as cauliflower-like

growth that is locally aggressive and destructive. Pruritus, malodourous vaginal discharge and contact bleeding are the common symptoms. Well-differentiated SCC is another differential.

Treatment
Standard treatment of VC is local excision with adequate margins.

Pearl
VC is a non-HPV-related well-differentiated form of vulvar SCC.

Recommended reading
1. Campaner AB, et al. An Bras Dermatol (2017). PMID: 28538888.
2. Dryden SM, et al. Cancer Rep (Hoboken) (2022). PMID: 35075817.

Basal cell carcinoma

Introduction
Vulvar basal cell carcinoma (BCC) accounts for 1–4% of all vulvar malignancies.

Epidemiology
Vulvar BCC is seen in post-menopausal women above 70 years of age. It commonly affects the outer labia minora, labia majora, mons and rarely affects inner labia, the clitoris and urethral orifice. It usually presents as a single lesion but can be multifocal, bilateral or disseminated.

Pathophysiology
Exact etiology is unknown. Ultraviolet radiation and sun exposure are not risk factors for vulvar BCC, unlike BCC elsewhere. Burn scars, chronic irritation, post radiotherapy, exposure to arsenic and certain genetic conditions like nevoid BCC syndrome and xeroderma pigmentosum are few risk factors for vulvar BCC.

Presenting complaints
Often asymptomatic but may occasionally complain of itching, discomfort, pain, swelling, bleeding and ulceration.

Clinical examination
Clinical picture has a wide variation. The lesion can be a simple erythematous papule or plaque, ulcer, nodule, vegetating growth, infiltrative or

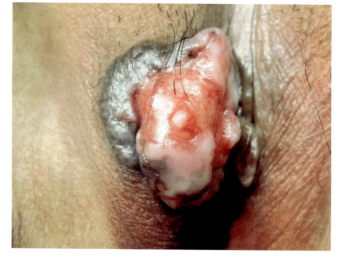

FIGURE 8.9 A case of BCC presenting as a large tumor with surface telangiectasia, depigmentation and rolled-out pigmented border at the periphery. (Photograph by Dr Ramapadma Namudri.)

morpheic plaque. Lesions in colored skin are usually pigmented, as are also reported in Chinese. Occasionally, some parts may be depigmented. Lymph node involvement may be part of the clinical spectrum (Figures 8.9–8.11).

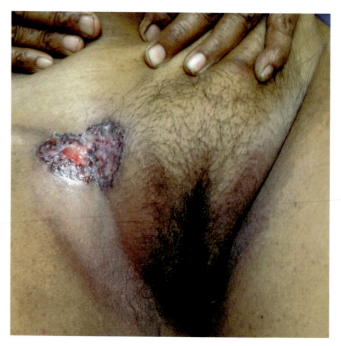

FIGURE 8.10 A well-defined, heart-shaped plaque in the right genito crural fold, encroaching onto the right labia majora. (Photograph by Dr Nina Madnani.)

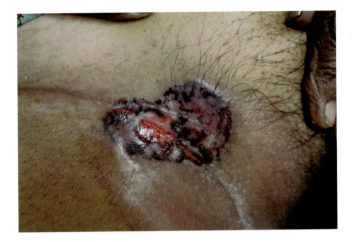

FIGURE 8.11 Close-up of the lesion showing typical BCE morphology. (Photograph by Dr Nina Madnani.)

Differential diagnosis

Vulvar BCC should be differentiated from benign lesions, mucous cysts, Paget's disease of the vulva, lichen simplex chronicus, LS, LP, VIN, SCC, melanocytic nevus and melanoma.

Extra mammary Paget's disease is usually well delineated or may present as weepy erosions or ulcerations.

Lichen simplex chronicus shows thickening of the skin, lichenified plaques and increased skin markings; pruritus is more severe in the night time.

Hypopigmented lesions of BCC should be differentiated from LS, which is characterized by loss of normal architecture and resorption of labia.

Differentiated VIN which commonly presents as a solitary lesion with a white or reddish ill-defined plaque or an ulcer.

Any persistent vulvar lesions not responding to treatment should be biopsied.

Dermoscopy

Presence of linear telangiectasias, fine, reddish, well-focused arborising vessels, blue ovoid nests, globules and leaf-like structures are the key features that aid in the diagnosis of BCC. Homogenous white shiny areas which correspond to peritumoral fibrosis are additional clues to indicate vulvar BCC.

Histopathology

Histological features of vulvar BCC are similar to BCC of the skin elsewhere. Histological subtypes are superficial, nodular, basosquamous, adenocystic, infiltrative and mixed types. The tumor cells in BCC are similar to normal basal cells of the epidermis and are composed of uniform cells with prominent palisading. The desmoplastic reaction is common in the stroma. Pigmented BCC has pigment in the dermal macrophages.

Course and prognosis

Vulvar BCC has a good prognosis and has fewer chances of metastases. If left untreated, lesions can become destructive. Potential risk factors for metastases are large size at the time of presentation, depth of involvement and aggressive histology. High recurrence rates are possibly due to inadequate surgical margins.

Treatment

The most common surgical treatment is local or WLE. Simple vulvectomy, hemi-vulvectomy, radical vulvectomy and MMS are other surgical methods.

Topical treatments like 5 fluorouracil, 5% imiquimod and photodynamic therapy are other options in early lesions.

Pearls

deep pigmentation, ulceration and a pearly border are important clues for the diagnosis of vulvar BCC

Recommended reading

1. Renati S, et al. Int J Dermatol (2019). PMID: 30506682.
2. Chokoeva AA, et al. Wien Med Wochenschr (2015). PMID: 25930015.

Malignant melanoma

Introduction

Malignant melanoma (MM) is the second most common vulvar malignancy. It constitutes about 5–6% of vulvar malignancies.

Epidemiology

The annual incidence rates of vulvar melanomas are found to be 0.87 in Blacks, 0.75 in American Indians and 1.03 in Asians per million female population. It predominantly occurs in older women in their sixth or seventh decade.

Pathophysiology

Melanoma is a multifactorial disease. Genetic factors like family history of melanoma and inherited dysplastic nevus syndrome are more likely causes, than UV radiation, in vulvar melanoma. LS is also found to be a precursor lesion of vulvar melanoma in a few case reports.

Presenting complaints

Early lesions are often asymptomatic, or patients may present with pain, pruritus, a palpable mass, bleeding or ulceration.

Clinical examination

Common sites involved are labia minora, clitoris and inner side of labia majora. Lesions vary from brown, red and black macules, asymmetrical in structure and color with polycyclic borders. Nodular and polypoidal lesions may be seen. The commoner variants among vulvar melanomas are mucosal lentiginous, nodular, superficial spreading and the unclassified type (Figures 8.12 and 8.13).

Dermoscopy

Dermoscopy shows a blue-white veil, irregular dots, multiple colors (blue, brown, black, pink and gray) atypical network of streaks and reticular depigmentation. Vessels are atypical with dotted and linear-irregular patterns. Vulvar melanoma should be differentiated from vulvar naevi, which

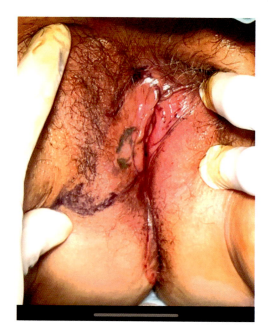

FIGURE 8.13 Melanomas can present as irregular or arciform, pigmented plaques. (Photograph by Dr Ramapadma Namudri.)

are characterized clinically by evenly pigmented red to dark colored papules or macules, with regular borders and <1cm size.

Laboratory examination

Local tumor extension is assessed by pelvic MRI. Whole-body PET or CT scans are done to assess distant metastases.

Histopathology

Biopsy should include the subcutaneous tissue so that the thickness can be measured. Excisional biopsy is considered the gold standard in the diagnosis of melanoma, and it has the advantage of providing accurate microstaging. Microscopic features of vulvar melanoma are increase in the number of atypical melanocytes throughout the epidermis with increased mitotic figures, cells arranged singly or as nests and pagetoid spread of melanocytes. Melanocytes are variable in size and shape and may become confluent and lack maturation. Atypical mitoses and increased apoptotic activity are seen.

Immunohistochemistry is used to differentiate from dysplastic naevi, Paget's disease and from undifferentiated carcinomas and sarcomas. Melanomas are immunoreactive for S100 and are carcinoembryonic antigen (CEA) negative.

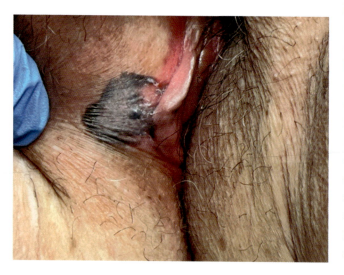

FIGURE 8.12 Pigmented lesions on the vulva must be viewed with suspicion, especially if they have a grayish-black hue. (Photograph by Dr Ramapadma Namudri.)

Differential diagnosis

Benign lesions like junctional, compound and intradermal naevi, dysplastic naevi, acanthosis nigricans, angiokeratoma and seborrheic keratosis are to be differentiated from MM. VIN, SCC and Paget's disease of the vulva are the other differentials.

Junctional, compound and intradermal naevi are tan to dark brown with uniform color throughout the lesion, sharp and regular borders and size of the lesion is less than 7mm.

Angiokeratomas are small, smooth papules and when solitary mimic nodular melanoma.

Course and prognosis

Untreated melanomas are notorious for metastasizing, giving a poor prognosis with a mean 5-year survival rate of less than 60%. Ulceration, tumor thickness and lymph node status are the most important prognostic markers. Adverse prognostic factors are advanced age at diagnosis, central location of tumor, ulceration, high mitotic rate and aneuploidy.

Treatment

Treatment of localized vulvar melanoma is WLE. The tumor free surgical margin required for WLE is 1 cm regardless of the depth of the tumor. Sentinel lymph node biopsy should be routinely done before doing a WLE in primary melanoma. In cases of invasion to adjacent structures or to regional lymph nodes, lymphadenectomy is advised.

Radiotherapy and chemotherapy are used as neoadjuvant treatments. Dacarbazine and temozolomide are the preferred drugs in vulvar melanoma.

Combination therapy of chemotherapy along with surgical excision or targeted therapy and radiotherapy is tried in individual cases with favorable outcomes.

Pearls

Dermoscopy is an important tool to diagnose a melanoma.

A pigmented nodule on the clitoris is highly suspicious of a melanoma

Recommended reading

1. Chokoeva AA, et al. Wien Med Wochenschr (2015). PMID: 25930015.
2. Wang D, et al. Am J Cancer Res (2020). PMID: 33414983.
3. Dobrică EC, et al. Biomedicines (2021). PMID: 34209084.

9

VULVAR MANIFESTATIONS OF SYSTEMIC DISEASES

Nina Madnani

Contents

Langerhans cell histiocytosis

Introduction

Langerhans cell histiocytosis (LCH) is a group of diseases characterized by clonal proliferation of Langerhans cells bone-marrow-derived. Involvement of the vulva is rare, and may be localized (LCH-single system) or multisystem (MS-LCH). The endometrium, cervix and vagina may be other sites of involvement.

Epidemiology

Although LCH is common in all age groups but mostly in children, vulvar involvement is uncommon, and less than 100 cases have been reported across the world.

Pathophysiology

The exact cause of this chronic disease is not known, but neoplastic or reactive theories have been put forth.

Presenting complaints

The patient may present with the complaint of itching, burning, pain, ulceration or even a blister or thickening of the labia, fourchette, perineum or perianal area.

Clinical features

The lesions may be indolent tender ulcers, usually multiple, involving the labia majora, minora, the perineum and extending to the perianal area (Figures 9.1 and 9.2).

Systemic findings

If the LCH is not pure genital only, but multisystem, the patient may have a history of headaches, excessive thirst or diuresis indicating diabetes

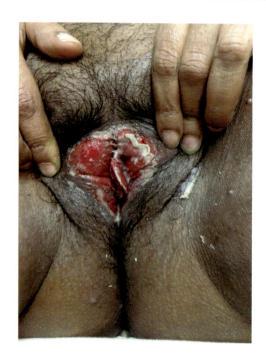

FIGURE 9.1 Large bright red ulcers involving the entire non-keratinized skin and mucosa with yellow slough at the periphery. (Photograph by Dr Nina Madnani.)

insipidus, bone pain seen as bone cysts or "hot spots" on imaging and/or deafness.

Lab investigations

If MS-LCH is suspected, imaging studies, bone-marrow biopsy and endocrine evaluation to rule out the bone, CNS and diabetes insipidus are required.

Histopathology

Skin biopsy is diagnostic. A hematoxylin and eosin staining reveal sheets of Langerhans cells in the dermis. Interspersed are eosinophils, neutrophils

DOI: 10.1201/9781003284116-9

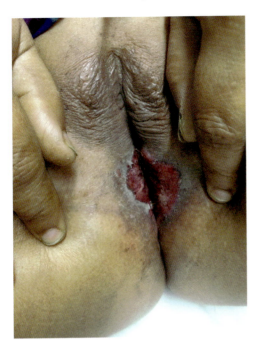

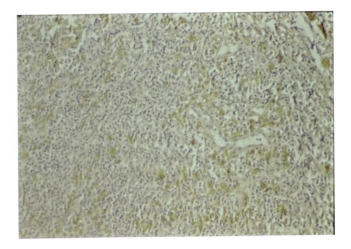

FIGURE 9.4 Langerhans cells staining positive with S 100 stain. ×200. (Photograph by Dr Nina Madnani.)

FIGURE 9.2 Perineal extension of the ulcer in the same patient. Early lesions may be erythematous papules. (Photograph by Dr Nina Madnani.)

and lymphocytes. Positive immunohistochemistry with CD1a, CD207 and S-100 stains clinches the diagnosis (Figures 9.3 and 9.4).

If MS-LCH is suspected, imaging studies, bone-marrow biopsy and endocrine evaluation to rule out the bone, CNS and diabetes insipidus are required.

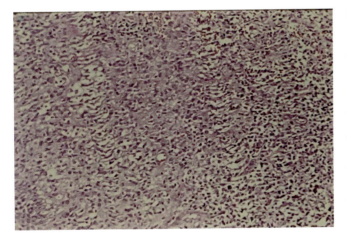

FIGURE 9.3 H & E, ×200. Sheets of Langerhans cells with their kidney-shaped nucleus and eosinophilic cytoplasm. (Photograph by Dr Nina Madnani.)

Differential diagnosis

Pure vulvar LCH should be distinguished from other chronic ulcers like Behcet's, tuberculosis, granuloma inguinale, Crohn's disease (CD) and malignancies.

Behcet's ulcers are multiple, extremely painful, round, with involvement of the ocular, and oral mucosa. Pathergy may be positive.

Tuberculosis and CD ulcers would be accompanied by fluctuant vulvar edema.

Granuloma inguinale can be ruled out by taking a biopsy, which shows the intracellular Klebsiella granulomatis.

Course and prognosis

The course of the disease cannot be exactly predicted, although some have a good response to topical or systemic corticosteroids. MS-LCH has a worse prognosis, especially if the bones or CNS is involved.

Treatment

Although there are no clear-cut guidelines, the Histiocyte Society guidelines include topical and oral steroids, vincristine, vinblastine, etoposide, thalidomide, radiation, tacrolimus, methotrexate and vulvectomy where indicated. Referral to a medical oncologist is recommended.

Pearl

A vulvar ulcer + diabetes insipidus, think of LCH.

Recommended reading

1. Wieland R, et al. Gynecol Oncol Rep (2017). PMID: 28932806.
2. Kurt S, et al. Case Rep Obstet Gynecol (2013). PMID: 24109536.
3. Zudaire T, et al. Int J Gynecol Pathol (2017). PMID: 27294606.
4. Histiocyte Society. Available from: http://www.histiocytesociety.org . [Last accessed on 2009 Sep 12].

Metastatic Crohn's disease

Introduction

Vulvar involvement in CD is rare and may extend from the gastrointestinal tract (GI) tract or have no connection with the GI tract (metastatic). Often as a solitary manifestation, appearing several years before the onset of GI involvement. In the Indian context where tuberculosis is so prevalent, many patients are misdiagnosed as vulvar tuberculosis and given anti-tuberculosis therapy, thus delaying the diagnosis and management of this chronic disease.

Epidemiology

Although CD is more prevalent in Western populations, the incidence has been increasing recently in India and Japan. One in four patients may have vulvar lesions before intestinal involvement. Very few cases of vulvar CD have been reported from India.

Pathophysiology

An interaction between genetics, immunologic dysfunction, gut bacteria and environmental factors has been considered in the pathogenesis of this chronic inflammatory disease.

Presenting complaints

Patients with vulvar CD may complain of swelling, pain, ulceration and discharge from the vulvar or perianal area. Some may have recurrent abdominal pain and diarrhea/constipation preceding the onset of vulvar involvement.

Clinical features

On clinical examination, the patient may have asymmetric edema of the labia majora, minora or clitoris. Fissures, knife-cut linear ulcers in the genito-crural, inter-labial or gluteal folds are the hallmarks of CD. Advanced disease presents as

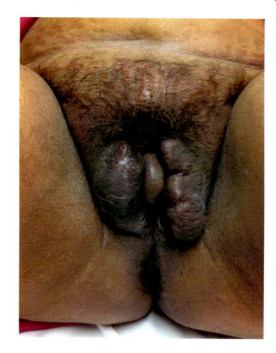

FIGURE 9.5   Crohn's disease is a diagnosis that needs to be considered in a patient with asymmetric vulvar edema. (Photograph by Dr Nina Madnani.)

multiple fistulae with foul-smelling discharge. The patient should be turned over to examine the perianal area for skin tags, fistulae, ulceration, abscesses or scarring. Other clinical findings include recurrent aphthous ulceration during periods of relapse and pyoderma gangrenosum (Figures 9.5–9.9).

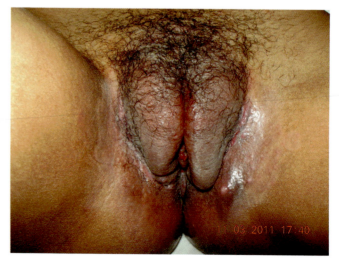

FIGURE 9.6   Fifteen years child with vulvar edema, knife-cut ulcers and fistulae. (Photograph by Dr Nina Madnani.)

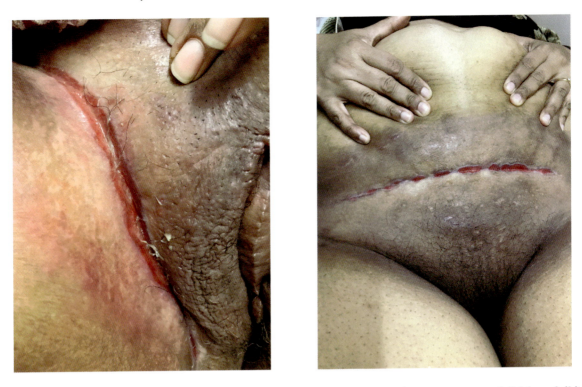

FIGURE 9.7 **(a)** Classic knife-cut ulcers described in CD seen in the genito-crural fold and **(b)** lower abdomen pendulous fold. (Photograph by Dr Nina Madnani.)

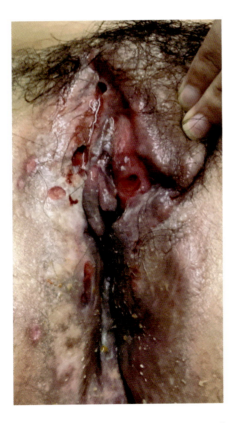

FIGURE 9.8 This young lady has multiple fistulous opening over the vulva and perineum. (Photograph by Dr Nina Madnani.)

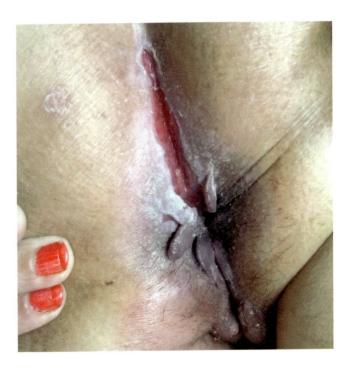

FIGURE 9.9 Presence of multiple perianal tags may be a clue to Crohn's disease. (Photograph by Dr Nina Madnani.)

Systemic findings

In some patients, the author has seen gingival hypertrophy as an associated finding, which on biopsy reveals non-caseating granulomas suggestive of CD. Intestinal CD may exist in most of the patients, as also rectovaginal fistulae or intestinal fistulae (Figures 9.10 and 9.11).

Differential diagnosis

These include granulomatous diseases like sarcoidosis, tuberculosis and others including hidradenitis suppurativa (HS), lymphogranuloma venereum (LGV), filariasis, syphilis, zirconium granulomas.

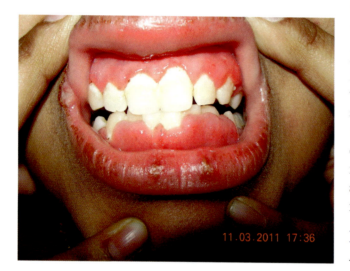

FIGURE 9.10   Gingival hypertrophy in a child with CD. (Photograph by Dr Nina Madnani.)

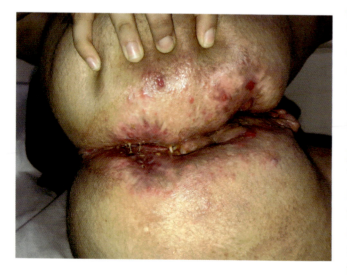

FIGURE 9.11   Recto-vaginal fistulae detected on MRI in this patient with CD. (Photograph by Dr Nina Madnani.)

Hidradenitis suppurativa can co-exist with vulvar CD. Comedones and bridged scars are hallmarks of HS.

Filariasis with a positive history of preceding fever and eosinophilia.

Vulvar TB strongly mimics vulvar CD; the diagnosis may be confirmed with a biopsy tissue culture, a Mantoux test or QuantiFERON gold TB test.

Sarcoidosis can be ruled out with a normal angiotensin-converting enzyme level and serum calcium.

LGV, besides the ulceration and edema, would have inguinal lymphadenopathy with the "groove sign". A positive history of exposure.

Investigations

Investigations must include stool for calprotectin to detect active disease. Other investigations such as inflammatory markers like C-reactive proteins (CRP), ESR, barium follow through and colonoscopy with mucosal biopsies to rule out intestinal involvement are advised. MRI/CT scan of the abdomen and pelvis may be required to detect the numbers and extent of sinuses.

Histopathology

A skin biopsy may show edema and non-caseating epithelioid cell granulomas, with a negative periodic acid-Schiff (PAS) and Ziehl Neelsen stain (Figure 9.12).

Course and prognosis

This is a chronic disease, and patients experience exacerbations interspersed with short periods of the quiescent disease. The edema leads to asymmetric deformity of the labial components. Rectovaginal, enterocutaneous, perianal and perivulvar fistulae can develop.

Management

Vulvar CD is a very difficult disease with recurrent flares, swelling, and distortion of the genitals. Metronidazole, azathioprine, infliximab and adalimumab are the therapy options. Systemic steroids give a rapid response. Intralesional corticosteroids or potent topical corticosteroids can help in reducing the edema.

Surgery is recommended only for cosmetic correction, but results are not too gratifying.

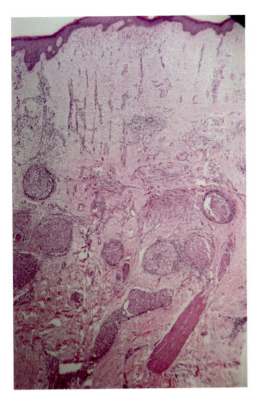
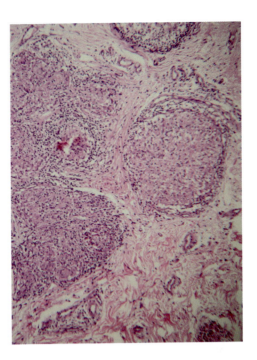

FIGURE 9.12 **(a)** H & E, 40×, upper dermal lymphedematous scar with granulomas in mid and lower dermis. **(b)** H & E, 400×, high-power view of epithelioid cell granulomas in the dermis. (Photograph by Dr Rajiv Joshi.)

Pearl
Asymmetric vulvar edema with knife-cut ulcers – Think of vulvar CD.

Recommended reading

1. Ananthakrishnan AN. Nat Rev Gastroenterol Hepatol (2015). PMID: 25732745.
2. Kedia S, et al. World J Gastroenterol (2019). PMID: 30700939.
3. Bhoyrul B, et al. J Gastroenterol Hepatol (2018). PMID: 29845642.
4. Feller ER, et al. Am Fam Physician (2001). PMID: 11759079.

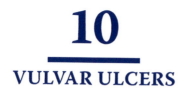

10

VULVAR ULCERS

Niti Khunger and Krati Mehrotra

Contents

Introduction

Vulvar ulcers are deep defects through the epidermis and into the dermis and can be acute, chronic or recurrent. They are mostly painful but rarely may be asymptomatic. The majority of acute vulvar ulcers are caused by sexually transmitted infections (STI), and noninfectious etiologies should be considered when STIs have been ruled out. Chronic or recurrent ulcers may be simple or complex and may be associated with systemic symptoms.

Ulcus acutum

Introduction

Lipschutz ulcer (LU), also known as ulcus vulvae acutum or acute vulvar ulceration, is a rare and underdiagnosed entity presenting as an acute painful vulvar ulcer in young women. It was first described by an Australian dermatologist, Lipschutz in 1913.

Epidemiology

According to recent data, LU comprises 30% of all vulvar ulcerations. The ulcers most frequently occur in young women of age group 14–20 years, out of which 70% of females are virgins. Although the exact etiology is unknown, LU has been linked to various microorganisms like Epstein-Barr virus (EBV) in 30% of cases, cytomegalovirus (CMV), *Mycoplasma pneumoniae*, *Mycoplasma fermentans*, mumps, *Toxoplasma gondii*, parvovirus B19, coinfection of influenza B and adenovirus and paratyphi.

Pathophysiology

LU develops from a hematogenous spread of a viral or bacterial infection resulting in a hypersensitivity reaction, leading to the deposition of immune complexes in the dermal vessels. This further activates the complement system, resulting in the formation of a microthrombus and subsequent tissue necrosis.

Presenting complaints

LU begins as a solitary painful ulcer of acute onset on the vulva with non-specific flu-like symptoms preceding it.

Clinical examination

LU classically presents as a well-defined large polycyclic ulcer in centimeters (>1 cm), shallow or deep, with a necrotic center covered by gray exudate, red granulation tissue on the floor and red-violaceous sharp margin. They are either single or multiple located over labia majora, minora, extending into the perineum, vagina, external urethral orifice, clitoris and posterior commissure with inguinal lymphadenopathy (Figure 10.1). LU when present symmetrically on the adjacent site is termed as "Kissing ulcer" (Figure 10.2). LU can present with different morphological patterns, such as pseudovesicles or herpetiform lesions. Ulcers with an eschar or gangrenous variation may also be seen. The patient can also develop other cutaneous manifestations like morbilliform-like rashes or erythema nodosum-like lesions. The revised criteria for diagnosing LU are given in

DOI: 10.1201/9781003284116-10

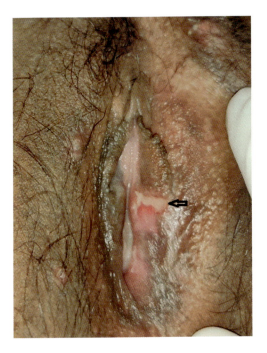

FIGURE 10.1 Irregular ulcer (black arrow) on the left labia minora. (Photograph by Dr Niti Khunger.)

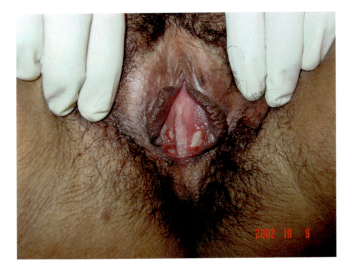

FIGURE 10.2 Sixteen years old girl presenting with punched-out "kissing" ulcers. (Photograph by Dr Nina Madnani.)

Table 10.1. If both of the major criteria and at least two of the minor criteria apply are fulfilled, then a diagnosis of LU is made.

Systemic findings
It can be associated with non-specific symptoms like fever, myalgia, headache, pharyngitis or tonsillitis.

TABLE 10.1: Revised Criteria for Diagnosis of Lipchitz Ulcer

Major Criteria:
- Acute onset of one or more painful ulcerous lesions in the vulvar region
- Exclusion of infectious and other non-infectious causes for the ulcer

Minor Criteria:
- Localization of ulcer at vestibule or labia minora
- No sexual intercourse ever (i.e. patient is a virgin) or within the last 3 months
- Flu-like symptoms
- Systemic infection within 2–4 weeks prior to the onset of vulvar ulcer.

Laboratory examination
Laboratory investigations suggested are complete blood count, STI panel to rule out herpes simplex virus (HSV) (by polymerase chain reaction), syphilis (by dark-field microscopy/serological tests), EBV and CMV IgM titers, human immunodeficiency virus (HIV) test and a skin biopsy from the ulcer edge for ulcers lasting longer than 3 or 4 weeks.

Histopathology
Cutaneous biopsy from the edge of the ulcer shows superficial edema, neutrophilic infiltration, ulceration and lymphocytic arteritis/leukocytoclastic vasculitis.

Differential diagnosis
The most important differentials to consider are discussed in Table 10.2.

Course and prognosis
LU is a self-limiting condition. There is no risk of transmission. Spontaneous healing is complete in 2–6 weeks.

Treatment
Patient care consists of pain control including topical and systemic analgesia and wound care. Patient and parents should be reassured that the disease is benign, its lack of recurrence and its self-limiting nature.

TABLE 10.2: Differential Diagnosis of Lipschutz Ulcer

Sexually Transmitted Infections
- Herpes simplex virus: multiple, painful ulcers with a history of sexual contact and detection of an etiologic factor on an investigation.
- Chancroid
- HIV

Hormone-Related
- Autoimmune progesterone dermatitis: they can also present as recurrent painful ulcers on the vulva during the late luteal phase
- Estrogen hypersensitivity

Non-Sexually Transmitted Infections
- Epstein-Barr virus
- Cytomegalovirus
- Influenza A
- Paratyphoid

Trauma
- Foreign body
- Caustic burns

Systemic Disease
- Crohn's disease
- Behçet's disease
- Pemphigus and childhood vulval pemphigoid
- Complex and simple aphthosis

Others
- Non-steroidal anti-inflammatory drugs
- Contact or irritant dermatitis
- Lymphoma/leukemia

The proposed approach:

- Correct hygienic treatment in all cases, including no soaps, specific emollients for the genito-anal region, sitting baths (Sitz bath) or wrappings with black tea.
- In case of painful LU, topical anesthetics along with oral non-steroidal anti-inflammatory drugs (NSAIDs) are prescribed.
- In the case of highly inflamed LU, high-potent topical corticosteroids or systemic corticosteroids (0.5 mg/kg of prednisolone for 1–2 weeks) are indicated. When flu-like symptoms or elevated inflammation parameters are present, broad-spectrum antibiotics (amoxicillin) are advised according to skin flora.

Pearl
The treating clinician should keep in mind LU as a differential of acute genital ulcer in non-sexually active young females.

Recommended reading

1. Bhat RM, et al. Indian J Sex Transm Dis (2007). DOI: 10.4103/0253-7184.39017.
2. Radhika SR, et al. Indian J Paediatr Dermatol (2021). DOI: 10.4103/ijpd.IJPD_80_20.
3. Huppert JS. Dermatol Ther (2010). PMID: 20868407.
4. Sadoghi B, et al. J Eur Acad Dermatol Venereol (2020). PMID: 31855308.

Chronic aphthosis

Introduction
Aphthous ulcers (sometimes called canker sores) are mucous membrane ulcerations that are extremely common on the oral mucosa, but less common over the genitalia. Chronic aphthosis is defined as ulcers lasting for more than 6 weeks and often followed by scarring.

Epidemiology
Aphthous vulvar ulcers may be reactive – following an infection (such as infectious mononucleosis) or trauma – or be related to an underlying systemic disease such as Crohn's disease, Behçet's disease (BD), gluten enteropathy (coeliac disease), systemic lupus erythematosus, HIV infection and myeloproliferative disorder.

Pathophysiology
Local mucosal injuries are the possible trigger factor. In addition, genetic factors and family history may be important factors. Neutrophilic chemotaxis and activity are known to play a significant role in the pathogenesis of complex aphthosis.

Presenting complaints
Chronic recurrent aphthosis may present as small, faster healing and less painful ulcers which recur annually 3–6 times. In complex aphthosis, it presents as long-standing, intensely painful ulcers with a short disease-free period on the vulva.

Clinical examination

Chronic aphthosis manifests as well-demarcated, small ulcerations covered by fibrinous exudate and surrounded by an erythematous halo on the lower vulvar region (either labia majora or minora) and oral mucosa. The types described are major/minor/herpetic (Figure 10.3).

Dermoscopy

Dermoscopy reveals three zones: a central yellowish-red area surrounded by a whitish structureless region and a rim of erythema.

Laboratory examination

Laboratory investigations suggested are complete blood count, STI panel to rule out HSV (by polymerase chain reaction), syphilis (by dark-field microscopy/serological tests), HIV test.

Systemic evaluation to be done for diseases like Crohn's disease, Coeliac disease and myeloproliferative disorder.

Differential diagnosis

Herpes genitalis can also present as recurrent genital ulcers but doesn't cause tissue destruction. BD should be ruled out. The investigation such as human leucocyte antigen-B51 (HLA-B51) level is more prevalent in BD than in chronic or complex aphthosis. But chronic aphthosis can evolve into BD.

Other causes of recurrent genital ulcers like Reiter syndrome are differentiated with the help of features of reactive arthritis, eye involvement and diarrhea and Crohn's disease which presents as vulvar edema or knife cut ulcers.

Course and prognosis

They have a longer course, and severe cases are refractory to management.

Treatment

Topical anesthetics such as 1% ligocaine, anti-inflammatory drugs (3% diclofenac gel) and topical corticosteriods are given as the first line of management in chronic vulvar aphthosis. Oral drugs such as corticosteroids (10–40 daily for short duration), colchicine (0.5–2 mg daily), thalidomide (100–300 mg daily with tapering to 50 mg daily for 3 months) and pentoxifylline (400 mg TDS) have been tried in refractory cases of vulvar aphthosis.

Pearls

Long-standing, recurrent ulcers can be idiopathic (primary) or secondary to systemic conditions.

A thorough clinical evaluation is done to label recurrent, multiple genital ulcers as chronic aphthosis.

Recommended reading

1. Altenburg A, et al. Dtsch Arztebl Int (2014). PMID: 25346356.
2. Aquino TM, et al. Case Rep Dermatol (2020). PMID: 32110204.
3. Kumar Jha A, et al. Dermatol Ther (2021). PMID: 33128323.

Behçet's disease

Introduction

BD, also known as Adamantiades-BD, is an auto-inflammatory disease with primary vasculitis and neutrophilic dermatosis affecting various systems. It causes oral aphthous ulcers, recurring genital ulcers, uveitis, retinal vasculitis and skin lesions (oculo-oro-genital syndrome). It can also lead to arthritis, neurological alterations and thrombophlebitis.

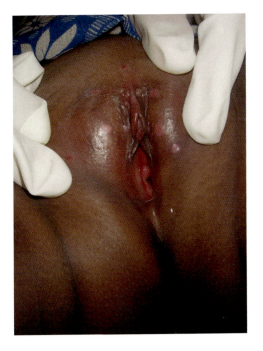

FIGURE 10.3 Chronic apthosis mimicing healing herpetic ulcers. Patient was HSV negative. (Photograph by Dr Nisha Chaturvedi.)

Epidemiology

BD is more common and often more severe along the ancient silk road, which occurs along eastern Asia to the Mediterranean. The prevalence is similar in men and women in the areas which are more endemic. It typically affects young adults of the age group 20–40 years but can be seen in children also. Most cases of Behçet's syndrome are sporadic, although familial clustering has been reported. Earlier onset of disease in successive generations, known as genetic anticipation, has been described. There is a combination of both environmental and genetic factors in the etiology.

Pathophysiology

Being a complex disease BD is related to more than one pathogenic pathway. A significant genetic association is documented with HLA-B51. Various viral and bacterial infections like HSV type 1 and streptococcus sanguinis have been proposed to trigger immune dysfunction.

Presenting complaints

Patients present with complaints of the first episode or recurrent episodes of painful oral ulcers most of the times (Figure 10.4), while 3.5% of patients start with genital ulcers. The patient can have associated eye complaints, arthritis and skin lesions with or without malaise, weakness, anorexia and headache at the time of presentation.

Clinical examination

Genital ulcers can affect any part of the genitourinary tract. They are common on the labia majora and minora and rare on the vagina and urethra. Genital aphthosis are well-defined round or oval, painful ulcers with yellowish-white necrotic base surrounded by erythema and fibrinous rim, with irregular borders (Figure 10.5). The ulcer measures 1–2 cm, usually multiple, deeper and take 4 days to months to heal. They heal with characteristic scar (64–88%) (Figure 10.6a and b).

Other systemic symptoms

The various other manifestations are posterior, anterior uveitis, cataract, glaucoma and neovascular lesions in eye (Figure 10.7). There can be coronary vasculitis, pericarditis, myocarditis, endocarditis along with pulmonary involvement. There can be glomerulonephritis or interstitial nephritis, non-erosive, asymmetrical and seronegative oligoarthritis. A patient can have neurological manifestations also. The diagnostic criteria are given in Table 10.3.

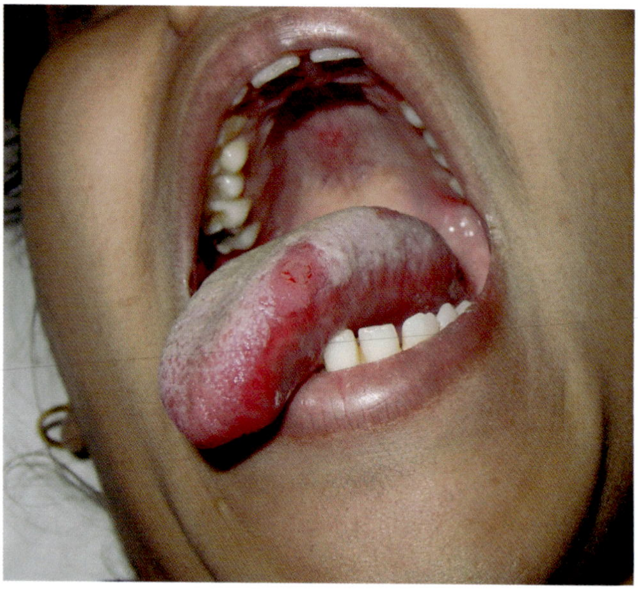

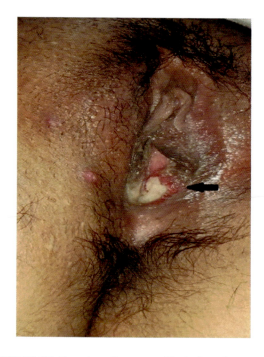

FIGURE 10.4 Palatal and tongue ulcers as part of oral manifestation in Behçet's disease. (Photograph by Dr Nina Madnani.)

FIGURE 10.5 A solitary well-defined, oval, tender, indurated, purulent ulcer, measuring 3×2 cm with a sloping edge on left labia majora lower 1/3rd. (Photograph by Dr Niti Khunger.)

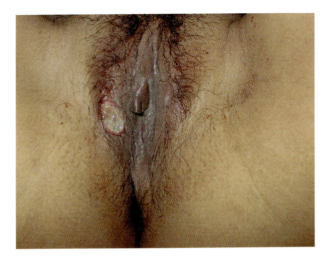

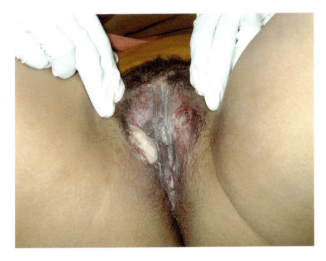

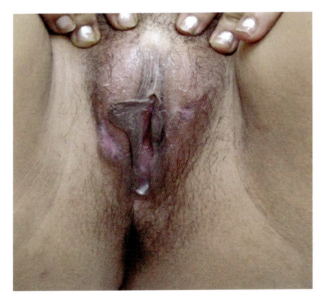

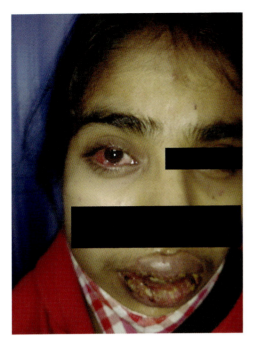

FIGURE 10.7 Ocular and oral involvement in Behçet's disease. (Photograph by Dr Niti Khunger.)

TABLE 10.3: The International Criteria for Behçet's Disease (2014)

Symptom	Score
Genital aphthosis	Two points
Ocular lesions	Two points
Oral aphthosis	Two points
Skin lesions (pseudofolliculitis, erythema nodosum, skin aphthosis)	One point
Vascular lesions	One point
Pathergy	One point
Neurological manifestation	One point

Note: Four points satisfy criteria for Behçet's disease.

FIGURE 10.6 **(a)** Punched-out ulcer with yellow slough on labia majora. **(b)** Enlargement of Ulcer post-biopsy showing pathergy positivity. **(c)** Ulcer healed with a characteristic scar. (Photographs by Dr Nina Madnani.)

Dermoscopy

Dermoscopy shows a characteristic white structureless area and the vascular component is less prominent. Half of the patients with genital ulcers showed a peripheral distribution of vessels. Dot and curved vessels were the most common pattern observed. The fiber sign, a dermoscopic sign associated with ulceration, is prevalent in genital lesions.

Laboratory examination

Diagnosis of BD is supported by clinical evidence of recurring genital ulcers along with oral ulcers after ruling out other mimickers of ulcers.

Vulvar biopsy is rarely performed to exclude other causes. Other routine investigations such as complete blood count, renal, liver profile, urine analysis have to be done along with a Pathergy test and skin biopsy with immunofluorescence.

Histopathology

Biopsy of genital ulcers shows a mixed infiltrate consisting of neutrophils, lymphocytes and macrophages at the ulcer base. The infiltrate is more of a perivascular type. Actual vasculitis and fibrinoid necrosis in the vessel wall are rare findings in a genital ulcer.

Differential diagnosis

Genital ulcerations should be differentiated from frequently seen venereal diseases such as herpes genitalis (small, multiple, painful ulcers of less duration), chancroid, syphilis and HIV.

Non-infectious conditions like fixed drug eruption, erythema multiforme, erosive lichen planus, autoimmune bullous dermatoses can also present as multiple painful ulcers on the vulva. Recurrent genital ulcerations may also be seen in MAGIC syndrome (mouth and genital ulcers with inflamed cartilage), Munchausen syndrome, hypereosinophilic syndrome, myelodysplastic syndrome and tuberculosis cutis.

In cases of long-standing ulcers, malignancy like vulvar squamous cell carcinoma, basal cell carcinoma and extramammary Paget's disease should be considered.

Course and prognosis

BD has a chronic, relapsing-remitting course. The disease significantly affects somatic and psychosocial wellbeing.

Treatment

As genital ulcers are extremely tender, they should be promptly treated for a week with strong analgesics, topical anesthetics (10% lidocaine spray or 2–5% gel), topical corticosteroid ointment or paste and oral antibiotics in case of secondary infection of the genital ulcer. Intractable ulcers can be treated with intralesional steroids (triamcinolone acetonide 0.1–0.5 mL/lesion) keeping in mind the risk of pathergy phenomenon, infection and pseudofolliculitis. Skin barrier can be maintained with emollients and avoiding the use of harsh soaps.

Patients with systemic features and resistance to topical therapy are treated with oral prednisolone (5–60 mg/day), colchicine (0.5–2 mg/day), dapsone (2–3 mg/kg/day) or azathioprine (2–3 mg/kg/day). Recently, tumor necrosis factor (TNF) alpha inhibitors and apremilast have also been tried.

Pearl

BD involving the vulva is a diagnosis of exclusion.

Recommended reading

1. Nair JR, et al. Clin Med (Lond). PMID: 28148585.
2. Leccese P, et al. Front Immunol (2019). PMID: 31134098.
3. Davatchi F, et al. Expert Rev Clin Immunol (2017). PMID: 27351485.
4. Singal A, et al. Indian J Dermatol Venereol Leprol (2013). DOI:10.4103/0378-6323.107636.

Amoebic ulcers

Introduction

Amebiasis is common, but rarely involves skin or genitalia. However, in the past few decades, more sexually transmitted amebiasis have been documented. Cutaneous amebiasis or amoeba cutis involving the genital is seen due to direct invasion of *E. histolytica* in previously damaged skin or through sexual intercourse. Female genital amebiasis is more prevalent in endemic areas of amebiasis.

Epidemiology

The etiologic agent *E. histolytica* and non-pathogenic *E. dispar* together infect 10% of the world's population. High rates of infection occur in India (15% of the population), Africa, Far east Asia, Mexican and South America. The primary mode of transmission of *E. histolytica* is waterborne, although genital involvement is seen in females of endemic areas through anal intercourse or invasion of perianal epithelial cells via rectovaginal fistula.

Age of presentation varies from 16 to 39 years old, and few case reports show the prediction for ages beyond 60 years. Risk factors identified include homosexual and heterosexual contact with infected partners and concomitant intestinal (also rectosigmoid) infection, poor genital hygiene and trauma.

Pathophysiology

Pathogenic *E. histolytica* strains from the intestine cause disruption of mucosal barriers and then adherence to perineal epithelial cells, followed by their lysis. Greater transmission among anal intercourse partners occurs due to asymptomatic infections.

Presenting complaints

Genital amebiasis usually presents with foul smelling and bloody vaginal discharge with raw area on vulva in mild cases. In cases of progressive disease, tender small pin head-sized ulcers on vulva (8.1%) along with abdominal pain and lower backache are seen. Genital amebiasis can also appear as long-standing ulcerative growth mimicking malignancy in severe cases.

Clinical examination

Multiple small, superficial and shallow, linear ulcers with irregular overhanging margins and grayish slough on floor present on the vulva, vaginal vault, perineal and anal region. Ulcers are painful, friable to touch with bleeding and show necrotic tissue. There is foul-smelling odor and profuse discharge from the ulcer.

Systemic findings

Most of the patients have features or a history of diarrhea because of its intestinal foci.

Laboratory examination

Genital amebiasis is diagnosed by direct smear (or Papaniculaou smear) of vaginal, cervical, or urethral discharge which shows the presence of *E. histolytica* on wet mount. Ulcerative lesions require biopsy to demonstrate invading trophozoite, in addition to inflammatory infiltrate and necrotic debris. The serological tests for the detection of amebiasis include immunofluorescent antibody test, radioimmunoassay, countercurrent immunoelectrophoresis and enzyme-linked immunosorbent assay.

Histopathology

Biopsy from the ulcer edge shows infiltration of mononuclear cells with spherical to oval (15–20 mm diameter) organisms known as trophozoites that have a single nucleus with a prominent nuclear border and karyosome. The cytoplasm can show vacuolation and erythrophagocytosis.

Differential diagnosis

Some important conditions which should be kept in mind when considering a diagnosis of amoebic ulcers include:

- Tubercular ulcer of vulva present as multiple small shallow ulcers with sinus tracts on vulva.
- Syphilitic ulcer is usually a solitary, painless, indurated ulcer overlying a firm papule on labia majora or minora, clitoris, urethral orifice or cervix.
- Vaginal carcinoma presents as ulcerative and necrotic ulcer on vulva. Cervical cytology, wet smear examination and biopsy helps in distinguishing it from amoebic ulcers.
- Metastatic Crohn's disease shows multiple, deep vulval abscess or "knife cut" ulcers.

Course and prognosis

Sexually transmitted amebiasis shows rapid and inexorable progression leading to organ destruction. But prognosis is good if treated effectively at an early stage in most of the cases.

Treatment

Oral or intravenous metronidazole (750–800 mg, three times a day for 5 days) followed by diloxanide furoate (500 mg three times a day) or paromomycin (30 mg/kg three times a day) for 10 days to clear luminal trophozoites is the usual treatment against amebiasis.

In case of genital organ mutilation, reconstructive surgery and autologous skin transplant are done.

Pearl

Recognizing this entity is essential to prevent unnecessary interventions.

Recommended reading

1. Musthyala NB, et al. J Midlife Health. 2019. PMID: 31391760.
2. Morán P, et al. Am J Trop Med Hyg. 2013. PMID: 23208883.
3. Fernández-Díez J, et al. Cutis. 2012. PMID: 23409482.
4. Holmes K. Sexually transmitted diseases. 4th ed. McGraw-Hill; 2008.
5. Sinha, A. A case of amoebic ulcer of vagina. J. Obstet. Gynec. Ind., 2: 323, 1961.

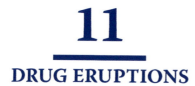

11

DRUG ERUPTIONS

Nisha Chaturvedi and Kaleem Khan

Contents

Erythema multiforme/ Stevens–Johnson syndrome/ toxic epidermal necrolysis

Nisha Chaturvedi

Introduction

Erythema multiforme (EM) and Stevens–Johnson syndrome (SJS)/toxic epidermal necrolysis (TEN) are immune-mediated blistering skin diseases commonly triggered by a drug or infection. EM and SJS/TEN often have overlapping clinical features but are now considered separate entities. SJS/TEN belong to the same spectrum of disease where SJS is defined as <10 percent of skin involvement and TEN as >30 percent of skin involvement. Around 10–30 percent represents an overlap between SJS and TEN.

Epidemiology

EM can occur at any age but is more frequently seen in young adults between 20 and 30 years of age. Many viral/fungal/bacterial infections, drugs, malignancies, immunizations, menstruation and autoimmune diseases have been implicated as the cause. The commonest cause of EM is herpes simplex also termed as herpes-associated EM (HAEM). In children, *Mycoplasma pneumoniae* infection is another important cause of EM.

SJS/TEN can affect all ages and races with higher predilection in elderly women. Drugs like antiepileptics, allopurinol, antivirals, non-steroidal anti-inflammatory drugs (NSAIDs) and sulfonamides are the commonest trigger for SJS/TEN in adults and the pediatric age group. People with HIV infection and certain genetic factors like human leukocyte antigen (HLA)-B*1502/HLA-B*5801 are at an increased risk of developing SJS/TEN.

Pathophysiology

The pathogenesis of EM and SJS/TEN are similar in that both involve cytotoxic lymphocyte responses against altered keratinocytes either via direct cytotoxicity or soluble mediators like Fas ligand and granzymes. The alteration in keratinocytes in EM in most cases is secondary to viral antigen, while in SJS/TEN, it is secondary to a drug.

Presenting complaints

Patients may present with an acute onset skin rash, redness and painful erosions on the mucous membrane. Occasionally, dysuria may be the presenting symptom. The skin rash may be preceded by fever, myalgia, malaise, photophobia and other symptoms mimicking viral flu. As the disease progresses in intensity, the patient may present with eye involvement and extensive blistering all over the body, the severity necessitating urgent admission. In herpes simplex virus (HSV)-associated EM, the patient may have had herpes simplex 2–17 days prior to getting a rash.

Clinical examination

Cutaneous lesions of EM are typically target lesions with 3 zones. An erythematous peripheral ring, an edematous clear middle ring, and an erythematous papule at the center with a blister or central necrosis. These lesions usually have an acral distribution.

TEN is the severe form of SJS, where the cutaneous lesions progress from erythema and blistering to skin necrosis. Skin tenderness and a positive

DOI: 10.1201/9781003284116-11

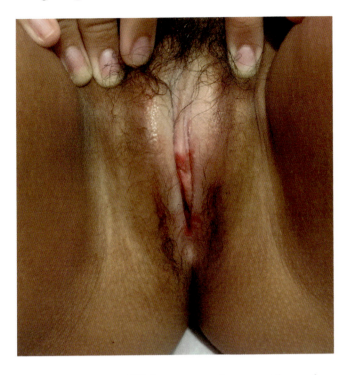

FIGURE 11.1 With two erosions on the vulva. (Photograph by Dr Nisha Chaturvedi.)

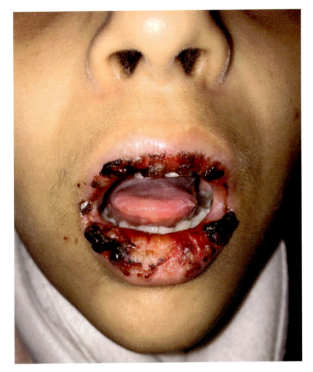

FIGURE 11.2 SJS with extensive oral involvement with ulceration and hemorrhagic crust. (Photograph by Dr Nisha Chaturvedi.)

Nikolsky sign are ominous findings. Vulvovaginal involvement includes erosive and ulcerative vaginitis (Figure 11.1). Urethritis can also develop, which may cause urinary retention.

Oral mucosa is involved with painful, hemorrhagic erosions with grayish-white slough (Figure 11.2).

Ocular changes include severe purulent conjunctivitis, corneal ulcerations, photophobia, anterior uveitis and panophthalmitis. In severe disease, sloughing of the mucosa may be seen.

Systemic findings
Patients with severe disease and extensive skin detachment may go into septic shock with electrolyte imbalance, renal failure and multiple organ dysfunction (Figure 11.3).

Histopathology
EM typically shows basal cell vacuolar degeneration, necrotic keratinocytes and lymphocytic exocytosis. SJS/TEN shows apoptotic keratinocytes, partial to full thickness epidermal necrosis, subepidermal bullae and perivascular lymphohistiocytic infiltrate with eosinophils.

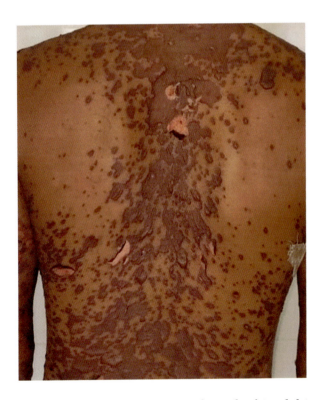

FIGURE 11.3 Extensive rash with skin dehiscence. (Photograph by Dr Bela Shah.)

Differential diagnosis

Differential diagnosis includes bullous pemphigoid, pemphigus vulgaris and staphylococcal-scalded skin syndrome.

Bullous pemphigoid is a chronic, autoimmune blistering disorder that clinically presents with erythematous and urticarial plaques and tense bullae, with or without mucosal involvement. Biopsy and immunofluorescence studies further help to distinguish this disorder.

Pemphigus vulgaris is a chronic, mucocutaneous autoimmune blistering condition with flaccid bullae and painful mucosal erosions and ulcerations. Histopathology and immunofluorescent tests are diagnostic.

Staphylococcal scalded skin syndrome is seen in neonates and children, caused by toxins produced by *Staphylococci*. Clinically, it presents as generalized erythema with flaccid blisters and desquamation without mucous membrane involvement.

Course and prognosis

EM usually resolves in a span of 2 weeks without any scarring. Post-inflammatory hyperpigmentation may remain, especially in dark skin patients.

In SJS/TEN re-epithelization may take 2–4 weeks. Cutaneous sequelae include scarring, post-inflammatory hyper or hypopigmentation, telogen effluvium, eruptive nevi and abnormal nail growth. Ophthalmic sequelae include keratitis, symblepharon and corneal scarring.

Patients with vulvovaginal involvement may develop strictures, vaginal adenosis and stenosis of the introitus with complete obliteration of the vagina.

Treatment

Suppressive therapy for HSV infection must be considered in HAEM patients.

For SJS/TEN, the offending drug must be discontinued. Milder disease can be treated with supportive care, prevention of infection and topical treatment. Severe disease requires multi-specialty care and the patient should be treated in a 'Burns Unit' where possible. Various therapies like systemic steroids, cyclosporine, TNF alfa-inhibitors, IVIG and plasmapheresis have been tried with varied responses. Supportive care, fluid and electrolyte management, wound debridement, pain

management and infection control are the mainstays of treatment.

Vulvovaginal care includes maintaining perianal hygiene, application of emollients and placement of catheter if required. Corticosteroid ointments can also be used. Suppression of menses must be considered in adolescent girls. Soft vaginal molds can be used as prophylaxis in the acute phase of illness. Tampons covered with petrolatum may be used to prevent vaginal adhesions. Vaginoscopy can be performed on a follow-up to detect any complications.

Pearls

Genital examination must be done in all patients with SJS/TEN even if asymptomatic, as lesions may develop during the course of the disease.

Menstrual suppression must be considered in menstruating women.

Recommended reading

1. Holtz M, et al. J Pediatr Adolesc Gynecol (2021). PMID: 33915265.
2. Pliskow S. J Reprod Med (2013). PMID: 23947089.

Fixed drug eruption

Kaleem Khan

Introduction

Fixed drug eruption (FDE) is a type of cutaneous adverse drug reaction that recurs at fixed locations on repeated exposure to the offending drug.

Epidemiology

FDE is the second most common presentation of cutaneous adverse drug reaction in the Indian population. No age is exempt, but it is most commonly reported between the second and fourth decade of life. In India, contrary to western literature, genital FDE is more prevalent in men than women. The common culprit drugs include antimicrobials, NSAIDs and anti-epileptics.

Pathophysiology

FDEs are considered a type of delayed hypersensitivity reaction (type IVc). The presence of CD8+ effector-memory T-cells along the epidermal side of basement membrane is key to the localization of this reaction on subsequent exposure to the offending drug. When the drug is withdrawn, the lesion resolves spontaneously with post-inflammatory pigmentation. Rarely, there may not be any residual pigmentation, and this is identified as non-pigmented FDE (NPFDE).

Presenting complaints

Within a few hours or days of consumption of the culprit drug, women complain of itching and discomfort, which may rapidly progress to burning sensation and pain. Women often give a history of similar episodes in the past.

Clinical examination

FDE may present as a symmetric erosive vulvitis involving the labia minora (Figure 11.4). This seems to be the predominant presentation in older Caucasian women. The vulva may be edematous, and occasionally a blister may be evident (Figure 11.5). The erosions may extend to the perianal region. In some patients, the buccal mucosa, lips and extra genital sites may be involved (Figure 11.6). The skin shows well-defined, dark red, dusky/violateous patches which may blister (Figure 11.7). In darker skin types, residual post-inflammatory pigmentation may be evident in healing.

Dermoscopy

Pigmented FDE may show coarse brown to black dots and globules.

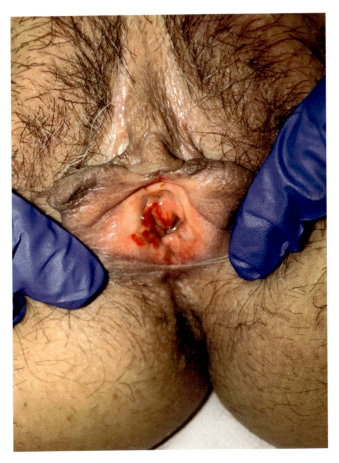

FIGURE 11.5 Bright red erosions at the introitus are seen following oral fluconazole, a common anti-fungal drug. (Photograph by Dr Nina Madnani.)

Laboratory examination

A modified patch testing is recommended, where the suspect medication (dissolved or in a paste form) is placed on lesional skin and the site is

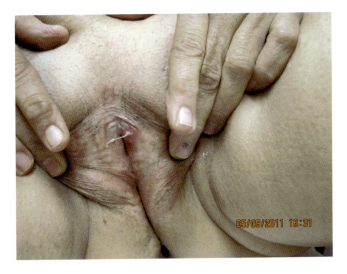

FIGURE 11.4 On the vulva, an FDE can present as an erosion. Here, you can see erosion on the left labia minora. (Photograph by Dr Nina Madnani.)

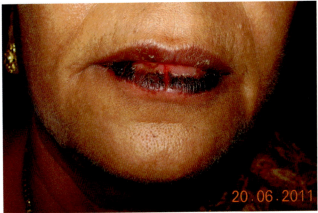

FIGURE 11.6 FDE to nitrofurantoin showing severe cheilitis. (Photograph by Dr Bela Shah.)

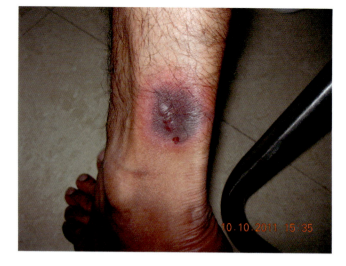

FIGURE 11.7 Repeated exposure to the same drug can lead to a bullous FDE. (Photograph by Dr Bela Shah.)

evaluated after 48 hours. This is not possible on the vulvar skin and needs to be done elsewhere. Hence, results are not so sensitive. Oral challenge has been recommended, but the ethics of doing so is questionable.

Histopathology
Biopsy reveals an interface dermatitis and a lympho-eosinophilic infiltrate with melanophages in the dermis. The epidermis has varying degrees of vacuolar change with necrotic keratinocytes. The NPFDE variant has subtle histologic findings and may be easily overlooked as non-specific dermatitis.

Differential diagnosis
Lichen planus: mucosal lichen planus presents with painful erosions involving labia minora and vestibule and progressing to scarring. Occasionally, a typical lacy pattern or violaceous flat-topped papules may be seen at the periphery of the lesions.

Desquamating inflammatory vulvovaginitis is a type of purulent vulvovaginitis seen in perimenopausal women and has non-specific signs and symptoms.

Contact dermatitis: Odematous vulva with erosion and a history of the application of a contact irritant.

Course and prognosis
Women experience recurrent episodes of vulvitis on repeated exposure to the offending drug. The reaction tends to worsen progressively. There is the faster onset of symptoms, existing lesions become more extensive and newer lesions develop on the body.

Upon withdrawal of the culprit drug, the lesions on keratinized skin may spontaneously resolve with significant post-inflammatory pigmentation, which may persist for months or even years (if intermittent exposure continues).

Treatment
It is imperative to identify and stop the offending drug. Most lesions resolve spontaneously, and topical application of mid/high-potent steroids will aid in faster resolution. Rarely, a short, tapering course of systemic corticosteroids may be required to control the symptoms.

Pearl
Erosive mucositis involving the labia may be the only presentation in NPFDE of the vulva.

Recommended reading
1. Fischer G. J. Reprod. Med (2007). PMID: 17393766.
2. Wain EM, et al. Clin Exp Dermatol (2008). PMID: 18681879.
3. Shalin SC, et al. Semin Diagn Pathol (2021). PMID: 32951943.

12

CYSTS AND NON-NEOPLASTIC SWELLINGS

Ashwini Bhalerao-Gandhi, Vrushali Kamale, and Anupkumar Tiwary

Contents

Introduction

The vulvar skin is lined by stratified squamous epithelium. The mons pubis and labia majora consist of fat, sebaceous, apocrine and eccrine sweat glands. Labia minora have no hair follicles but contain sebaceous glands and few sweat glands. The epithelium of the vestibule is rich in eccrine glands. These glands are a source of lumps, cysts and abscesses. The common vulvar cysts are Sebaceous cyst, Epidermoid cyst, Bartholin's cyst and Skene's duct cyst.

There are various non-neoplastic pathologies that can develop on vulvar skin. The ability to identify such benign entities can not only reduce patient anxiety but also minimize unnecessary diagnostic workup. Many of the vulvar lesions remain unreported, undiagnosed or misdiagnosed because of less patient-doctor interaction or lack of optimum clinical knowledge, which results in the patient's psychological and physical suffering.

Epidermoid cyst

Ashwini Bhalerao-Gandhi
and Vrushali Kamale

Introduction

Epidermoid cyst is a benign, cutaneous cyst of the vulva which originates from the epidermis or pilo-sebaceous follicle.

Epidemiology

Epidermoid cysts are seen in all ages of women; however they are more common in adolescence and reproductive age, probably due to hormonal interplay. Women with steatocystoma multiplex, an autosomal inherited disorder, have multiple epidermoid cysts in the axilla and femoral folds.

Pathophysiology

The epidermoid cyst can develop primarily directly from the infundibulum of an inflamed hair follicle. Secondary epidermal cysts result from traumatic implantation of the superficial epidermal tissue into the dermal/subcutaneous plane following trauma or surgical procedure. The vulvar epidermoid cysts occur mostly following episiotomy. These cysts can also be seen in women of ethnic origin following cultural practices of female circumcision.

Presenting complaints

Majority of the cysts are small and asymptomatic. Patients with large and inflamed cysts may experience pain and difficulty in walking. Some cysts may rupture during physical activity. History of trauma may not always be present.

Clinical examination

The lesions may be solitary or multiple (Figure 12.1) and presents typically as a freely mobile, firm, dome-shaped cyst with a central punctum (Figure 12.2).

DOI: 10.1201/9781003284116-12

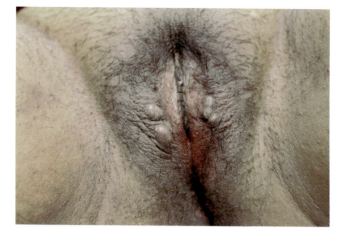

FIGURE 12.1 Multiple, yellowish, dome-shaped papules with a central punctum on the labia majora. (Photograph by Dr Nina Madnani.)

On palpation, it is felt as a nodule just beneath the skin. The size varies from a few millimeters to several centimeters. Vulvar epidermoid cysts are frequently seen on the clitoris, labia majora and perineum. Through a punctum, on pressure, rancid-smelling yellow pasty material can be expressed; the wall of the epidermoid cyst is thin and may rupture easily. Inflammation may lead to an increase in size. Giant vulvar epidermoid cysts may be encountered including lesions that may result in pseudo clitoromegaly.

Dermoscopy

It shows a punctum which typically appears in an epidermoid cyst. Occasionally seen are bluish discoloration and the presence of arborizing vessels (Figure 12.3).

Laboratory examination

Detailed history, physical examination and clinical appearance can confirm the diagnosis of a typical epidermoid cyst. However, in the pediatric population and in a large vulvar cyst in adults, to confirm the diagnosis and extent of the lesion, trans-labial ultrasound is advisable. Magnetic resonance imaging (MRI) is also a good modality for the differentiation of large vulvar masses. Laboratory investigations are not typically advised unless the cyst is infected with abscess collection.

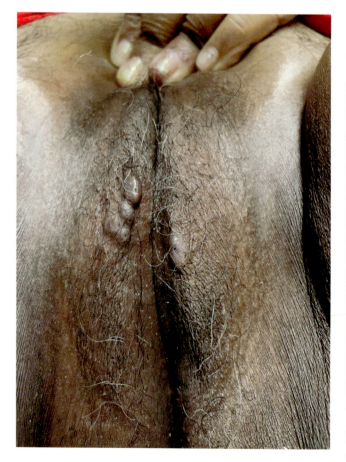

FIGURE 12.2 Epidermoid cyst may be mistaken for molluscum contagiousum due to the central opening. (Photograph by Dr Nina Madnani.)

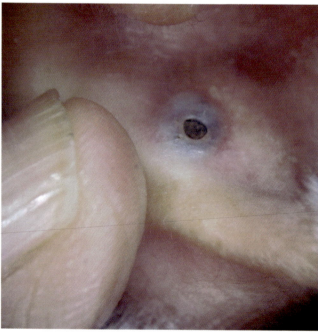

FIGURE 12.3 Dermoscopy of epidermoid cyst showing pore sign, bluish-white veil and periphery arborizing vessels. Dinolite digital microscope WF-20, polarized, 10x. (Photograph by Dr Nina Madnani.)

Histopathology

The diagnosis is confirmed by histologic examination, which shows epidermoid cysts lined by stratified squamous epithelium with the cavity filled with keratin.

Differential diagnosis

Sebaceous cyst: While clinical differentiation can be difficult, the histology is distinct and characteristic. Classification is based on the pathogenesis, nature of cyst contents which are oily and the wall lining.

Cyst of the canal of Nuck is a painless or mildly painful, reducible or irreducible mass in the inguinal region, which typically extends to the labia majora.

Lipoma is a soft, painless, slow-growing vulvar nodule, histopathologically composed of mature adipocytes.

Vulvar endometriosis is an uncommon condition; however, in women with persistent tender bluish nodules located at labia majora with complains of dyspareunia and an increase in lesions during menstruation, diagnosis of endometriosis should be considered.

Skene's duct cyst is an interlabial bulging mass on either side of the urethral meatus, usually seen in neonates.

Inguinal hernia is painless, reducible swelling. With the impulse to cough, it can slowly increase in size. However, it is rare in females.

Vulvar syringoma is seen in young adults with multiple small, firm, skin-colored papules bilaterally on the vulva. It may be asymptomatic, but pruritis is prominent. Histopathology shows that the duct lining is of two layers of cuboidal cells.

Among malignant tumors of the vulva, rarely liposarcoma should be kept in mind.

Course and prognosis

Usually excellent. However, rupture of cyst, hematoma, localized cellulitis, infection and rarely carcinoma can develop in some untreated women.

Treatment

Non-infected small vulvar epidermoid cysts may not require any treatment. If symptomatic, slowly growing, and for cosmetic reasons, surgical excision of the cyst with its wall intact is the definitive treatment. The best time for excision is when the cyst is not acutely inflamed. Fluctuant inflamed cyst is incised and drained after oral antibiotic coverage. In case of inflamed cysts, intralesional triamcinolone acetonide injection potentially reduces the need for surgical excision.

Pearl

Epidermoid vulvar cysts occur due to inflammation of hair follicles typically following trauma or surgical procedures.

Recommended reading

1. Birge O, et al. J Med Case Rep (2019). PMID: 31027516.
2. Mahmoudnejad N, et al. Urol J (2020). PMID: 33159314.
3. Ghigliotti G, et al. Clin Exp Dermatol (2014). PMID: 24708085.
4. Aggarwal SK, et al. J Indian Assoc Pediatr Surg (2010). PMID: 21180500.

Bartholin's cyst

Ashwini Bhalerao-Gandhi
and Vrushali Kamale

Introduction

Bartholin's glands are a pair of small, pea-shaped mucous glands that lie posterior to the bulbs of the vestibule on each side of the vaginal opening. The duct of each gland opens into the vestibule along the posterolateral margin of the vaginal opening. Normally, Bartholin's gland are not seen or felt unless infected or swollen.

Epidemiology

Literature reviews reveal that symptomatic Bartholin's cysts and abscesses account for 2% of all gynecologic visits per year. Bartholin's cyst and abscess are often seen at the onset of puberty, child-bearing age, and their incidence decreases after menopause.

Pathophysiology

Obstruction of the Bartholin duct causes accumulation of mucus, leading to cystic dilatation of the gland. Obstruction may occur due to trauma to the area, during episiotomy or childbirth; however, it may also occur without an identifiable cause. Generally, a cyst is very sterile. If this cyst becomes infected, abscess is formed. The most common pathogen is *E. coli*, followed by *Staphylococcus aureus*, Group B *Streptococci*, *N. gonorrhea*, Chlamydia trachomatis or polymicrobial. Bartholin gland carcinoma is rare.

Presenting complaints

Usually, a Bartholin's cyst is painless, unilateral, asymptomatic and detected incidentally during a routine gynecological examination or by the patient herself. Large cysts may cause discomfort while walking or a sexual intercourse. Bartholin's cyst abscess presents with severe pain and swelling. It causes intense pain while walking, sitting and during sexual intercourse. It is necessary to ask the history of previous Bartholin's cyst/abscess, sexually transmitted infection and purulent drainage of the cyst. With an abscess, a patient may give a history of fever.

Clinical examination

The vulvar inspection and palpation of the Bartholin gland is performed. Typically, the gland is palpated by holding the labia majora between the index finger inside the vagina and the thumb outside. A small Bartholin's cyst is often detected incidentally. A cyst averages 1–3 cm and is usually unilateral (Figure 12.4). A Bartholin abscess is unilateral, tender, warm, soft, fluctuant mass felt in the lower medial, posterior aspect of the vaginal introitus (Figure 12.5). The overlying skin is thin, red and edematous (Figure 12.6). The pus may burst through the thin layer of skin at a pointing area.

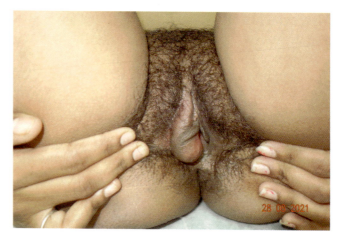

FIGURE 12.5 Sometimes, the Bartholin cyst may enlarge to involve the entire length of the labia minora. (Photograph by Dr Yogesh Bhingradia.)

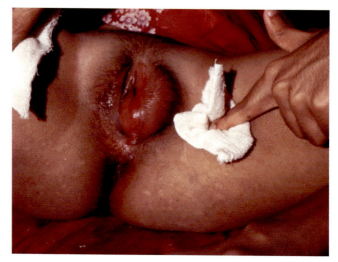

FIGURE 12.6 An infected Bartholin cyst can form a huge abscess. (Photograph by Dr Janak Maniar.)

Laboratory examination

A proper medical history and pelvic examination are adequate to diagnose Bartholin's cyst or abscess. Fluid culture and biopsy are performed during incision and drainage. Imaging studies are not required in the evaluation of a Bartholin's cyst mass. There is no role of blood tests, if a systemic infection is not suspected.

Histopathology

The Bartholin's gland is composed of several epithelial types; the body is mucinous acini, the duct is the predominantly transitional epithelium, and the orifice is the squamous epithelium.

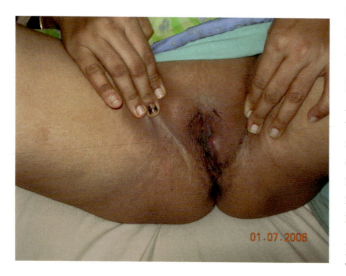

FIGURE 12.4 Bartholin cyst typically presents as a cystic swelling on the lower one-third of labia minora. (Photograph by Dr Nina Madnani.)

Differential diagnosis

Some important differentials to keep in mind when suspecting Bartholin gland cyst include Skene's duct cyst: This is seen anteriorly, whereas Bartholin cyst is present posterolaterally near the introitus.

Canal of Nuck cyst is painless or mildly painful, reducible or irreducible mass in the inguinal region, which typically extends to the labia majora.

Vaginal prolapse: The swelling is usually seen inside the vagina, and there is an associated dragging sensation or something coming down. The Bartholin gland is mostly posteriolateral, whereas prolapse can be from any corner of the vaginal vault.

Vulval hematoma and lipoma can be differentiated based on history and examination.

Syringoma, adenocarcinoma, squamous cell carcinoma and endometriosis are other differential diagnoses that are quite rare.

Course and prognosis

Asymptomatic cysts do not require treatment. Some cysts or abscesses may spontaneously drain. If a cyst is aspirated, high recurrence rate of 2–13% has been reported.

Treatment

Asymptomatic Bartholin's cyst does not require any treatment. In some cases, the cyst or abscess ruptures and drains spontaneously, or may need analgesics and warm compresses. Large cyst and abscess' of Bartholin's gland are treated with incision and drainage. Material obtained at the time of incision & drainage (I&D) or spontaneous rupture should be sent for culture. Antibiotic therapy should also be considered in patients with systemic symptoms like fever, chills, suspected sepsis and those considered at high risk of complicated infection.

Other less common procedures include silver nitrate ablation, carbon dioxide laser vaporization and Jacobi ring placement.

Pearls

Bartholin mass should be biopsied if it has a solid component, is adherent to surrounding tissues, or is unresponsive to treatment and in all post-menopausal women.

Recommended reading

1. Marzano DA, et al. J Low Genit Tract Dis (2004). PMID: 15874863.
2. Illingworth B, et al. BJOG (2020). PMID: 31876985.
3. Kroese JA, et al. BJOG (2017). PMID: 27640367.

Periurethral cyst

Ashwini Bhalerao-Gandhi
and Vrushali Kamale

Introduction

Periurethral gland/Skene's gland is situated anteriorly, near the external urethral meatus, in the vestibule of the vulva. The ducts of Skene's gland open into the vestibule, one on each side of the lateral margin of the urethra. Skene's glands are considered the female homologue of the male prostate. Skene's glands secrete fluid on sexual stimulation.

Epidemiology

The actual incidence of the Skene's gland cyst is not known, probably due to underreporting. Most commonly, Skene's duct cyst or its abscess is found in middle-aged women.

Pathophysiology

The exact cause of the cyst is unknown. However, obstruction of the paraurethral duct as a result of infection or inflammation or cystic degeneration of embryonic remnants of the paraurethral glands has been postulated. Very rarely, Skene's duct cyst can present as an interlabial mass in neonates.

Presenting complaints

Generally, the Skene's duct cyst presents with an asymptomatic interlabial bulging mass. Rarely, it may be associated with pain, dysuria, dyspareunia, urinary tract infection and voiding dysfunction.

Clinical examination

Examination shows interlabial mass on either side of the urethral meatus. One can notice the displacement of the urethral meatus by the bulging mass.

Laboratory examination

The swelling itself is assessed by ultrasound examination. In cases with symptoms related to infection or dyspareunia, complete blood count, renal function test, urine analysis, pelvic ultrasound, voiding cystourethrogram and cystoscopy are required. MRI may be needed in doubtful cases.

Histopathology
The cyst wall is lined with transitional epithelium.

Differential diagnosis
Depending upon the age of the female. Some important differentials include:

- Imperforate hymen, Mullerian duct cyst, urethral polyp, urethral diverticulum and congenital lipoma are to be considered during evaluation in newborns. Condyloma needs to be ruled out, in pre-pubertal girls. Hymenal imperforation presents as a smooth mass that fills the vaginal introitus.
- Periurethral cystic lesions are rare even in adults and need to be differentiated from urethral diverticulum, urethral prolapse, prolapsed ectopic ureterocoele, rhabdomyosarcoma of vagina. In the latter, an introital grape-like cluster of masses will be seen.

Course and prognosis
Most Skene's cysts are < 1 cm and are asymptomatic. Cancerous transformation is extremely rare.

Treatment
Management is conservative in an asymptomatic case. Particularly in a newborn, it can show spontaneous resolution. Surgical excision of the cyst or marsupialization is the treatment in young adults in case of an abscess.

Pearls
Although periurethral cysts are asymptomatic, when enlarged, they can cause urethral obstruction and urinary retention.

Recommended reading
1. Moralioğlu S, et al. Urol Ann (2013). PMID: 24049387.
2. Nickles SW, et al. J Pediatr Adolesc Gynecol (2009). PMID: 19232290.
3. Nussbaum AR, et al. AJR Am J Roentgenol. (1983). PMID: 6602532.
4. Kusama Y, et al. J Gen Fam Med. (2017). PMID: 29264050.

Vulvar lipoma
Anupkumar Tiwary

Introduction
Lipomas are very common, benign, mesenchymal tumors of mature fat cells located mostly in the subcutaneous layer. The common sites are nape of the neck, upper back, shoulders, abdomen, buttocks and proximal part of the limbs. Lipoma on vulva is a multilobulated subcutaneous tumor which needs careful diagnostic work up.

Epidemiology
Lipoma on the vulva is very rare. Usually appear between the 4th to the 6th decade. The etiology is not known, but trauma has been implicated in some cases. Genetic predisposition is seen in only 2–3% of patients with multiple lipomas.

Pathophysiology
Local trauma leading to cytokine release triggering pre-adipocyte differentiation and maturation has been hypothesized as a mechanism for lipoma formation.

Presenting complaints
Patient comes with the complaint of painless swelling on the vulva. Difficulty in urination and sexual intercourse would be a concern if the size was excessively large.

Clinical examination
The swelling may be single or multiple, slowly growing, painless, ill-defined, mobile, with a characteristic doughy feel. The overlying skin is usually normal (Figure 12.7).

Histopathology
It demonstrates a thin capsule surrounding a lobular proliferation of mature lipocytes interspersed with strands of fibrous connective tissue.

Differential diagnosis
It includes Bartholin cyst, inguinal hernia and cyst of canal of Nuck. Radiologic evaluation by ultrasound, computed tomography and MRI are useful in differentiating lipomas from other cysts and inguinal hernias.

Ultrasound shows the hypoechoic cystic appearance of Bartholin's cysts or other vulvar cysts. Peritoneal lining and hernial contents are clearly

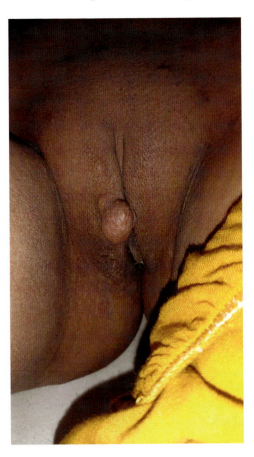

FIGURE 12.7 Ill-defined, skin-colored lipomatous swelling on the right side of the vulva. (Photograph by Dr Nina Madnani.)

seen in the case of inguinal hernias, whereas vulvar lipomas appear as nonspecific homogenous lobular structures with homogenous echogenicity consistent with fat deposition.

Course and prognosis
It runs a benign clinical course. The size increases slowly causing cosmetic concerns. A larger size can also have a negative impact on sexual life.

Treatment
Complete surgical excision is the treatment of choice. Steroid injections for small lipoma and liposuction for larger lipoma can also be effective. Intralesional deoxycholine can also be done to debulk the size of lipomas.

Pearl
A radiologic investigation is mandatory to confirm the diagnosis of vulvar lipoma as it is often misdiagnosed as an inguinal hernia.

Recommended reading
1. Odoi AT, et al. Ghana Med J (2011). PMID: 22282580.
2. Oh JT, et al. J Pediatr Surg (2009). PMID: 19853747.

Pyogenic granuloma
Anupkumar Tiwary

Introduction
Pyogenic granuloma (PG) or lobular capillary hemangioma is an acquired hemorrhagic benign vascular lesion of the skin and mucous membranes. Though common throughout gastrointestinal tract, nasal mucosa, larynx, conjunctiva and cornea, vulval involvement is rare.

Epidemiology
PG can be seen in all age groups and gender. Mucosal lesions are more common in females, but vulval involvement is rare. PG is frequently observed in the second decade with a female predilection of 2:1. Usual age presentation in females is in the thirties and forties. Post-menopausal cases are even rarer. In the pediatric age group, the average age at diagnosis is 6–10 years. Onset is usually linked with trauma or itching.

Pathophysiology
It is considered to be a reactive hyperproliferative vascular response to a variety of stimuli rather than a true hemangioma. Stimuli could be minor trauma – due to sexual interaction, itching due to underlying cutaneous disease, hormonal influences, viral oncogenes, underlying microscopic arteriovenous malformation and excessive local production of tumor angiogenesis factor/cytokines.

Presenting complaints
Patients usually present with a reddish growth which can increase with time (rapidly or slowly). It may have a foul smell and ulceration, or bleeding is commonly noted. Occasional pain is often documented. The extent of discomfort corresponds to the size of the lesion.

Clinical examination
The PG presents as a single, glistening, cherry-red/skin colored, variably sized, pedunculated or sessile, smooth, mostly non-tender, friable papule or nodule on labia majora either or both sides,

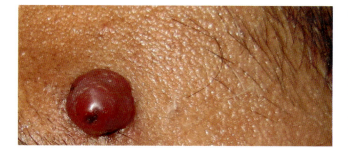

FIGURE 12.8   Smooth, friable, cherry red nodule on an extra genital site. (Photograph by Dr Bela Shah.)

at the point of intersection of labia majora or clitoris (Figure 12.8). The border is usually irregular. In large lesions, ulcerations and bleeding are frequently observed.

Systemic findings

Mostly, PG involves mucous membrane and rarely the vulva. Hence, the involvement of other sites must be looked for.

Dermoscopy

It shows homogeneous, reddish or white-red areas surrounded by a whitish collarette in almost 85% of cases. The white-red areas correlate with the proliferating blood vessels. The collarette corresponds to the epidermal collarette surrounding the blood vessels. Lesions showing lobular appearance have fibrous septa surrounding the lobules, which appear as white lines in dermoscopy examination.

Laboratory examination

An infectious cause needs to be ruled out by Gram's stain and culture.

Histopathology

It reveals an ulcerated polypoidal structure with hyperkeratotic epidermis and extensive vascular proliferation lined by a single layer of endothelium. The intervening stroma consists of collagen infiltrated by mononuclear cells.

Differential diagnosis

It includes poroma, hidradenoma papilliferum (HP), syringocystadenoma papilliferum and angiokeratoma. First three looks are similar but do not bleed on trivial trauma. Angiokeratoma is usually small, multiple, reddish/purple unlike PG.

Course and prognosis

It is benign in nature and grows gradually over a few months to years. Ulceration or bleeding can occur due to trauma as its size increases. Recurrence is rare after adequate removal.

Treatment

Wide excision under local anesthesia has been the most effective treatment. Other options are electrocautery, cryotherapy, laser ablation and sclerotherapy.

Pearl

Complete excision of PG is curative and recurrences are rare.

Recommended reading

1. Mahmoudnejad N, et al. Case Rep Urol (2021). PMID: 34395016.
2. Abreu-Dos-Santos F, et al. Case Rep Obstet Gynecol (2016). PMID: 28127485.
3. Jha AK, et al. Indian Dermatol Online J (2017). PMID: 29204415.

Milia

Anupkumar Tiwary

Introduction

Milia are benign, subepidermal, small keratinous cysts that probably arise from blockage of pilosebaceous/eccrine ducts. Primary forms arise spontaneously, probably due to embryonic abnormality in the epithelial bud. Secondary milia occur after an injury to the skin.

Epidemiology

Milium is a very common entity, but it is so rare to find on the vulva. Previous cases have been reported in both young and elder women. Ultraviolet light, external mechanical injury, burn, blistering disorders and procedures like dermabrasion are common triggering factors.

Pathophysiology

Subsequent to any external injury mentioned above, eccrine/pilosebaceous structures get damaged and blocked, leading to the development of milia.

Presenting complaints

These are completely asymptomatic. A patient only feels some bumpy surfaces on the touch. Sometimes, it may have an impact on sexual life, causing emotional distress.

Clinical examination

Milia are usually seen as multiple, small, firm, yellowish-white or skin-colored, domed papules with smooth surfaces of usually 1–2 mm diameter.

Dermoscopy

It shows yellowish-white structureless areas to globules, mixed flower pattern of vessels and absence of a central orifice.

Histopathology

It reveals a small dermal cyst lined by stratified squamous epithelium and filled with eosinophilic keratinous debris.

Differential diagnosis

It includes molluscum contagiousum, lichen nitidus, steatocystoma, syringoma, colloid milia, milia-like idiopathic calcinosis cutis, trichoepitheliomas, comedonal acne and skin tags.

The absence of a central orifice rules out molluscum contagiosum. The shiny/waxy, yellowish-white color differentiates milia from steatocystoma, trichoepithelioma, comedonal acne, skin tags and syringoma. Lichen nitidus does not express out keratin after deroofing as seen in milia. Rest can be further differentiated on histopathology in case of any clinical dilemma.

Course and prognosis

These are completely benign lesions and may clear sometimes spontaneously without any medical intervention.

Treatment

Usually not required. The smaller lesions may subside with topical retinoid application. Larger milia need curettage, electrodessication or extraction.

Pearl

Vulvar milia is so rare that it can be easily misdiagnosed on clinical grounds. In case of any doubt, deroofing of a single non-umbilicated lesion can be done to express the keratin, which confirms the diagnosis.

Recommended reading

1. Adotama P, et al. Dermatol Online J (2014). PMID: 24746302.

Hidradenoma papilliferum

Anupkumar Tiwary

Introduction

HP is a rare, painless, slow-growing, cystic, benign tumor arising from mammary-like anogenital glands (MLAGs) in the vulva and perianal region.

Epidemiology

It is a rare entity that mostly affects white women in their 4th–7th decade of life, although 5 cases of vulvar HP have been reported from India. Lack of histopathologic examination has been a reason for underdiagnosis.

Pathophysiology

The origin of HP is disputed. An earlier concept suggested its origin from apocrine glands derived from rudiments of the embryonic milk lines or mammary ridges in the vulva. Recent observations showed that primordia of the mammary glands do not extend beyond the axillary-pectoral area. Now it is evident that vulvar MLAGs, the source of HP, are distinct anogenital glands which have mammary-like features and cannot be derived from the mammary ridges or milk lines.

Presenting complaints

Most of the cases are asymptomatic and the patient only complains of slow-growing, smooth, erythematous vulvar swelling. However, some may become ulcerated and painful or tender.

Clinical examination

It is usually seen as solitary, erythematous or reddish-brown, non-ulcerated, firm, nodular swelling of size mostly between 1 cm and 2 cm in diameter, generally located on the lower aspect of labia majora/minora or but may also occur on the clitoris, interlabial sulcus or the fourchette (Figure 12.9). The plaque form is rare, and ulceration may develop in some cases (Figure 12.10).

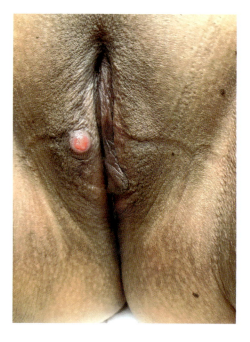

FIGURE 12.9 A well-circumscribed encapsulated swelling on Rt Labia majora. (Photograph by Dr Nina Madnani.)

Dermoscopy

It shows polymorphous vascular pattern composed of lacunae (red globular structures), elongated telangiectasias, serpentine and glomerular vessels and shiny white area on a red background (Figure 12.11).

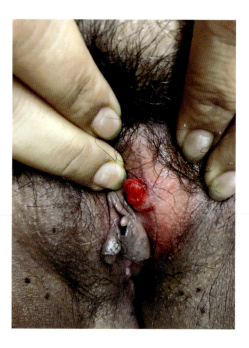

FIGURE 12.10 An eroded, fleshy swelling, on the non-keratinized surface of left labia majora. (Photograph by Dr Nina Madnani.)

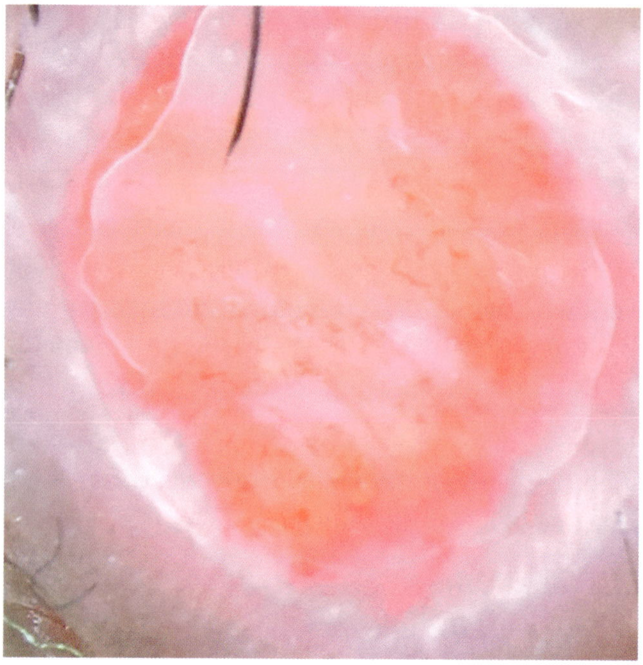

FIGURE 12.11 Dermoscopy findings reveal a pinkish-white background with arborizing vessels. Dinolite digital microscope WF-20, polarized, 10×. (Photograph by Dr Nina Madnani.)

The capsule is evident at the periphery. Grayish blue homogeneous pigmentation has also been described.

Histopathology

It demonstrates a well-circumscribed dermal adenoma with stromal pseudocapsule, apocrine differentiation and no connection to the overlying epidermis (Figure 12.12a and b). Tubular and papillary folds projecting into the cystic spaces are present. The lumina consists of an inner layer of secretory cells and an outer cuboidal layer with surrounding myoepithelial cells.

Differential diagnosis

Clinically, it can be mistaken for many entities, but the closely mimicking examples are PG, Bartholin cyst, eccrine poroma and hidradenocarcinoma papilliferum of vulva. As the clinical picture may be misleading, only histopathology can help to differentiate from above.

Course and prognosis

The course is usually benign with an excellent prognosis. Malignant transformation to adenocarcinoma is very rare.

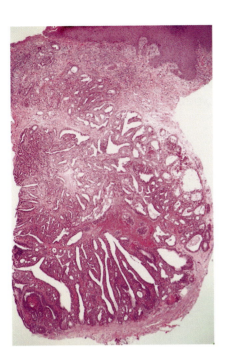
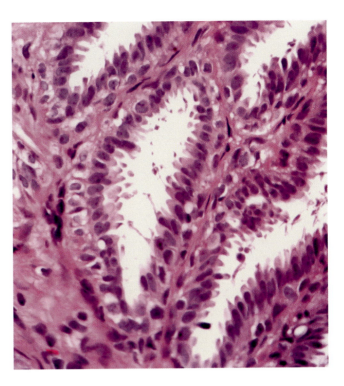

FIGURE 12.12 **(a)** Hidradenoma papilliferum 1: H & E, 40×, proliferation of glandular epithelium in the lower dermis. **(b)** Hidradenoma papilliferum 4: H & E, 400×, apocrine cells with decapitation secretion. (Photograph by Dr Rajiv Joshi.)

Treatment

Simple surgical excision is adequate. Wide-margin excision is done if there is rapid progression or dysplastic histopathology.

Pearl

HP should be suspected when dealing with a red, fleshy vulvar nodule which does not bleed on touch.

Recommended reading

1. El-Khoury J, et al. J Am Acad Dermatol (2016). PMID: 26944596.
2. Duhan N, et al. Arch Gynecol Obstet (2011). PMID: 21132312.
3. Tosti G, et al. Clin Exp Dermatol (2020). PMID: 32356582.

13

DISORDERS OF BLOOD VESSELS AND LYMPHATICS

Archana Singal and Rishi Goel

Contents

Hemangioma

Introduction

Hemangiomas are benign vascular neoplasms characterized by proliferative endothelium. They are rarely found in the female genital tract, and vulvar involvement is more common than that of the cervix and vagina.

Epidemiology

Hemangiomas of the vulva are uncommon and mostly acquired. They may present in infancy or more commonly in adulthood. Though mostly sporadic, genetic susceptibility is suggested in infantile forms and autosomal dominant inheritance may be seen.

Pathophysiology

Hemangiomas are vascular tumors characterized by increased cell turnover, unsuppressed proliferation and abnormal angiogenesis. Infantile forms have a rapid proliferative phase followed by slow involution.

Presenting complaints

Hemangiomas present as asymptomatic/painful bright red-colored elevated lesions that are usually solitary but can sometimes be multiple. Hemangiomas occurring in adulthood may present with red raw eroded lesions. Complaints like dyspareunia, intermittent bleeding may be reported.

Clinical examination

Superficial forms present as bright red-colored localized firm, rubbery, slightly raised plaques on the vulva (Figure 13.1), while deep/subcutaneous hemangiomas are skin to blue-colored, elevated

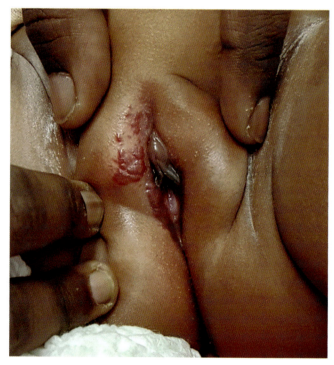

FIGURE 13.1 Bright red grouped papules and plaques over the right labia majora. (Photograph by Dr Archana Singal.)

plaques that show secondary changes like telangiectasias, atrophy, fibrofatty replacement and scarring. Hemangiomas occurring in adulthood commonly present as genital ulcer/s, which may bleed profusely, with no associated regional inguinal/femoral lymphadenopathy, unless secondarily infected.

Systemic findings

Multifocal and multiple (more than 5) hemangiomas may be associated with visceral hemangiomas in the liver, gastrointestinal tract and brain.

DOI: 10.1201/9781003284116-13

Thyroid abnormalities, i.e., hypothyroidism may be seen. Vulvar hemangiomas occurring in infancy/childhood may occur as part of PELVIS syndrome.

Dermoscopy

Vascular structures (globular, linear, corkscrew and comma vessels) are seen, separated with fibrotic bands.

Laboratory examination

Excision biopsy under local anesthesia is both diagnostic and therapeutic. It is especially helpful in ruling out vulvar malignancies in adult-onset atypical cases.

In acquired cases presenting as genital ulcers, sexually transmitted infections (STIs) have to be ruled out using serological tests for HIV, hepatitis B and C, venereal disease research laboratory test (VDRL), herpes simplex virus 1 and 2 IgM and IgG antibodies.

Transvaginal ultrasound, color Doppler and pelvic MRI can detect concealed hemangiomas in the vagina, transabdominal ultrasound search for gastrointestinal and hepatic hemangiomas and renal ultrasound is very important in case of perineal hemangiomas occurring in infancy to rule out PELVIS syndrome.

Histopathology

Proliferative, tortuous vessels of various sizes in the submucosa, filled with red blood cells and lined by a single layer of flattened endothelial cells. These are present in the papillary dermis in superficial hemangiomas and deep dermis/subcutaneous tissue in deep-seated hemangiomas.

Differential diagnosis

Genital ulcer – Adult-onset hemangioma presenting as a genital ulcer should be differentiated from STIs, by its potential for profuse bleeding.

Vulvar/vaginal malignancies – They may present as late onset, rapidly enlarging single asymptomatic lesion with ulceration/episodes of bleeding. Excision biopsy with tumor markers is indicated for disease confirmation.

Arterio-venous malformations – Congenital fast-flow malformations, red colored, warm temperature, with a thrill on palpation. Histology shows direct communications between arteries and veins, with no endothelial proliferation.

Course and prognosis

Overall prognosis of most infantile hemangiomas is excellent with spontaneous involution, but vulvar/perineal hemangiomas carry a high risk of ulceration and scarring (Figure 13.2). There may be a significant functional, emotional and psychosexual disability. Late-onset hemangiomas may rapidly increase in size in pregnancy with the risk of life-threatening post-partum hemorrhage. Large genital tract hemangiomas can complicate normal vaginal delivery due to obstruction of the birth canal.

Treatment

Timolol 0.5% drops twice daily for 4–8 weeks can be curative for small, slow-growing lesions. Alternatively, imiquimod cream 5% thrice weekly for 4–8 weeks has been tried with variable success. Oral propranolol in the dose of 1.5–3 mg/kg/day, divided over 2–3 times/day, may be needed for at least 6 months, especially in case of infantile hemangiomas. Monitoring of heart rate, blood pressure and blood sugar is important because of the risk of hypotension and hypoglycemia. Intralesional corticosteroids (10–40 mg/ml) every 2–3 weeks for 4–8 weeks have been tried. Sclerotherapy may be useful but intralesional bleomycin should be avoided because of the risk of scarring and hyperpigmentation.

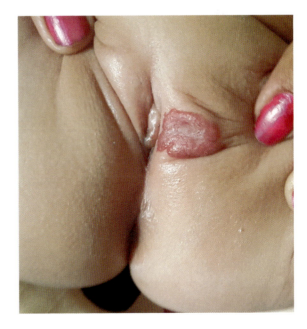

FIGURE 13.2 Large red plaque on left labia majora. (Photograph by Dr Archana Singal.)

Excision is needed in cases refractory to medical treatment and for large hemangiomas. Circular excision followed by purse-string closure and reconstruction of labia majora is done.

Pearl

Vulvar hemangiomas, unlike hemangiomas on other cutaneous sites, need prompt medical/surgical intervention because of the risk of scarring, ulceration and psycho-sexual dysfunction.

Recommended reading

1. Silva JMD, et al. Rev Bras Ginecol Obstet (2018). PMID: 29980161.
2. Mutyala P, et al. Indian J Paediatr Dermatol (2021). DOI: 10.4103/ijpd.IJPD_36_20.
3. Oakley A. Australas J Dermatol (2016). PMID: 25754966.

Angiokeratoma

Introduction

Angiokeratomas are benign cutaneous lesions characterized by the presence of vascular ectasia in the papillary dermis. Vulvar involvement is quite common and is analogous to scrotal skin involvement seen in angiokeratoma of Fordyce.

Epidemiology

Angiokeratomas of the vulva are mostly acquired and present between the age of 20–50 years. The genetic association is not seen. The precise incidence is unknown because of misdiagnosis as they closely mimic many other dermatological conditions affecting the female genital tract (Figures 13.3 and 13.4). The primary inciting factor leading to their formation is the presence of local venous hypertension attributable to a significant number of causes like trauma, obesity, hernias, pregnancy and post-partum, post hysterectomy, genital tract/urinary system tumors, following irradiation, venous abnormalities like varicosities/malformations, infection with human papillomavirus, use of contraceptive pills, etc.

Pathophysiology

The blood vessels of labia majora and the perivascular elastic and smooth muscle fibers are highly sensitive to local venous pressure changes, inflammation and obstruction, which then leads to vascular stasis with subsequent vascular dilatation.

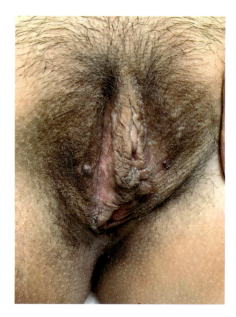

FIGURE 13.3 This lady's angiokeratoma was clinically mistaken as a vulvar nevus because of its deeply pigmented appearance. (Photograph by Dr Nina Madnani.)

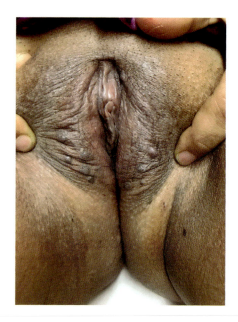

FIGURE 13.4 Angiokeratomas may mimic usual vulvar intraepithelial neoplasia (uVIN). (Photograph by Dr Nina Madnani.)

Presenting complaints

Patients present with multiple, elevated, asymptomatic/itchy/painful, unilateral (less commonly bilateral), red/blue/black/purple-colored lesions on the labia with intermittent bleeding (Figure 13.5).

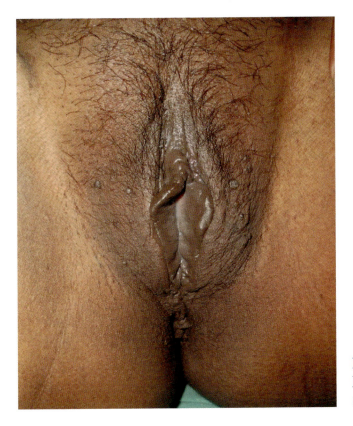

FIGURE 13.5 Scattered round pigmented papules on both labia majora. (Photograph by Dr Archana Singal.)

A cyclical increase in the size of the lesions may be seen during menstruation. Dyspareunia can also occur rarely with larger lesions.

Clinical examination
Multiple, small (2–5 mm), grouped, well-defined red/blue/black hyperkeratotic papules (less commonly plaques), with a slightly rough surface, are present unilaterally/bilaterally over labia majora and/or labia minora (Figure 13.6). Some lesions may have a nodular/verrucous appearance. Lesions do not blanch on pressure.

Systemic findings
Involvement of other mucosal sites like oral mucosa and tongue can occur with similar presentation. Moreover, in the presence of an extensive number of lesions not limited to the vulva, the possibility of Fabry's disease has to be kept in mind where lesions may present in bathing trunk distribution (affecting umbilicus, genitals, buttocks, lower abdomen, sacrum and inner thighs), albeit less commonly than in males.

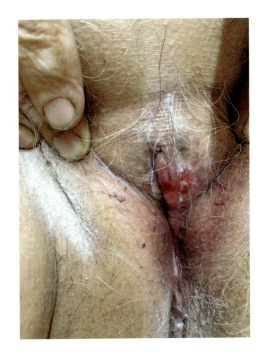

FIGURE 13.6 Incidental finding of angio-keratoma in this lady with vulvar malignancy. (Photograph by Dr Nina Madnani.)

Dermoscopy
Well-demarcated round lacunae are seen (Figure 13.7). The presence of dark-blue lacunae suggests vessel thrombosis. A white veil representing epidermal hyperkeratosis may also be seen.

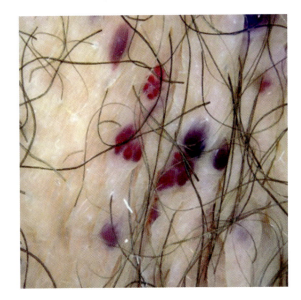

FIGURE 13.7 Non-contact polarized dermoscopy showing bluish purple lacunae representing non-trombosed vessels. Dinolite digital microscope WF-20, polarized, 10×. (Photograph by Dr Nina Madnani.)

Laboratory examination

Only histopathology is sufficient in isolated lesions. However, when the age of presentation is childhood and multiple lesions are distributed elsewhere too, Fabry's disease has to be ruled out, for which genetic testing may be required.

Histopathology

H & E section of the lesion shows epidermal acanthosis, hyperkeratosis, papillomatosis and elongated rete ridges. Dilated blood-filled vascular spaces are seen in the papillary dermis, without significant endothelial proliferation, sometimes with organized thrombus in the vessel lumen (Figure 13.8).

Differential diagnosis

Genital warts – pale/dull red colored papules with verrucous/cauliflower appearance, usually multiple in number, not associated with bleeding. They may be seen at other sites like perianal, lower abdomen, thighs, etc. History of contact with multiple partners/unprotected intercourse/presence of other sexual tract infections may be present.

Pyogenic granuloma – red fleshy papule/nodule, typically 5–10 mm, usually solitary, with a smooth surface that can become verrucous or ulcerate with subsequent crusting. Lesion bleeds profusely on minor trauma.

Melanoma – Usually, late age of onset (above 50 years), rapidly growing, dark/black colored, solitary, asymptomatic lesion with/without other site/s involvement (nail, eyes, etc.)

Cherry angioma – asymptomatic, multiple, round to oval, bright red, dome-shaped papules and pinpoint macules that increase in number with age and are seen at other places too like upper trunk, arms, etc.

Seborrheic keratosis – asymptomatic, pale/black/brown/mixed color growths with waxy, scaly, stuck-on appearance. Sometimes, they have a verrucous appearance.

Course and prognosis

Lesions are benign but may/may not resolve spontaneously. Trauma can cause bleeding and thrombosis.

Treatment

Conservative management is sufficient in asymptomatic/non-progressive lesions. For symptomatic/large/multiple/rapidly growing lesions, treatment options include surgical excision, ablative lasers like CO_2, erbium-doped yttrium aluminum garnet. However, potassium titanyl phosphate (KTP) laser or 800-nm diode laser gives best cosmesis because of the minimal risk of scarring. Superficial and small lesions can be removed using curettage and cryotherapy/electrocautery/radiofrequency ablation or even chemical cauterization with 70–90% trichloroacetic acid.

Pearls

In darker skin types, the angiokeratomas appear deeply pigmented instead of the red/blue/violaceous color.

Angiokeratomas occurring on the vulva can be confused with many benign/malignant conditions like seborrheic or viral warts, melanoma, and hence, an elaborate clinical, dermoscopy and histopathological examination is warranted.

Recommended reading

1. Deo K, et al. Indian J Sex Transm Dis AIDS (2018). PMID: 30623188.
2. Dhawan AK, et al. J Obstet Gynaecol India (2014). PMID: 25404845.

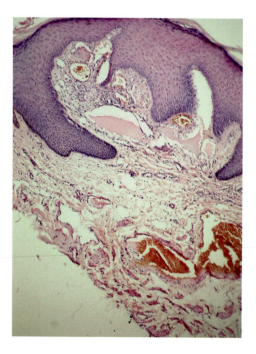

FIGURE 13.8   H & E, 100×, dilated, blood-filled vessels in upper dermis, partially encircled by the hyperplastic epidermis. (Photograph by Dr Rajiv Joshi.)

Varicocele

Introduction
Varicosities of the vulva refer to the dilated veins of labia majora and labia minora (Figure 13.9). They are quite rare as compared to scrotal varicosities. They are most commonly seen in pregnancy, where they may/may not undergo spontaneous resolution in the post-partum period but are also reported in non-pregnancy states secondary to lower limb varicosities and very rarely pelvic malignancies.

Epidemiology
Overall incidence of varicosities in the vulva is not known. However, 4–10% of pregnant women develop varicocele. With each subsequent pregnancy, there is an earlier appearance and greater dilatation of vulvar veins (Figure 13.10). A major contributing factor is local venous hypertension which can occur due to increased abdominal/thoracic pressure, dysfunction of the venous system, venous occlusion and venous compression.

Pathophysiology
Varicosities of the vulva may/may not co-exist with pelvic varicosities. Vulval veins drain into external and internal pudendal veins, which drain

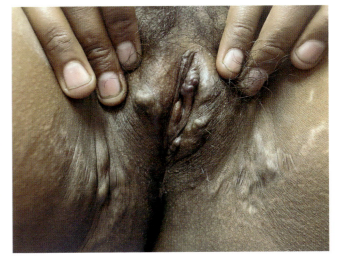

FIGURE 13.10 Varicosities developed in this pregnant woman during her second trimester. (Photograph by Dr Rashmi Mahajan.)

into a great saphenous vein (GSV) and internal iliac vein, respectively. Compression of renal veins or inferior vena cava (IVC) by renal tumors can lead to pelvic varicosities. In pregnancy, pelviperineal blood reflux can occur under the influence of hormones, especially progesterone, that reduce venous tone.

Presenting complaints
Varicocele presents as an asymptomatic/dull aching, painful mass in the labia with visible veins around the vulva or inner thigh. There can be pelvic discomfort, heaviness in the vulva, dyspareunia and vulvodynia (vulval pain), which gets worsened after standing, sexual/physical activity.

Clinical examination
Inspection reveals dilated vulvar veins, with swelling of vulvar lips and perineum. There may be erythema and superficial cutaneous ulceration. Impulse on coughing may be seen. The varicosities are soft on palpation and usually get reduced on lying down except when they occur secondary to malignancies like renal cell carcinoma, where they become irreducible (Figures 13.11 and 13.12).

Laboratory examination
Duplex ultrasound (venous doppler) of veins of the pelvis and lower extremities is useful to look for retrograde blood flow and accurately measure vein diameter. Dilated veins seen on ultrasound can be

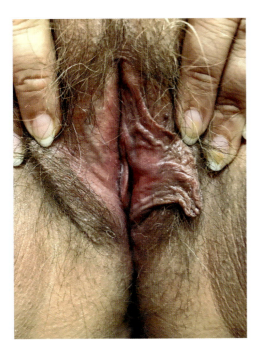

FIGURE 13.9 Dilated veins in the labia minora. (Photograph by Dr Nina Madnani.)

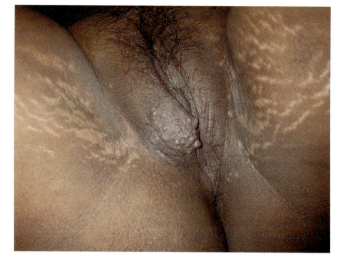

FIGURE 13.11 Although mimicing a lymphangioma, palpation gave a "bag of worms" feel. (Photograph by Dr Nisha Chaturvedi.)

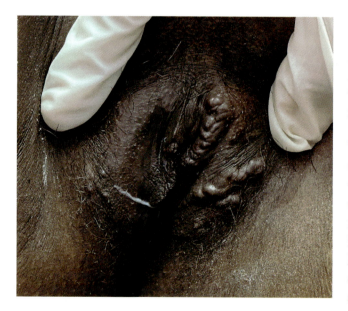

FIGURE 13.12 Vulvar varicocities may be seen with compression of the pudendal veins by a tumor. (Photograph by Dr Rashmi Mahajan.)

compressed with a probe and may be associated with phleboliths. Transvaginal/transabdominal duplex ultrasound also helps in ruling out vulval and pelvic vein thrombophlebitis. Pelvic CT/MRI/Contrast CT angiography also shows dilated veins in the vulva and/or pelvis. Moreover, MRI can help in ruling out pelvic malignancies.

Histopathology

Histopathology shows narrowing/obliteration of vein lumen, occasional thrombi, fragmentation of internal elastic lamina, invagination of the intima, thickening of the vein wall, hypertrophy of smooth muscle fibers and deposition of collagen bundles. Endothelial cells stain positive with CD31.

Differential diagnosis

Bartholin duct cyst – Slowly growing fluid-filled swelling on one of the Bartholin's glands that may be asymptomatic/associated with erythema, swelling or discomfort during sexual activity. They can get secondarily infected and lead to pus draining from the cyst, along with fever, chills and difficulty in walking.

Lymphangioma/lymph varix – Multiple, ill-defined, grouped, 2–4 mm raised pseudo-vesicular/warty lesions over vulva that resemble frogspawn and weep clear fluid (lymphorrhea).

Course and prognosis

Most varicoceles formed during pregnancy resolve spontaneously 6–8 weeks after delivery. In very few cases, they may persist and even increase in size and number with subsequent pregnancies.

Treatment

Conservative treatment is sufficient in asymptomatic, small, non-progressive varicosities, especially those seen in pregnancy. It includes general measures, i.e., avoid prolonged squatting, straining, standing, physical activity and wearing high heels. Intermittent resting, leg elevation, cold compresses, supportive underwear with gusset and double sanitary pads are helpful. In addition, pelvic floor exercises are recommended as they improve blood circulation and strengthen supporting tissues around pelvic veins.

Sclerotherapy of vulvar veins can be tried provided there is no obvious connection between a dilated vulval vein and large tributary of internal iliac vein on duplex ultrasound.

Pelvic congestion syndrome needs referral to the gynecology department for appropriate medical management (progestins/danazol/hormone replacement therapy/gonadotropin-releasing hormone agonists) or surgical management (hysterectomy and surgical ligation of ovarian veins).

Pearl

Development of a late onset left-sided varicocele in a non-pregnant female should alert dermatologists to evaluate and investigate the patient for pelvic/renal malignancies.

Recommended reading

1. Kim AS, et al. Dermatol Surg (2017). PMID: 28005626.
2. Basile A, et al. Semin Ultrasound CT MR (2021). PMID: 33541587.
3. Jindal S, et al. Indian J Dermatol (2014). PMID: 24700962.
4. Henry F, et al. Am J Clin Dermatol (2006). PMID: 16489843.

Lymphangioma circumscriptum

Introduction

Lymphangiomas are benign congenital lymphatic malformations that can involve skin, subcutaneous tissue and may extend deep to underlying muscle and viscera. Lymphangiomas are classified into either superficial/microcystic lymphatic malformations (lymphangioma circumscriptum [LC]) or deep-seated/macrocystic lymphatic malformations (cavernous lymphangioma and cystic hygroma).

LC is prominently seen over proximal extremities, trunk, axilla and oral cavity, and primary vulval involvement is quite uncommon.

Epidemiology

Precise incidence of LC is unknown. LC of the vulva is a microcystic (size < 1 cm) lymphatic malformation that can be classified as

- Primary/congenital LC
- Secondary/acquired LC (also known as lymphangiectasia)

Etiology

The unifocal nature and lack of familial forms of LC suggest that they originate from localized somatic mutations. Primary LC occurs due to aberrant development of lymphatic vessels and presents in early childhood (infancy or within 5 years of age). Sometimes, they may not be noted till puberty, after which they may increase in size or number or both.

Acquired LC is overall more common and occurs following the obstruction of lymphatics secondary to many underlying physiological/pathological conditions. These include pregnancy, old age, infections (e.g. tuberculosis, recurrent erysipelas), inflammatory causes (e.g. Crohn's disease, systemic sclerosis). Besides, neoplastic and surgical can also lead to acquired LC via intra-lymphatic metastases (e.g. melanoma, breast cancer) or through regional lymph node dissection, after surgical resection of pelvic malignancies, and sometimes also as a side effect of radiotherapy (done in malignancies of prostate, bladder, cervix, breast etc).

Pathophysiology

In LC, there are marked distended lymphatic channels in the papillary dermis, which can sometimes extend into the subcutaneous and even deeper tissues In lymphangiectasias, deep collecting lymph channels are disrupted due to underlying causes like regional lymph node dissection, radiotherapy, infections etc that cause lymph stasis, backflow and ultimately distension of papillary dermal lymphatics. Lymphatic malformations in LC are disconnected from surrounding normal lymphatic vessels. For this reason, they are called truncular lymphatic malformations and are not usually associated with lymphedema.

Presenting complaints

Patients present with multiple asymptomatic/itchy raised lesions that may discharge clear watery fluid (lymphorrhea) or may be associated with recurrent minor bleeding episodes. They may enlarge in response to fever, infection or trauma (causing intracystic bleeding). When persistent, they can be a cause of chronic vulvar edema (Figure 13.13).

Clinical examination

Multiple, ill-defined, grouped, 2–4 mm raised pseudovesicular/warty lesions are present over vulva, mons pubis, often distorting or obliterating the normal vulvar anatomy (Figures 13.14 and 13.15). The grouped fluid-filled pseudo vesicles resemble frogspawn and may weep clear fluid (lymphorrhea) or can rarely bleed (in the presence of blood vascular component) (Figure 13.16).

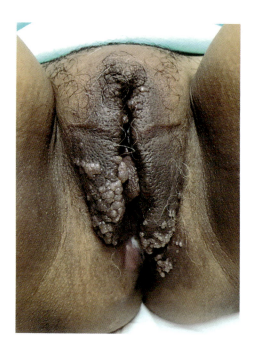

FIGURE 13.13   Older lesions may cause vulvar lymphodema with post-inflammatory pigmentation. (Photograph by Dr Nina Madnani.)

Excoriation/crusting is infrequent. Secondary infection can lead to localized cellulitis. On palpation, they are firm, non-compressible with no local rise of temperature.

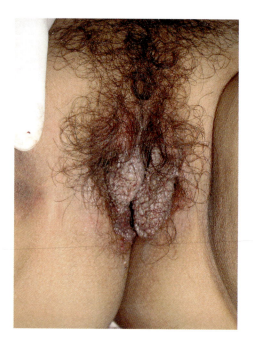

FIGURE 13.14   Extensive involvement of both labia with pseudovesicles and warty lesions obliterating the normal vulvar anatomy. (Photograph by Dr Archana Singal.)

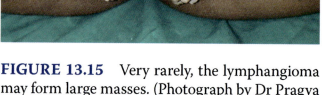

FIGURE 13.15   Very rarely, the lymphangioma may form large masses. (Photograph by Dr Pragya Nair.)

Systemic findings

Rare systemic findings that can occur in mixed lymphatic malformations (having both microcystic and macrocystic elements) include chylothorax, chylous ascites, elephantiasis, protein-losing enteropathy, hypoalbuminemia etc.

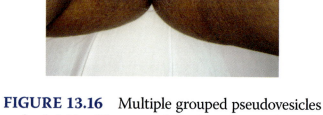

FIGURE 13.16   Multiple grouped pseudovesicles on both labia. (Photograph by Dr Nina Madnani.)

Dermoscopy

Dermoscopy shows two distinct patterns: Yellow lacunae surrounded by pale septa without the inclusion of blood represent dilated lymphatic vessels filled with lymph (Figure 13.17). The other pattern is yellow to pink lacunae alternating with dark-red or bluish lacunae is due to the inclusion of blood. Red/blue lacunae represent variable concentrations of red blood cells, and this has been described as a "hypopyon-like feature."

Laboratory examination

Duplex ultrasound shows slow flow malformation. MRI must always be done before proceeding with any therapy to rule out the extension of lymphatic malformation into muscle/bone. Lymphoscintigraphy study is abnormal only in truncal lymphatic malformations.

Histopathology

H and E sections show the presence of acanthosis, hyperkeratosis and elongated rete ridges. In the papillary dermis, markedly distended lymphatic channels lined by flattened endothelial cells are

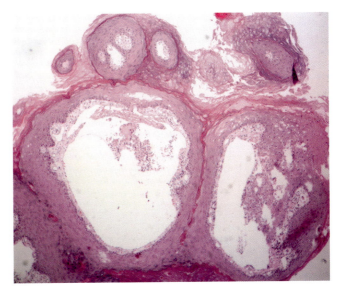

FIGURE 13.18   H & E, 200×, many dilated lymphatics in upper dermis with papillated epidermis. (Photograph by Dr Rajiv Joshi.)

seen that may extend into subcutaneous and deeper tissues (Figure 13.18). Superficial perivascular lympho-histiocytic infiltrate and red blood cells (due to intracystic hemorrhage) may also be seen.

Differential diagnosis

Genital warts – Papular warty lesions are seen that do not weep clear fluid/blood upon puncture, and might be associated with lesions elsewhere (e.g. perianal, palmar, plantar surfaces etc). History of contact with multiple partners, co-existence of other STIs can be present.

Molluscum contagiosum – Discrete, papular, lesions with central umblication are observed. Lesions can be present elsewhere too like face, trunk, proximal arms, etc. History of contact with multiple partners and co-existence of other STIs can be present.

Herpes zoster – Painful, grouped vesicles on an erythematous base along the affected dermatome are seen. Constitutional symptoms may be present.

Genital Herpes – Painful, grouped vesicular lesions occur 4–7 days after sexual contact; progressing to vesicles/erosions are seen in primary genital herpes. In recurrent genital herpes, symptoms are mild and lesions are more often asymptomatic.

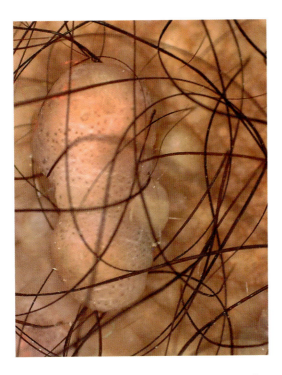

FIGURE 13.17   Multiple pinkish yellow lacunae separated by septae. Dinolite Digital Microscope WF-20 polarized, 10×. (Photograph by Dr Nina Madnani.)

Course and prognosis

Most common complications are discharge of clear fluid (lymphorrhea), ulceration and secondary infection leading to cellulitis. Recurrence is quite common following surgery due to incomplete excision and is especially common in lesions with both microcystic and macrocystic components (size more than 7 cm). Very occasionally, squamous cell carcinoma can arise within the lesion.

Treatment

Treatment of underlying cause is of paramount importance in acquired lymphangiectasias. The best therapeutic outcome is seen with sclerotherapy (after doing MRI to know the depth of the lesion). Sclerosants used include bleomycin, polidocanol and sodium tetradecyl sulfate.

Laser therapy – Neodymium yttrium aluminum garnet laser (NdYAG), CO_2 laser and pulse due laser (PDL) are useful for superficial lesions. For superficial pseudo-vesicles, other useful modalities include cryotherapy, superficial radiofrequency ablation and electrocautery.

Topical rapamycin, an mTOR inhibitor, 1% cream applied twice daily for 8–12 weeks has shown good therapeutic results, suggesting the role of somatic mutations in AKT/PIK3CA/mTOR pathways in the pathogenesis of LC. The most common side effect of topical rapamycin is local irritation, which may be a treatment-limiting factor in some patients.

Pearls

Due to poor cosmetic appearance, there is associated psychosexual dysfunction.

With all treatment modalities, follow-up till 1 year has to be done in view of the higher incidence of recurrence, especially in lesions more than 7 cm size.

Recommended reading

1. Kokcu A, et al. J Low Genit Tract Dis (2015). PMID: 24886872.
2. Gude G, et al. Australas J Dermatol (2019). PMID: 30812056.
3. Yoon G, et al. Arch Gynecol Obstet (2016). PMID: 26156111.

14

DISORDERS OF VULVAR SKIN APPENDAGEAL TUMORS

Nina Madnani and Sharmila Patil

Contents

Steatocystoma multiplex

Introduction

Steatocystoma multiplex (SCM) is known as a polycystic disease of the epidermis and sebocytes. The literal meaning of SCM is "a bag of fat." Although the disease is considered rare, it is possibly under-reported.

Epidemiology

SCM has an autosomal dominant mode of inheritance, with few sporadic cases. The exact origin of the cysts is still unknown, but multiple theories which suggest their origins are: they result from sebaceous retention cysts of a nevoid or they are a variety of dermoid cysts. SCM limited to the vulva is a very rare condition as there are only five known cases in literature.

The average age of onset is 26 years old, with no sex predilection. It's a common presentation at puberty, which suggests a hormonal trigger for the lesion growth.

Pathophysiology

The causative factors of SCM remain unclear, but trauma, infection or immunologic events might be responsible. SCM is associated with a mutation in the keratin 17 gene in the areas which are identical to the mutations which are found in patients with pachyonychia congenita.

Presenting complaints

Often asymptomatic. Patients/spouse/caregiver may casually notice multiple, small, raised, painless, yellowish lesions over the vulvar area.

Clinical examination

Lesions limited to the genital area may present as multiple white to yellowish firm papules or nodules on the labia majora measuring about 2–3 mm, rarely larger (Figures 14.1 and 14.2). They occasionally rupture to ooze a yellow oily liquid or may get secondarily infected. Other non-genital sites include upper anterior portion of the trunk, upper arms, axillae and thighs. Sometimes a small central punctum can be identified, and they may contain one or more hairs (eruptive vellus hair cysts).

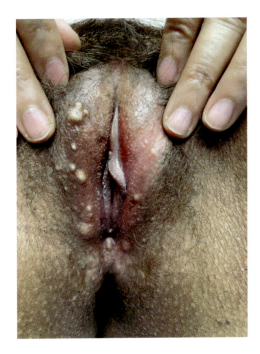

FIGURE 14.1 Scattered yellowish firm papules on the labia and perineum. (Photograph by Dr Nina Madnani.)

DOI: 10.1201/9781003284116-14

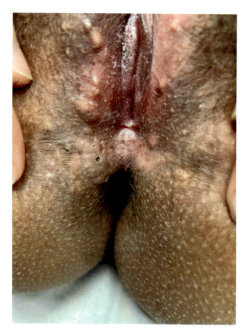

FIGURE 14.2 This lady presented with multiple yellow papules of Steatocystoma. Note the sebaceous cyst in the perineum. (Photograph by Dr Nina Madnani.)

A few syndromes associated with SCM are pachyonychia congenita, Gardner syndrome, Noonan syndrome or LEOPARD syndrome, Alagille-Watson syndrome and Favre-Racouchot syndrome.

Dermoscopy
Polarized dermoscopy of a papule shows a uniform yellow color with surrounding pseudoreticular pigment network.

Histopathology
Biopsy of a papule shows a convoluted cyst wall lined with several squamous epithelial layers. The granular layer is usually absent. Sebaceous glands may be seen adjacent or attached to the cyst wall.

Differential diagnosis
Syringomas, eruptive vellus cysts and milia are the closest differentials.

Syringoma presents as small (1–3 mm), multiple, non-regressing, bilaterally firm, skin colored to yellow papules present on the labia majora as well as non-genital sites like the eyelids, axillae. They may occasionally be itchy.

Eruptive vellus hair cysts present with multiple asymptomatic skin-to-black-colored papules, probably due to occlusion of the infundibulum of vellus hair follicles with resultant cystic dilatation and retention of keratinous material and hairs.

Milia presents as tiny, discrete, whitish papules.

Course and prognosis
SCM generally tends to remain as is, though occasionally may get secondarily infected.

Treatment
SCM can be left alone, but if the patient is keen to get them removed, minor procedures like radiofrequency/CO_2 laser ablation, cryotherapy or minor incision and drainage with the removal of cyst wall can be done. Systemic isotretinoin has not had very successful results, albeit with minor shrinkage. Counseling about the benign nature of this condition is essential.

Pearl
SCM is a benign condition of cosmetic concern and can be left alone unless secondarily infected.

Recommended reading
1. Rongioletti F, et al. Clin Exp Dermatol (2002). PMID: 12372080.
2. Kartal S, et al. JAMMR (2016). DOI: 10.9734/BJMMR/2016/27081.
3. Park J, et al. Indian J Dermatol Venereol Leprol (2014). PMID: 24448142.

Vulvar syringoma

Introduction
Syringoma are common appendageal tumors of intraepithelial eccrine sweat ducts. Friedman and Butler classified syringoma into four types – localized, generalized, associated with Downs syndrome and familial. Vulvar syringomas are usually associated with extragenital lesions. Three clinical forms of vulvar syringoma are described viz multiple flesh colored or brownish papules, cystic and lichenoid.

Epidemiology
Syringomas are common in adolescence but generally seen between 10 and 60 years of age. The exact incidence is not clear as under-reporting is common as the lesions are usually asymptomatic and unrecognized by the patient and clinician. Familial syringomas are also reported.

Pathophysiology

The histogenesis of syringomas is most likely related to eccrine elements or pluripotential stem cells. The growth of syringoma is under hormonal influence. Positive staining of progesterone marker may be seen in these patients.

Presenting complaints

Vulvar syringoma are generally asymptomatic and may be casually noticed the first time after a hair-removal procedure. Rarely itching may be the first complaint. Itching may increase during warmer months or during menstruation, pregnancy, with the use of oral contraceptive pills and during puberty.

Clinical examination

Syringomas appear as small, multiple, stable, bilaterally symmetrical, firm, skin colored to yellow papules of 1–3 mm in diameter on both labia majora. Giant syringomas have been reported where the lesions are much larger and form plaques (Figure 14.3).

Extragenital areas are often affected simultaneously especially the eyelids and malar areas and should be looked out for in women with vulvar syringomas (Figure 14.4).

Dermoscopy

Dermoscopy shows whitish areas on an erythematous base and a faint pigment network.

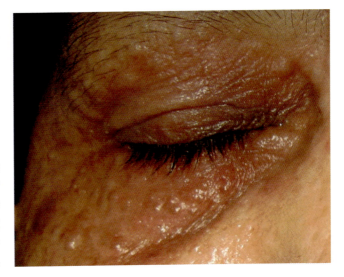

FIGURE 14.4 Closely grouped, skin colored to yellowish papules around the eyelid. A typical site for syringomas. (Photograph by Dr Bela Shah.)

Histopathology

The upper dermis contains multiple ducts and cyst-like structures, some having a tail-like extension (Figure 14.5). These are lined by 2 layers of cells and some lumen contains a pinkish material. These are situated in a fibrous stroma.

Differential diagnosis

Syringomas have to be differentiated from SCM and Fox-Fordyce disease.

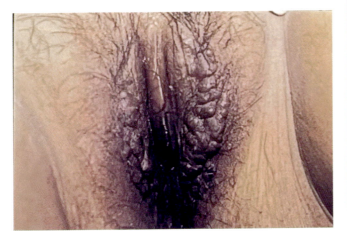

FIGURE 14.3 Giant syringomas can present as these pigmented grouped papules almost form verrucous plaques. (Photograph by Dr Nina Madnani.)

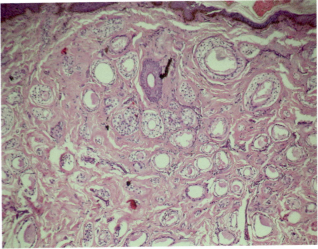

FIGURE 14.5 H & E, 100×, numerous ductal structures seen in the dermis lined by cells with clear cytoplasm, some with a comma-like tail. (Photograph by Dr Rajiv Joshi.)

Steatocystoma multiplex presents with multiple, uniform, yellowish, soft to firm cystic papules, usually 2–6 mm in diameter. The lesions do not have a punctum.

Fox-Fordyce disease has symmetrically distributed, flesh-colored to mildly erythematous monomorphic, dome-shaped papules (1–3 mm) that are typically follicular based.

Course and prognosis
Syringomas are benign tumors and can be left untreated. Occasionally, some may get calcified. Malignant transformation if reported in few cases to syringocarcinoma.

Treatment
Usually, treatment is not needed except for the itchy ones or for cosmetic reasons. Removal of lesions can be done by excision, electrodessication, carbon dioxide laser ablation and 50% trichloroacetic acid chemical peeling. Cryotherapy is a minimal aggressiveness treatment and heals without scarring.

Pearl
Vulvar syringomas are generally associated with syringomas at other sites such as eyelids, so people with eyelid syringomas should be checked for vulvar involvement.

Recommended reading
1. Shalabi MMK, et al. Proc (Bayl Univ Med Cent) (2021). PMID: 34970057.
2. Huang YH, et al. J Am Acad Dermatol (2003). PMID: 12734503.
3. Mendiratta V, et al. Indian J Dermatol (2007). DOI: 10.4103/0019-5154.35353.

Fox-Fordyce disease

Introduction
Fox-Fordyce disease is a chronic, uncommon, itchy condition affecting the apocrine gland-bearing areas of the integument. It is often referred to as "apocrine miliaria."

Epidemiology
Fox-Fordyce disease usually occurs on the axillae, peri areolar and very rarely on the pubic area, mostly in females. This disease occurs commonly post-adolescence, and most cases remit after menopause; hence, hormonal factors are thought to be responsible. Alterations in follicle-stimulating hormone, estrogen and premenstrual urinary gonadotropin have been noted in case reports. Thermal changes and emotional factors are the other precipitators.

The disease has been described in monozygotic twins, and familial occurrence has occasionally been reported.

Pathophysiology
It is hypothesized that the obstruction of the intraepidermal portion of the apocrine gland ducts is necessary for the development of the disease. The intraluminal obstruction leads to glandular distension and eventual ductal rupture. The subsequent expulsion of glandular contents into the surrounding dermis then causes an inflammatory response that manifests clinically.

Presenting complaints
The patient is distressed by an itchy rash on her vulva which gets worse when she is stressed, in hot humid weather, and often premenstrually. She may also mention a similar itch in her underarms and around her breasts (Figures 14.6 and 14.7).

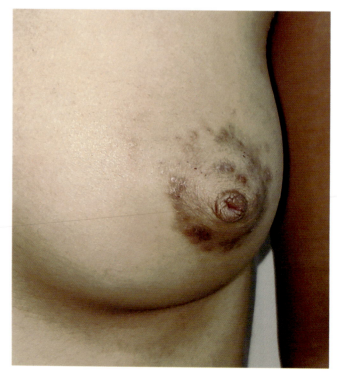

FIGURE 14.6 Follicular papules of Fox-Fordyce on the areola. (Photograph by Dr Rashmi Mahajan.)

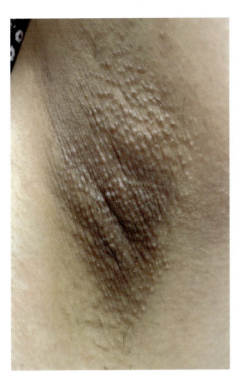

FIGURE 14.7 A common site for involvement in Fox-Fordyce disease. (Photograph by Dr Nina Madnani.)

Clinical examination

The affected hair-bearing areas, commonly the pubis and labia majora, show grouped, symmetrically distributed, monomorphic, dome-shaped papules (1–3 mm) that are typically follicular-based, flesh-colored to mildly erythematous. In darker skin types, erythema may be difficult to visualize and the papules are dark brown. The area may also show post-inflammatory hyperpigmentation (Figure 14.8a and b).

Dermoscopy

Polarizing dermoscopy shows multiple brown follicular structureless areas and keratin plugs in the follicles (Figure 14.9).

Histopathology

Histopathologic features of Fox-Fordyce lesions are variable. The most consistent finding is hyperkeratosis of the infundibular epithelium with dilatation, focal spongiosis of the upper infundibulum along with perifollicular lymphohistiocytic infiltrate and adventitial fibrosis (Figure 14.10). Perifollicular and periductal xanthomatosis cells are frequently seen.

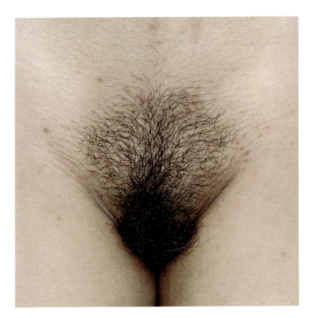

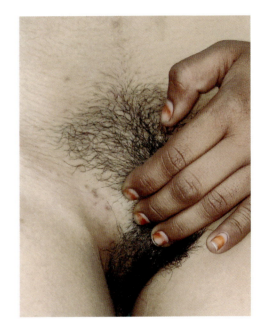

FIGURE 14.8 (a) Fox-Fordyce may present as these tiny, itchy, folliculo-centric papules. (b) Close-up of the papules mimicking those of scabies. (Photograph by Dr Rashmi Mahajan.)

Differential diagnosis

Fox-Fordyce disease is often misdiagnosed as lichen nitidus, syringomas, lichen simplex chronicus or lichen planus.

Lichen nitidus presents with multiple 1- to 2-mm, discrete, smooth, round, skin-colored papules. Lesions may be umbilicated. Scaling may be present. Associated pruritis is present. Koebner's phenomenon may be observed.

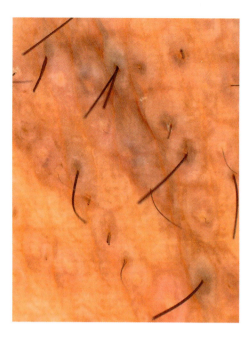

FIGURE 14.9 Yellowish-gray, structureless areas (folliculo-centric) with follicular plugs seen in some. Dinolite digital microscope WF-20 polarized, 10×. (Photograph by Dr Nina Madnani.)

Eruptive syringoma often present as multiple, 1- to 3-mm, flesh-colored, sometimes yellow, papules on the labia majora.

Scabies usually presents with severely pruritic red-brown colored papules with excoriations. Other family members will give a similar history. Web spaces may show the scabietic burrows.

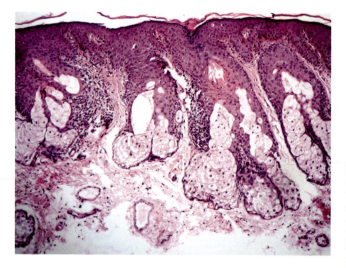

FIGURE 14.10 H & E, 200×, higher power view of sebaceous glands that open onto the surface of the epidermis. (Photograph by Dr Rajiv Joshi.)

Lichen planus papules are more violaceous and polygonal, affecting the labia majora, genito crural folds or extended sites. Other parts of the body may show similar lesions. Oral mucosa is to be checked for typical lacy pattern of the papules.

Lichen simplex chronicus shows more lichenification with accentuation of skin markings.

Course and prognosis

This condition is very refractory to treatment, and patients with Fox-Fordyce disease are often debilitated and embarrassed by the constant itching.

Treatment

Conservative and symptomatic management includes stress reduction and heat avoidance. Topical short-term steroids, calcineurin inhibitors, adapalene and clindamycin have been tried with some effect. Ultraviolet light – 4–6 weekly doses – has proven helpful in many cases. Oral antihistamines and low-dose doxepin are given for the control of pruritis. In resistant cases, systemic retinoids and oral contraceptives have been tried.

Intralesional steroids and botulinum toxin injection have also proven effective in recurrent cases.

Pearl

Intralesional botulinum toxin has been reported to induce remission in refractory cases.

Recommended reading

1. Mahajan R, et al. Indian J Sex Transm Dis AIDS (2012). PMID: 23188940.
2. Gurusamy L, et al. Indian J Sex Transm Dis AIDS (2016). PMID: 27190415.
3. Singal A, et al. Skin Appendage Disord (2020). PMID: 32903893.

Hidradenitis suppurativa

Introduction

Hidradenitis suppurativa (HS) is a debilitating, chronic, recurrent, inflammatory disease of follicular occlusion characterized by painful, deep-seated inflamed nodules, sinuses, fistulae and scarring. Sites commonly involved are the axillary, inguinal, inframammary and anogenital regions. South-East Asians and East Asians with HS are reported to have higher metabolic disease.

Epidemiology

This disease has its onset post-puberty with a peak between 20 and 30 years of age and improves after menopause. Family history is positive in 30–40% of family members. A higher incidence is reported in women, obese individuals, smokers and those with the polycystic ovarian disease.

Pathophysiology

Although the exact pathogenesis is still not certain, we know that the pilosebaceous follicle is involved with occlusion, rupture, dermal spill of follicular contents and recruiting of inflammatory cells and cytokines. Dysbiosis of gut bacteria and biofilm formation which perpetuates inflammation are some of the other hypotheses put out. The role of sex hormones is supported by the onset at puberty when androgen production increases, premenstrual and post-partum flares when progesterone levels are high, the spontaneous remission post-partum and the good response to contraceptive pills containing estradiol and cyproterone acetate.

Presenting complaints

The post-pubertal women commonly present with recurrent painful "boils" on one or more folds which last for weeks and some may rupture to ooze a foul-smelling discharge. There may be a pre-period flare. The women also complain about ugly scarring and disfigurement of the folds, and often depression may have suicidal ideation with a poor quality of life (QoL).

Clinical examination

The areas involved include the genito crural folds, inter-gluteal cleft, buttocks and often extend to the upper thighs. The axillary, inframammary and/or infra-abdominal may or may not be involved depending on the severity of the disease. The lesions may be painful boils with no head, sinuses, fistulae and cord-like bridge scars. Submarine comedones are early clues. Extensive and severe scarring leads to woody edema of the labia majora and contractures of the folds making abduction difficult. It is important to check for pilonidal sinus and fistulae in the perianal and gluteal folds. To plan treatment and monitor

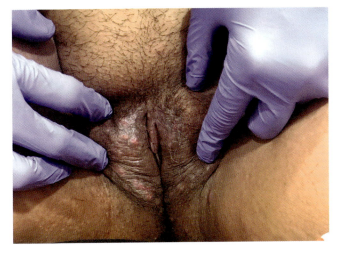

FIGURE 14.11 Multiple inflammatory nodules on the inner surface of both labia majorae. (Photograph by Dr Nina Madnani.)

response, a patient's disease can be classified by Hurley's staging system.

Stage I: Solitary or multiple isolated abscess formation without scarring (Figures 14.11 and 14.12a and b).
Stage II: Recurrent abscesses, single or multiple widely separated lesions, with sinus tract formation and cicatrization (Figure 14.13).
Stage III: Diffuse or broad involvement across a regional area with multiple interconnected sinus tracts and abscesses, without intervening normal skin (Figure 14.14).

Systemic findings

Obesity is a common co-morbidity in HS patients. Hypertension, diabetes, dyslipidemias and depression are other associations. Nine percent of HS patients may have polycystic ovarian syndrome (PCOS). Other comorbidities include inflammatory bowel disease (IBD), pyoderma gangrenosum and as a part of follicular occlusion triad. Patients are often anemic and hypoalbuminemic. Amyloidosis is a complication in long-standing cases.

Laboratory examination

Blood work up for metabolic syndrome. Pus swab from the discharging sinus if the patient is not responding, or if one suspects pseudomonas or a resistant bacterium. Ultrasound or MRI screening

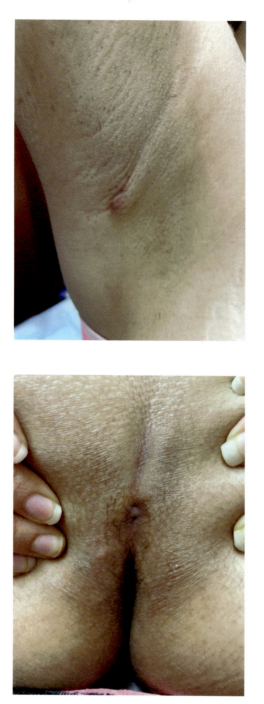

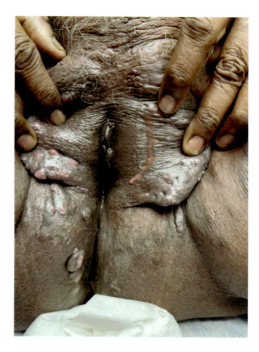

FIGURE 14.13 Moderately severe HS with inflammatory nodules with serosanguinous discharge. (Photograph by Dr Nina Madnani.)

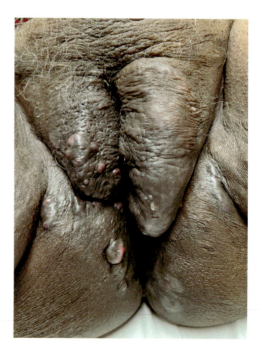

FIGURE 14.12 **(a)** Solitary inflammatory nodule with comedones suggestive of early HS. **(b)** Early pilonidal sinus in the same patient. (Photographs by Dr Nina Madnani.)

may be recommended in advanced disease or pre-surgery. Sinogram may be performed to determine the depth of the sinuses.

Histopathology
The follicles show hyperkeratosis, follicular occlusion with dilatation. Follicular rupture with debris

FIGURE 14.14 Late state of HS with intense labial edema with fibrosis. (Photograph by Dr Nina Madnani.)

in dermis and a dense perifollicular infiltrate of inflammatory cells. The dermis may show fibrosis in long standing cases. Foreign body granuloma may be seen.

Differential diagnosis

Recurrent furunculosis and an inflamed sebaceous cyst are commonly misdiagnosed as HS.

Furuncles may start off as a follicular pustule which then enlarges to form an inflamed nodule with a center.

Sebaceous cysts have the typical yellowish appearance with a giant comedone at the center.

Metastatic Crohn's disease can also present with vulvar edema, painful swellings, sinuses and fistulae. Typical knife-cut ulcers are an important clue. A history of IBD may or may not be present.

Course and prognosis

HS has a chronic, recurrent course, which if untreated, leads to debilitating scarring, impairment in physical activities and a significant decrease in the QoL. Chronic inflammation and ulceration can lead to malignancy.

Treatment

Therapy is dictated by the Hurley staging.

Obese individuals and those with metabolic changes would require diet and lifestyle modification. Cessation of smoking is beneficial. Hair reduction lasers have shown some benefits. Metformin to increase insulin sensitivity.

General skin care by washing the areas with chlorhexidine or benzoyl peroxide washes. Topical clindamycin 1% or dapsone 5% gel twice a day in very early cases. Intralesional corticosteroids in small nodules may help in the early stages.

Systemic antibiotics such as tetracyclines, minocycline, clindamycin-rifampicin combination for more advanced cases. For unresponsive, IV ertapenem for 3 weeks may be a good option. Systemic spironolactone, oral contraceptive pills for those with premenstrual flares have been reported to help. Severe cases may require TNF alfa inhibitors like infliximab or adalimumab. Surgical interventions

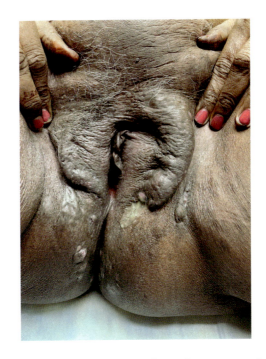

FIGURE 14.15 HS significantly improved with treatment with residual lymphedema. The same patient as in Figure 14.13. (Photograph by Dr Nina Madnani.)

like opening out sinuses, scraping out the contents, fistulectomies, or wide excision with primary closure or secondary healing.

Pearls

HS is a disease which is either missed or misdiagnosed.

TNF alfa inhibitors like adalimumab and infliximab are strongly indicated in Hurley stage II and to calm down the disease before surgery in Hurley stage III.

Recommended reading

1. Goldburg SR, et al. J Am Acad Dermatol. 2020. PMID: 31604104.
2. Zouboulis CC, et al. Exp Dermatol. 2021. PMID: 34085333.

15

IMMUNOBULLOUS DERMATOSES

Vidya Kharkar and Shreya Singh

Contents

Pemphigus vulgaris

Introduction

Pemphigus is a common autoimmune blistering disease affecting the skin and mucous membranes with a chronic relapsing course. It affects middle-aged (40–60 years) females and genital involvement is reported in almost half of the patients (35–51%) with pemphigus vulgaris (PV).

Etiology

Pemphigus in India tends to occur at a younger age and is more severe as compared to Western countries with 34% having a recurrent disease. Genetic predisposition along with triggers such as drug intake, viral infections, physical agents (UV radiation), contact allergens, diet (rich in thiols, polyphenols, tannins) and emotional stress initiates the autoimmune pathway.

Pathogenesis

Autoantibodies directed against desmogleins (Dsg1 & 3) expressed on the epithelial cells of the skin and mucosa, resulting in acantholysis.

Presenting complaints

The patient presents with blisters that rupture easily and result in raw areas (Figure 15.1), which have little/no tendency to heal but rather extends at their periphery. There is an associated itching or burning sensation, genital discharge (foul smelling & often blood stained), pain on micturition, discomfort or pain on intercourse (among those sexually active) and adherence of undergarments to the raw areas.

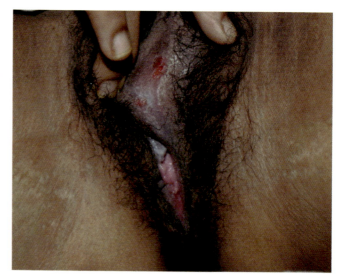

FIGURE 15.1 Erosions on labia minora. (Photograph by Dr Vidya Kharkar.)

Clinical examination

Multiple flaccid vesicles and bullae are seen, which rupture easily to form erosions and crusts with little or no tendency to heal (Figure 15.2). They eventually heal with hyperpigmentation but no scarring. Nikolsky's sign is positive. Genital involvement in women occurs either concurrently with other affected sites (mucosal-oral cavity, conjunctivae, larynx, esophagus, urethra, anal canal or non-mucosal) or when other involved sites have been in remission. Vulvar lesions occur more commonly than vaginal lesions. Sites most commonly affected are the labia minora (92%), labia majora (28%), vagina (36%) and cervix (15%).

DOI: 10.1201/9781003284116-15

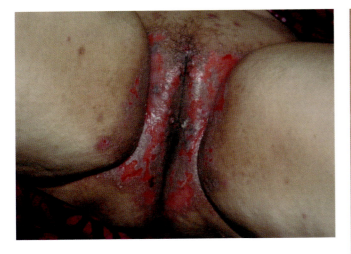

FIGURE 15.2 Erosions on vulva and medial thighs. (Photograph by Dr Vidya Kharkar.)

The most common site for labial involvement reported is the inferior portion of the labia minora and for vaginal involvement was the distal one-third of the vagina. Clinical types which might show vulvar involvement are Pemphigus foliaceus (PF), Pemphigus vegetans & Paraneoplastic pemphigus. Pemphigus vegetans presents as a vegetating and hyperkeratotic lesion in the groins.

Investigations

Diagnostic tests include Tzanck smear (acantholytic cell seen), cervicovaginal Pap smears, dermoscopy, lesional biopsy, perilesional direct immunofluorescence (DIF) which reveals intercellular staining with IgG and C3 in a net-like pattern within the epidermis, indirect immunofluorescence (IIF) which reveals circulating IgG autoantibodies against Dsg 1and/or 3 and enzyme-linked immunosorbent assay (ELISA) helps detects IgG autoantibodies to Dsg 1 and Dsg 3.

Dermoscopy

Vesicles show a yellowish translucent background with an absent pigment network and white linear folds (Figure 15.3a and b). Erosive areas with irregular and/or angulated borders and peripheral epidermal remnants, corresponding to intraepidermal cleft with detached epidermis, have also been reported.

Histopathology

A supra-basal cleft is seen in the case of PV ("row of tombstones" appearance) and a subcorneal cleft

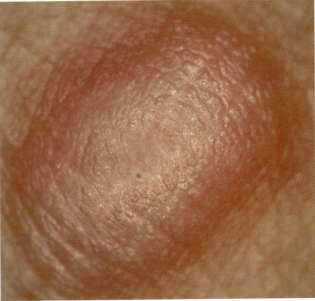

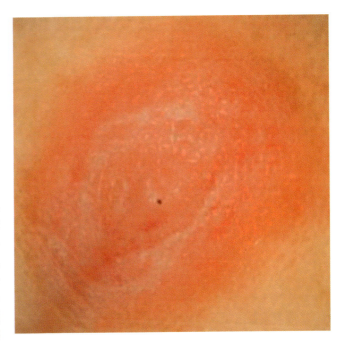

FIGURE 15.3 Dermoscopy of a flaccid bulla: non-polarized (**a**); polarized (**b**) showing whitish areas corresponding to subclinical epidermal detachment with multiple irregular elongated blood vessels in the adjacent skin. Dinolite Digital Microscope AM413ZT×10 magnification. (Photograph by Dr Vidya Kharkar.)

in the case of PF. The blister cavity may contain inflammatory cells including eosinophils and rounded acantholytic cells with intensely eosinophilic cytoplasm and a perinuclear halo (Figure 15.4 a and b).

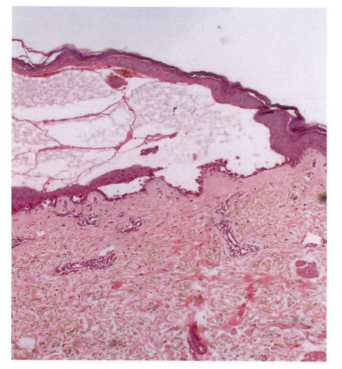

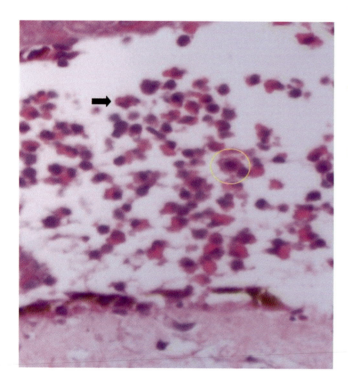

Differential diagnosis

The common differentials to keep in mind are the ones which present with erosion on the vulva such as lichen planus, fixed drug eruptions, mucus membrane pemphigoid and erythema multiforme.

Erosive lichen planus has a characteristic lacy pattern at the periphery.

Mucus membrane pemphigoid heals with scarring.

Fixed drug eruption may be blistering and recurs at a fixed site upon repeated exposure to the offending drug.

Erythema multiforme has diagnostic target lesions.

Course and prognosis

Complications include secondary bacterial/fungal infection (Figure 15.5) or, rarely, the severely affected vulva may exhibit resorption of the labia majora and a scarred clitoris. The mortality rate is 3.58% and the extent of cutaneous involvement is the single most important factor leading to death in pemphigus patients, secondary to sepsis due to the entry of bacteria through the raw areas.

Treatment

Local care of the affected areas includes Sitz bath with potassium permanganate ($KMnO_4$) (light pink color dilution) which facilitates easy removal

FIGURE 15.4 (a) Histopathology picture (H&E; 10×) showing a suprabasal cleft with the "Row of tombstone" appearance of basal cells at the floor of the cleft. (b) (H&E; 100×) showing inflammatory infiltrate composed predominantly of eosinophils (black arrow) and acantholytic cells (yellow circle) in the suprabasal cleft. (Photographs by Dr Vidya Kharkar.)

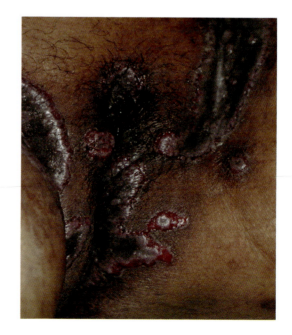

FIGURE 15.5 Erosions on the vulva with secondary infection. (Photograph by Dr Vidya Kharkar.)

of crusts, sterile Vaseline gauze sheets to prevent friction and Lignocaine gel to relieve burning or pain. Topical steroids can be applied to the active lesions (the vesicles/bullae) and intralesional steroids can be injected into thick crusted plaques. Antibiotic and antifungal creams may be applied to erosions to prevent secondary infection.

Systemic therapy includes corticosteroids like prednisolone (1–2 mg/kg/day with slow tapering over a prolonged period of time of 1–2 years) with or without steroid-sparing immunosuppressants like cyclophosphamide/azathioprine/mycophenolate mofetil (MMF). Intravenous rituximab (2 doses, 1 gm each, separated by 15 days). IVIg and dapsone are other options.

Pearl
Female patients with PV must be subjected to vaginal examination to look for mucosal involvement.

Recommended reading
1. Akhyani M, et al. Br J Dermatol (2008). PMID: 18070212.
2. Malik M, et al. Obstet Gynecol (2005). PMID: 16260519.
3. Fairbanks Barbosa ND, et al. J Am Acad Dermatol (2012). PMID: 22153790.
4. Edwards, L. Genital Dermatology Atlas and Manual. Third ed., (Wolters Kluwer, 2017).

Bullous pemphigoid

Introduction
It is the most common subepidermal autoimmune blistering disease affecting the elderly (40–70 years) with slight female preponderance. The prevalence is 7.2 per million per year and genital involvement is uncommon (10%). Vulvar involvement is described in 9% of adult patients with BP and in 40% of children. Localized vulval pemphigoid of childhood (LVPC) has also been described.

Etiology
The facilitating factors in genetically predisposed individuals are drug intake, physical agents and viral infections.

Pathogenesis
Autoantibodies are directed against two components of the hemidesmosome, BP 230 kD (BPAg1) and BP 180 kD (BPAg2). More than 70% have serum IgE directed against both the NC16A and non-NC16A domains of BP180, as well as against the BP230 antigen.

Presenting complaints
Patients present with severe pruritus (which is the hallmark) along with red raised lesions in the early stages. Later, they present with clear fluid-filled blisters or painful raw areas (Figure 15.6).

Clinical examination
Cutaneous lesions are polymorphic. Early stages may be papular or urticarial which may progress to tense blisters on normal skin or erythematous base. Excoriations, erosions and crusting may be the outcome of severe itching. The lesions heal with dyspigmentation and occasionally with milia formation but without scarring.

Blisters are seen at the introitus. Extra genital sites commonly involved are the flexures of limbs and lower trunk, followed by intertriginous zones.

Investigations
Tests include Tzanck smear (absence of acantholytic cells, presence of eosinophils), dermoscopy, biopsy and DIF (shows linear staining of basement membrane zone (BMZ) with C3 and IgG). Further investigations that can be done are IIF from serum or urine, salt-split skin technique where immunoreactants are seen on the roof ("n-serrated" pattern) and ELISA (detects anti-BP180, NC16 antibody and their level correlates with the disease activity).

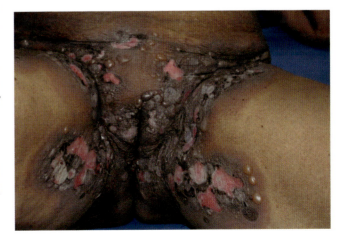

FIGURE 15.6 Tense bullae and erosions over vulva, medial thighs, inguinal region and lower abdomen. (Photograph by Dr Vidya Kharkar.)

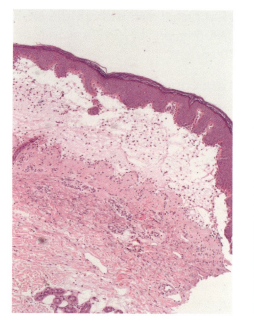
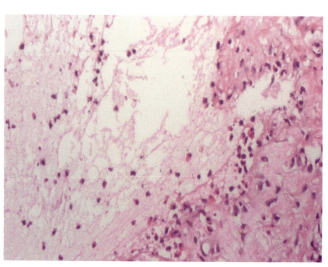

FIGURE 15.7   **(a)** Histopathology pic showing subepidermal split with inflammatory infiltrate in the upper dermis (H&E ×40). **(b)** Abundance of eosinophils within the blister. (H&E ×100). (Photographs by Dr Vidya Kharkar.)

Dermoscopy

Yellowish-pink translucent areas with distorted pigment network are seen with prominent follicular and eccrine openings and perifollicular as well as peri-eccrine pigmentation.

Histopathology

The split is subepidermal, and the blister cavity is filled with plenty of eosinophils (Figure 15.7a and b).

Differential diagnosis

Blisters and erosions on the vulva must be differentiated from the following:

- Herpes simplex presents as grouped vesicles on an erythematous base and has a history of recurrence.
- PV has flaccid blisters that rupture easily, and biopsy will reveal an intraepidermal split. Intercellular staining is seen on DIF.
- Mucus membrane pemphigoid shows a predominant mucosal involvement and heals with severe scarring.

Course and prognosis

BP is often a self-limiting disease but may last for months to years with exacerbations and remissions. Relapses are more frequent in patients with extensive disease. The average disease duration is 3–6 years and the mean mortality in the first year is 12.9%

Management

Local care includes Sitz bath with dilute KMnO4, 4% Lignocaine gel (to relieve burning or pain), topical antibiotics (for erosions) and potent topical steroids (for vesicles/bullae). Topical tacrolimus 0.1% can be used as a steroid-sparing agent for localized lesions.

Systemic therapy includes oral corticosteroids (prednisolone 0.3–0.5 mg/kg/day with slow tapering), steroid-sparing immunosuppressants (cyclophosphamide/azathioprine/MMF) and others (dapsone, doxycycline, tetracycline, nicotinamide).

Pearl

LVPC has a good prognosis and responds well to topical corticosteroids.

Recommended reading

1. Iwata Y, et al. Arch Dermatol (2008). PMID: 18209167.
2. Schumann H, et al. Br J Dermatol (1999). PMID: 10354084.
3. Kirtschig G, et al. Br J Dermatol (1994). PMID: 8204469.
4. Nayak S, et al. Clin Dermatology Rev (2017). DOI: 10.4103/cdr.cdr_9_17.

Cicatricial pemphigoid

Introduction
Cicatricial pemphigoid (CP) or benign mucous membrane pemphigoid (MMP): It is a rare autoimmune subepidermal blistering disorder that affects 60 to 80-year-old individuals with a female predominance. There is a predominant involvement of mucosae where the incidence of genital involvement is 20–50%. It is characterized by a chronic course and a tendency towards scarring.

Etiology
The human leukocyte antigen (HLA) haplotype may be important in the presentation of specific epitopes on target antigens in the generation of an autoimmune response. HLA D2w7 is associated with both oral and ocular forms of the disease.

Pathogenesis
Autoantibodies (IgG/IgA) are formed against various proteins of dermoepidermal junction including BP180 (C-terminal epitopes), BP230, Type 7 collagen, Laminin 332 (laminin-5 or Epiligrin), Integrin $\alpha6\beta4$ & Laminin-6, leading to its disruption and subsequent blister formation.

Presenting complaints
Patients present with persistent painful raw areas in the mouth, eyes and genitalia sometimes with blood-tinged discharge. One-third of the patients present with itchy tense blisters on the vulva that may heal with scarring. There is associated genital discomfort, dysuria and sexual dysfunction.

Clinical examination
On the genitalia, painful erosions involving the clitoris or labia may be seen. Perianal involvement manifests as perianal blisters and erosions.

On the skin, tense blisters or erosions may be seen on either normal-appearing skin or erythematous plaques. In patients with active disease, erosions may be persistent and difficult to heal. Scarring and milia are frequently encountered. The eye can also be involved in this disease often causing blindness.

Investigations
Tzanck smear (absence of acantholytic cells), biopsy, DIF (shows linear staining of BMZ with IgG and/or C3, and sometimes IgA), IIF (on salt-split normal human skin substrate, it shows immunoreactants on the roof as well as a floor) and immunoprecipitation with human keratinocytes (the most sensitive test for detection of anti-laminin 5 antibodies).

Dermoscopy
Findings have not been standardized yet.

Histopathology
Histology is similar to bullous pemphigoid, which shows subepidermal cleft without acantholysis with a mixed inflammatory infiltrate composed primarily of mononuclear cells. Older lesions show upper dermal fibrosis. The vulvar lesion infiltrate may be composed of some plasma cells as well.

Differential diagnosis
Other conditions with vulvar erosions and scarring must be ruled out when considering a diagnosis of CP.

Erosive lichen planus does not have associated blisters, and histopathology and immunofluorescence help to reach the diagnosis.

Lichen sclerosus is associated with scarring, and it may resemble the late stage of CP, but the cigarette-paper wrinkling or hypertrophic lesions, petechiae, are not seen in CP.

Behcet's disease has similar involvement of the mucosae but has deeper genital ulcers, while ocular involvement is in the form of uveitis.

Contact mucositis usually has a history of a topical allergen or application.

Course and prognosis
Blistering and subsequent scarring can result in severe structural changes to the vulva, including resorption of the labia minora, stenosis of the introitus, stenosis of the urethral meatus and phimosis of the clitoris (clitoral burial). This can eventually lead to sexual and urinary problems. It has a chronic relapsing course and rarely goes into spontaneous remission. Patients with both IgG and IgA have severe diseases. Involvement of genital mucosa is associated with a less favorable prognosis.

Management

A multidisciplinary approach is required. Local care includes Sitz bath with dilute $KMnO_4$, 4% Lignocaine gel (to relieve burning or pain), topical anti-inflammatory antibiotics (for erosions) and potent topical steroid (for vesicle/bulla/early scar).

Systemic therapy includes corticosteroids like prednisolone with or without steroid-sparing immunosuppressants like cyclophosphamide/azathioprine/MMF and drugs like dapsone.

Surgical interventions include dilators for vaginal/urethral meatal stenosis or scar excision/revision.

Pearls

A cost-effective topical treatment is tacrolimus solution (1 g capsule in 500 ml of water) applied twice a day.

Vulvar scarring should prompt the physician to examine other mucosal sites.

Recommended reading

1. Rashid H, et al. JAAD Case Rep. 2021. PMID: 34179323.
2. Loyal J, et al. Int J Womens Dermatol. 2017. PMID: 29234717.
3. Belzile E, et al. Pediatr Dermatol. 2019. PMID: 30762244.

Linear IgA bullous dermatosis (LABD)

Introduction

LABD or chronic bullous disease of childhood (CBDC) is a rare, immune-mediated, subepidermal blistering disease in adults (> 60 years) and children (mean age of 4.5 years) characterized by linear deposits of IgA in the BMZ. It is the most frequent autoimmune blistering disease in children with slight female preponderance and can have overlapping features with bullous pemphigoid, mucus membrane pemphigoid and epidermolysis bullosa.

Etiology

There is an association with HLA B8, Cw7, DR3, lymphoproliferative disorders, non-lymphoid malignancies and ulcerative colitis. Precipitating factors include drugs (vancomycin, non-steroidal anti-inflammatory drugs [NSAIDs], penicillin), preceding illnesses (typhoid, brucella, tuberculosis, varicella, herpes zoster, certain gynecologic and upper respiratory infections), trauma, vaccination and ultraviolet radiation.

Pathogenesis

In drug-induced variants, the implicated drug stimulates the immune system to produce the IgA class of antibodies in predisposed individuals. Antibody deposition leads to complement activation and neutrophil chemotaxis, which results in loss of adhesion at the dermal–epidermal junction and blister formation.

Presenting complaints

Children present with an abrupt onset of fluid-filled lesions and painful raw areas on the genitalia and medial thighs associated with itching/burning. Adults present with abrupt/insidious onset of red raised lesions or blisters associated with itching/burning and painful raw areas with genital discomfort and foul-smelling discharge.

Clinical examination

Mucosal involvement is seen in 60–80% in the form of oral/vaginal ulcers and erosions. On the vulvar skin and thighs, tense clear/hemorrhagic vesicles and bullae are seen on normal or erythematous skin. New lesions arise around the resolving lesions forming arciform or annular bullae surrounding the central crust. This is called "string of pearls" or "cluster of jewels" or "rosette pattern" and is more commonly seen in children (Figure 15.8).

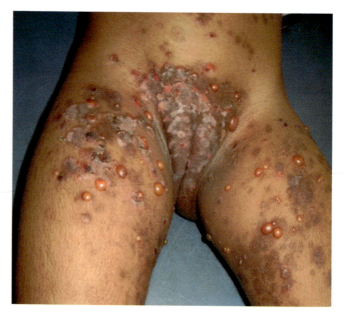

FIGURE 15.8 Multiple tense vesicles and bullae with central crusting. (Photograph by Dr Vidya Kharkar.)

Investigations

Tzanck smear (absence of acantholytic cells), dermoscopy, biopsy, DIF (gold standard for diagnosing LABD reveals linear deposits of IgA and rarely IgG, IgM and C3 along the basement membrane at the dermo-epidermal junction), western immunoblotting and immunoelectron microscopy.

Dermoscopy

A yellowish translucent background (corresponding to the serum inside the vesicles), brown or gray-brown rim around the lesions (owing to post-inflammatory pigment and hemosiderin deposition) and a distorted pigment network (due to subepidermal vesiculation, papillary dermal edema and mild spongiosis) have been observed.

Histopathology

In the early urticarial stage with papules and plaques, neutrophils are seen along the BMZ with vacuolar change in the epidermis, whereas in a fully developed lesion, a subepidermal split is seen along with neutrophils in the dermis either alone or with eosinophils (Figure 15.9a,b).

Differential diagnosis

Itchy plaques with blisters or erosions of LABD in children must be differentiated from:

- Bullous impetigo, which almost always has honey-colored crust and a simple Gram stain and culture can be diagnostic.
- Epidermolysis bullosa simplex, which presents with tense blisters but on trauma-prone sites.
- Rarely, child abuse may have a similar presentation, but there will be a history of abuse and signs of trauma elsewhere.

Important differentials to consider in adults include:

- Dermatitis herpetiformis (DH), which presents as grouped papulo-vesicles & excoriations, which are present symmetrically on the elbows, knees, buttocks, back or scalp.
- Bullous pemphigoid is seen in older females and has tense, large bullae, with bulla spread sign positive.

Course and prognosis

LABD responds well to treatment and relapses are characterized by less severity. Adult LABD

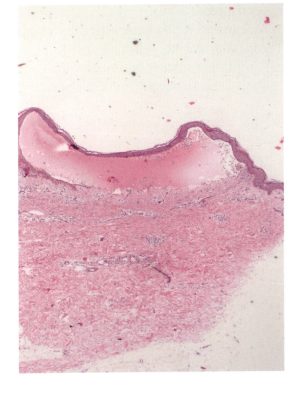

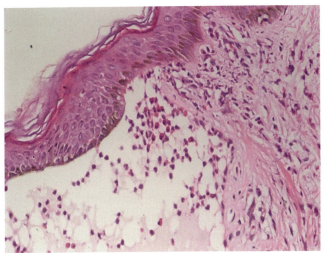

FIGURE 15.9 **(a)** Subepidermal blister (H&E 25×). **(b)** Blister cavity filled with a mixed inflammatory infiltrate (H&E; 400×). (Photographs by Dr Vidya Kharkar.)

goes into remission within 3–6 years, while in children, the disease remits spontaneously after several months to 4 years. It may follow a waxing and waning course but remits before puberty. Drug-induced LABD heals within 4–8 weeks after discontinuation of the drug.

Management

Local care includes Sitz bath with dilute KMnO$_4$, 4% Lignocaine gel (to relieve burning or pain), topical anti-inflammatory antibiotics (for erosions) and potent topical steroid (for vesicle/bulla/early scar).

Systemic treatment options include dapsone (1–1.5 mg/kg/day) with very potent topical steroids with or without systemic steroid (prednisolone 0.25–0.5 mg/kg/day), other sulpha drugs and anti-inflammatory antibiotics like tetracycline, doxycycline with or without nicotinamide & MMF. Omalizumab can provide a safe and effective alternative to other existing therapies.

Pearl

Dapsone is extremely effective in managing this disabling condition and should be the first line of therapy.

Recommended reading

1. Lammer J, et al. Acta Derm Venereol. 2019. PMID: 30809685.
2. Haulrig MB, et al. Clin Case Rep. 2022. PMID: 35280104.
3. Chaudhari S, et al. J Clin Aesthet Dermatol. 2015. PMID: 26557220.

Hailey-Hailey disease

Introduction

Hailey-Hailey disease (HHD) or familial benign chronic pemphigus is an autosomal dominant genodermatosis characterized by vesicular and erosive lesions in the intertriginous areas. Thirty-three percent of cases are sporadic. It presents in the second to a fourth decade but improves with age.

Etiology

The triggering factors are friction, heat, sweating, constrictive clothing, physical trauma, stress and menstruation in a predisposed individual.

Pathogenesis

Mutations in the ATP2C1 gene, which encodes Ca^{2+}/Mn^{2+} ATPase protein 1 (hSPCA1) localized to the Golgi apparatus, lead to impaired calcium sequestration.

Presenting complaints

Patients complain of intense itching/burning on the vulva and intertriginous areas, with aggravation in summer and partial relief in winter. They also complain of a bad odor emanating from the affected areas.

Clinical examination

Moist, malodorous plaques with painful fissures are seen over labia majora, minora, extending over the perineum and perianal area (Figures 15.10a and 15.10b). Genito-crural folds are also involved (Figure 15.11). Some lesions may be keratotic/scaly/

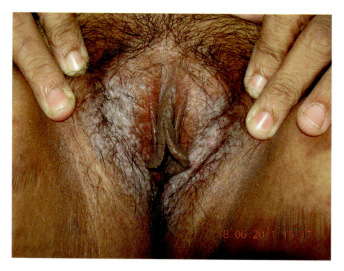

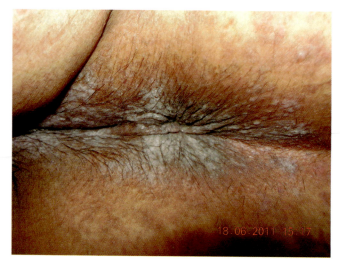

FIGURE 15.10a, 15.10b Flat-topped grayish white papules over the labia minora, extending backwards to the perianal area. (Photograph by Dr Nina Madnani.)

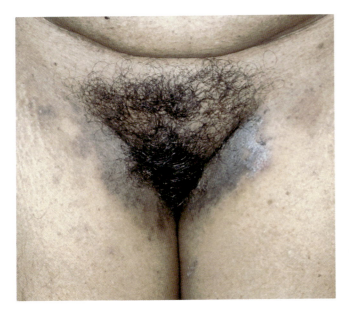

FIGURE 15.11 hyperpigmented eczematous plaques in bilateral crural folds. (Photograph by Dr Vidya Kharkar.)

condylomatous/hypertrophic/hyperpigmented (Figure 15.12).

Extra genital sites include flexures, neck axillae, inframammary areas and groins (Figures 15.13 and 15.14). Rare presentations include isolated vulvar, perianal, perineal, segmental, extensive, mucosal and photo-exposed areas (Figure 15.15).

Investigations

Tzanck smear (absence of acantholytic cells), dermoscopy and histopathology.

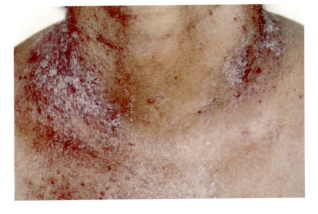

FIGURE 15.13 Neck involvement in a patient with HH disease. (Photograph by Dr Nina Madnani.)

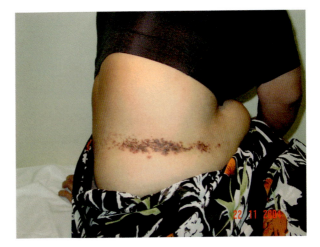

FIGURE 15.14 Waist folds also need to be checked in patients with HH disease. (Photograph by Dr Nina Madnani.)

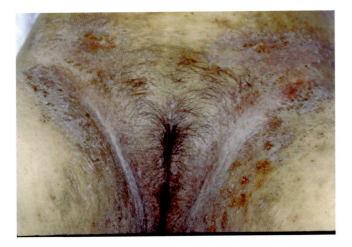

FIGURE 15.12 This lady presented with extensive, whitish scaly lesions and excoriations. (Photograph by Dr Nina Madnani.)

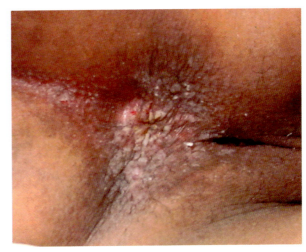

FIGURE 15.15 Perianal pruritus can be the first sign of HH disease.

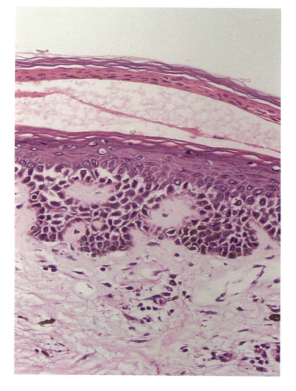

FIGURE 15.16 Histopathology showing the classical "Dilapidated brick wall" appearance. (Photograph by Dr Rajiv Joshi.)

Dermoscopy

Dermoscopy reveals irregular pinkish-white areas separated by pink furrows with whitish areas in an occasional cloud-like arrangement. The term "Crumpled fabric" pattern has been used to describe the grouped arrangement of vesiculopustules.

Histopathology

Biopsy shows a suprabasal split with partial loss of intercellular bridges giving rise to "dilapidated brick wall appearance" (Figure 15.16).

Differential diagnosis

The important dermatoses which must be considered when evaluating a patient with suspected HHD include:

Inverse psoriasis is characterized by well-demarcated, erythematous plaques with minimal scaling; biopsy is confirmatory.
Candidiasis presents as macerated intertriginous lesions with characteristic peripheral satellite pustules. KOH mount is confirmatory.

PV/PF can pose a diagnostic challenge, but desmoglein levels and biopsy can help differentiate. Darier's disease presents as greasy hyperkeratotic papules in seborrheic areas of the body.

Course and prognosis

HHD is a chronic disease that easily gets secondarily infected and is especially troublesome in obese individuals. Response to treatment is unpredictable.

Management

The frequency of exacerbations may be reduced weight reduction, wearing loose clothing, use of anti-perspirants and avoiding intense physical activities. Bleach baths twice weekly help to reduce superficial infections.

Local care includes the use of topical agents like corticosteroids, antibiotic, antifungal, retinoids, calcipotriol, tacrolimus or zinc oxide as per indication.

Systemic therapy includes corticosteroids, antibiotics/antifungals (for infection), retinoids, dapsone, cyclosporine, methotrexate or biologics. Magnesium and low-dose naltrexone have been found to be effective. Refractory cases can be treated with intralesional steroids, phototherapy (narrowband-UVB) or cosmetic/surgical options (Botulinum toxin-A, dermabrasion, CO_2 laser, Er:YAG laser).

Pearl

OnabotulinumtoxinA (OnA) injections can be an efficient therapeutic option for refractory cases of HHD.

Recommended reading

1. Vasudevan B, et al. Indian J Dermatol Venereol Leprol (2015). PMID: 25566918.
2. Lemieux A, et al. SAGE Open Med Case Rep (2020). PMID: 32110406.
3. Sousa Gomes M, et al. Arch Gynecol Obstet (2020). PMID: 32776297.
4. Kelati A, et al. J Am Acad Dermatol (2017). PMID: 28087023.

Dermatitis herpetiformis

Introduction

DH or Duhring-Brocq disease is a chronic autoimmune blistering disease characterized by polymorphic and intensely pruritic skin lesions in patients with gluten-sensitive enteropathy (GSE). The mean age of presentation is 44.35±15.52 years.

Etiology
Associations include GSE (clinically silent/mild), small bowel lymphoma, rheumatoid arthritis, auto-immune thyroid disease, type 1 diabetes mellitus, Addison's disease and vitiligo.

Pathogenesis
A genetic predisposition for gluten sensitivity, coupled with a diet high in gluten, leads to the formation of IgA antibodies which cross react with epidermal transglutaminase (e-TG) triggering an immunologic cascade.

Presenting complaints
Patients present with intensely itchy rashes with a premonitory sensation of burning and tingling, immediately preceding it. Blisters are rarely seen because the lesions are immediately excoriated.

Clinical examination
Polymorphic lesions, including grouped excoriations, erythematous urticarial plaques and papules are seen distributed on the vulva and buttocks (Figure 15.17a and b). Recurrent genital ulceration is sometimes seen. Similar lesions are seen in a symmetrical distribution over elbows and knees. Lesions eventually heal with post-inflammatory hypo- and/or hyper-pigmentation.

Investigations
Diagnostic tests include Tzanck smear, dermoscopy, lesional biopsy, perilesional DIF (**IgA** deposits are seen at dermal papillary tips in granular/fibrillar pattern), IIF (IgA endomysial antibodies found on using monkey esophagus) and ELISA (IgA anti-eTG antibody). Additional workup includes gastroduodenoscopy, anti-thyroid peroxidase and blood sugar level.

Dermoscopy
Extravasations, yellow hemorrhagic crusts and characteristically clustered dotted vessels.

Histopathology
Subepidermal vesicles and blisters with an accumulation of neutrophils at the tips of dermal papillae (papillary microabscesses) with relative sparing of the lower tips of rete ridges (Figure 15.18).

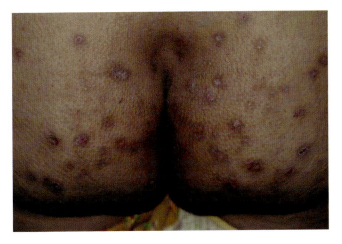

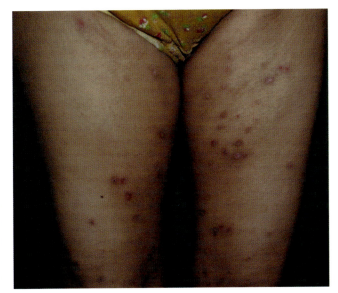

FIGURE 15.17 Multiple excoriations seen over bilateral buttocks (a) and over thighs (b). (Photograph by Dr Vidya Kharkar.)

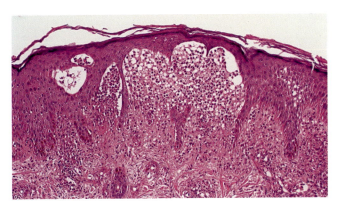

FIGURE 15.18 Histopathology (H&E, 400×) showing papillary tip microabscess consisting of neutrophils. (Photograph by Dr Vidya Kharkar.)

Differential diagnosis

The intensely itchy lesions of DH must be differentiated from the following:

- Scabies: Here, the itching is maximal in the areas of burrows and is more peripherally like finger webs, axilla and toes.
- Atopic dermatitis presents with eczematization over the vulva with severe itching, but features of atopic dermatitis in other folds may be present.
- Linear IgA bullous dermatosis presents with vesicles arranged in an annular pattern.

Course and prognosis

The disease has a chronic relapsing course, but remission is common in adults above 40 years. GSE results in malabsorption, leading to anemia, weight loss, osteoporosis and short stature in children. Long-term gluten-free diet (GFD) is required for better results.

Management

Local care includes topical corticosteroids for the vesicles, antibiotics for excoriations/erosions and antihistamines for the itch. A GFD is the treatment of choice. Systemic drug options are dapsone (100–400 mg/day), sulphapyridine (3 gm/day) and sulphamethoxypyridazine (0.5–1.5 gm/day). Systemic corticosteroids are ineffective.

Pearls

All patients of DH should be screened for autoimmune thyroid disease (5–20%).

Patients should be counseled to avoid iodine exposure, vitamin supplements and adulterated oats.

Recommended reading

1. Handa S, et al. Int J Dermatol (2018). PMID: 29752728.
2. Antiga E, et al. Clin Cosmet Investig Dermatol (2015). PMID: 25999753.
3. Reunala T, et al. Am J Clin Dermatol (2021). PMID: 33432477.

16

PEDIATRIC VULVAR DISEASE

Nisha Chaturvedi

Contents

Introduction

The pediatric vulvar disease is not uncommon but is often missed as the child is unable to express her discomfort. Due to the lack of estrogen and the raised pH, the skin becomes susceptible to bacterial infections and irritant contact dermatitis. The high pH also discourages candidial infection.

Pediatric vulvar dermatoses can be broadly grouped into the following categories:

- *Congenital vulvar abnormalities* – Ambiguous external genitalia, labial adhesions, congenital labial hypertrophy, hymenal abnormalities, hemangioma, melanocytic nevi
- *Infections* – Bacterial (impetigo, streptococcal infection), viral (herpes simplex, molluscum contagiosum, genital warts), fungal (candidiasis, tinea) and infestations (scabies, pinworms)
- *Inflammatory dermatoses* – Diaper/seborrheic/irritant/allergic contact dermatitis, psoriasis, atopic dermatitis, lichen planus, lichen sclerosus, vitiligo
- *Bullous disorders* – Erythema multiforme, linear IgA disease
- *Nevoid/Segmental dermatoses* – Linear psoriasis, linear morphea, lichen striatus, segmental vitiligo
- *Nutritional dermatosis* – Acrodermatitis enteropathica

Caveat

This chapter is a representation of many common/uncommon vulvar diseases in children but does not encompass the entire spectrum.

Congenital vulvar abnormalities

Fifteen-month-old girl with fused labia minora with a midline raphe was noticed while examining the depigmented patch (Figure 16.1).

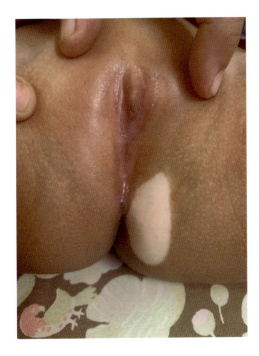

FIGURE 16.1 Labial adhesion with vitiligo. (Photograph by Dr Nisha Chaturvedi.)

DOI: 10.1201/9781003284116-16

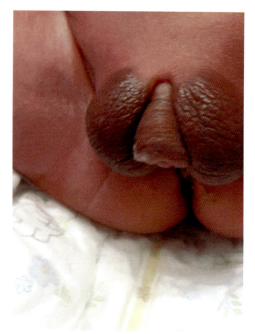

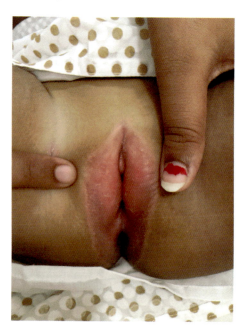

FIGURE 16.2 Ambiguous external genitalia in a child. (Photograph by Dr Nandkishor Kabra.)

The exact etiology of this condition is unknown, but poor hygiene, local irritation and lack of estrogen may be contributing factors. Labial adhesions primarily affect infants and young girls. The condition is usually asymptomatic and may resolve spontaneously. Topical estrogen creams to be applied twice a day is recommended. Surgical adhesiolysis can also be done if the previously mentioned treatment fails.

A rare condition in which the external genitals of an infant are not clearly male or female (Figure 16.2). The majority of the ambiguous genitalia are due to female pseudohermaphroditism. Congenital adrenal hyperplasia, androgen-producing tumors or ingestion of androgens (drugs) can cause virilization of a female fetus. Male pseudohermaphroditism is less common and is caused due to lack of gonadotropins, enzyme defect in testosterone synthesis or androgen receptor defect.

Vulvar infections

A 3-year-old child with well-demarcated erythema around the vulva and perianal area. This condition may be associated with dysuria and painful defecation. Differentials for this are sexual abuse, eczema, psoriasis or candidiasis. Systemic antibiotics like erythromycin or penicillin with a

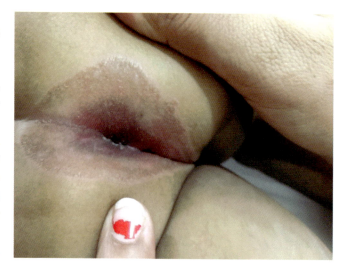

FIGURE 16.3 (**a and b**) Vulvar and perianal streptococcal dermatitis. (Photograph by Dr Nisha Chaturvedi.)

topical antibiotic cream like mupirocin are used for treatment (Figure 16.3a and b).

A 14-month-old with annular, symmetrical, erythematous plaques with central clearing seen on the mons pubis, inner thigh and labia. Parents and siblings had similar lesions. Topical antifungal creams like 1% clotrimazole, miconazole and 1% terbinafine are generally the first-line treatment (Figure 16.4).

A 1-year-old with multiple skin colored to pearly white, firm, dome-shaped, umbilicated papules on her labia. Genital molluscum can spread via fomites and autoinoculation. It may show spontaneous

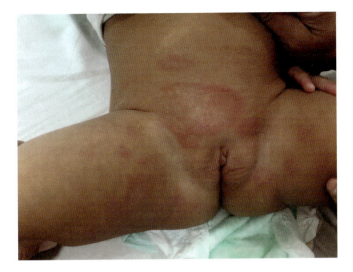

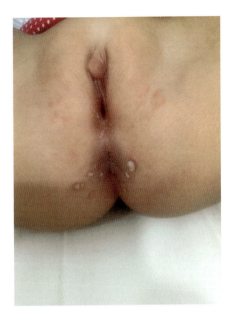

FIGURE 16.4 Tinea cruris. (Photograph by Dr Nisha Chaturvedi.)

resolution in 6–12 months. Electrocautery, chemical cautery, cryotherapy or mechanical removal are various modalities that can be used (Figure 16.5).

An infant with multiple, small rough, skin colored to grayish papules located peri-anally. The virus can be transmitted during vaginal delivery or autoinoculation from an infected individual (mothers, caretakers) (Figure 16.6a and b).

A 4-month-old child with vegetative lesions perianally. The presence of condyloma acuminata in a child should raise suspicion of the possibility of sexual abuse.

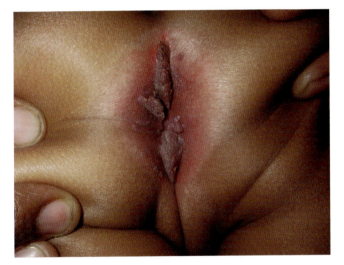

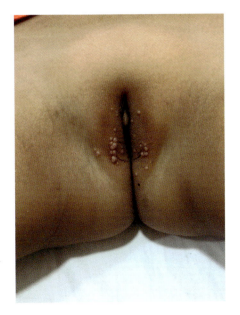

FIGURE 16.6 **(a)** Perianal genital warts. **(b)** Condyloma acuminata. (Photographs by Dr Nisha Chaturvedi.)

Spontaneous resolution of genital warts can occur. Cryotherapy, electrocautery, chemical cautery, podophyllin solution and imiquimod have been used to treat genital warts in children.

Inflammatory dermatoses

An 11-month-old baby with glazed erythema, scaling and crusting seen on the convex surface of labia majora and thighs (Figure 16.7a).

Diaper dermatitis is caused due to repeated contact with irritants like urine, feces, wet wipes and friction. Secondary infection with candida may occur. Frequent diaper changes, diaper-free time,

FIGURE 16.5 Molluscum contagiosum. (Photograph by Dr Nisha Chaturvedi.)

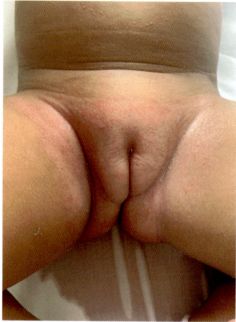

avoiding wet wipes and use of barrier creams containing zinc oxide, topical antifungal creams and 1% hydrocortisone cream help in the management of diaper dermatitis (Figure 16.7b and c).

A 6-month-old with well-defined erythematous scaly plaques seen on the vulva and the inguinal folds (Figure 16.8a).

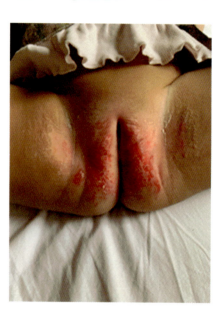

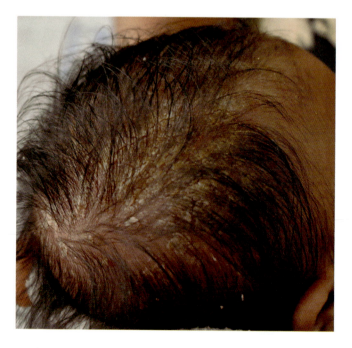

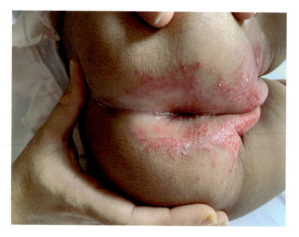

FIGURE 16.7 **(a)** Diaper dermatitis. **(b and c)** The papular erosive type of diaper dermatitis. Note the characteristic sparing of the inguinal folds. (Photographs by Dr Nisha Chaturvedi.)

FIGURE 16.8 **(a)** Seborrheic dermatitis. (Photograph by Dr Nisha Chaturvedi.) **(b)** Greasy yellow scaly plaques are seen on the scalp. (Photograph by Dr Bela Shah.)

Pediatric Vulvar Disease

Seborrheic dermatitis is usually seen in the first 3 months of life. Other areas like the scalp, retro auricular crease and trunk may be involved (Figure 16.8 b).

The proposed etiology is an immune reaction to Malassezia species. Topical antifungal creams like 1% clotrimazole/miconazole with a mild topical corticosteroid like 1% hydrocortisone cream are useful in the management.

A 2-year-old with a well-defined, erythematous scaly plaque on the labia and inner thighs (Figure 16.9a and b).

A 7-month-old with involvement of inguinal folds and labia with minimal scaling.

Diagnosis of psoriasis in infants is often difficult as it can mimic seborrheic dermatitis and candidiasis. It may present as chronic, bright red, well-defined plaques on the labia majora and mons pubis or as erythematous non-scaly plaques in the inguinal and gluteal fold. In infants, diaper dermatitis, which is resistant to treatment and chronic, must arouse suspicion of psoriasis. Psoriatic plaques may be seen on other areas like elbows, knees, scalp, nails and other body folds. Treatment includes emollients like white soft paraffin, topical calcineurin inhibitors: pimecrolimus, tacrolimus and mild topical corticosteroids like 1% hydrocortisone cream/desonide cream.

A 4-year-old child with a well-defined, shiny, hypopigmented area involving the labia majora, clitoral hood and extending onto the perianal area forming a "figure of eight" pattern (Figure 16.10a).

Pediatric lichen sclerosus usually begins before 7 years of age. These children may be asymptomatic or may complain of itching or severe constipation. Erosions, excoriations, purpura, bleeding and bruising as an outcome of pruritus may be mistaken for sexual abuse (Figure 16.10b).

Eight-year-old child with lichen sclerosus showing the classic "cigarette paper" crinkling (Figure 16.10c).

Treatment of choice in childhood lichen sclerosus consists of the application of a potent to super potent topical steroid (clobetasol propionate 0.05% cream/mometasone furoate 0.1% cream) for 6–12 weeks and then tapered off to the minimum requirement. If untreated, these patients are at risk of scarring, labial absorption or squamous cell carcinoma. Long-term regular follow-up is recommended.

A 4-year-old with depigmented macules and patch extending over the mons pubis, labia majora, inner thighs, perineum and buttocks, without any atrophy or sclerosis (Figure 16.11).

Vitiligo patches may also be present on extra-genital sites. Topical corticosteroids and calcineurin inhibitors have been used for the treatment of genital vitiligo.

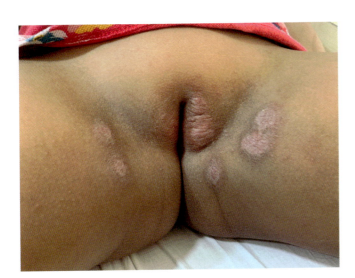
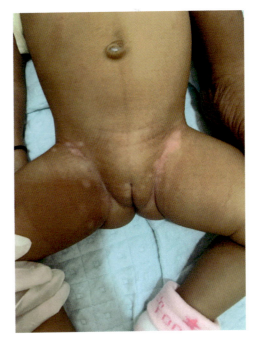

FIGURE 16.9 **(a and b)** Psoriasis. (Photograph by Dr Nisha Chaturvedi.)

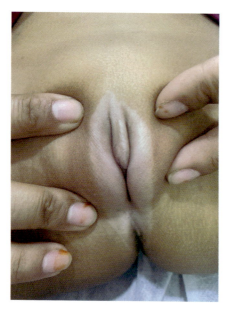

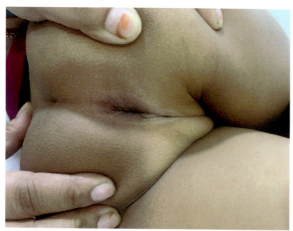

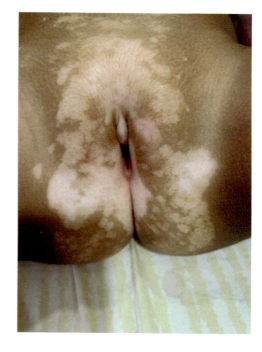

FIGURE 16.11   Vitiligo. (Photograph by Dr Nisha Chaturvedi.)

Nevoid/segmental dermatoses

A 16-year-old with a unilateral, depigmented patch in a linear distribution involving the vulva and medial thighs. Leukotrichia is seen on the pubic area (Figure 16.12).

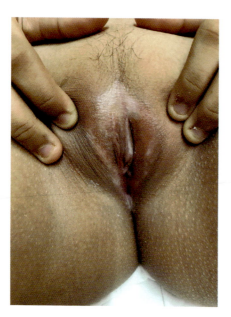

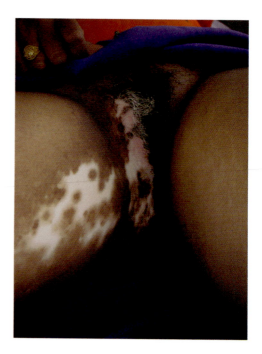

FIGURE 16.10   (a–c) Lichen sclerosus. (a and b – Photograph by Dr Nisha Chaturvedi. c – Photograph by Dr Nina Madnani.)

FIGURE 16.12   Segmental vitiligo. (Photograph by Dr Nisha Chaturvedi.)

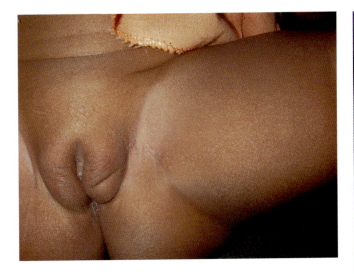

FIGURE 16.13 Lichen striatus. (Photograph by Dr Nisha Chaturvedi.)

Topical corticosteroids, calcineurin inhibitors, narrow band-UVB and surgical therapy viz NC-MCT (non-cultured melanocyte cell transfer) are the recommended treatment options in segmental vitiligo.

A 5-year-old child with multiple, grouped, pinhead sized, skin colored to whitish papules in a linear pattern along the Blaschko's line (Figure 16.13).

Lichen striatus is an asymptomatic self-limiting condition, which completely resolves within 1–3 years. Diagnosis is mainly clinical and parents must be counseled that no treatment is required.

A 10-year-old child with an erythematous scaly plaques in a band-like distribution over the mons-pubis extending down the medial aspect of her leg (Figure 16.14).

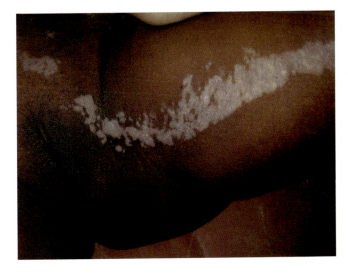

FIGURE 16.14 Linear psoriasis. (Photograph by Dr Nisha Chaturvedi.)

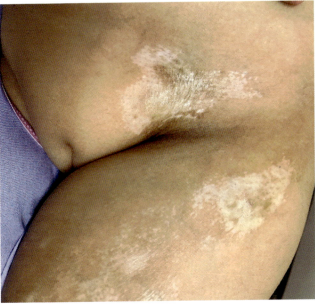

FIGURE 16.15 Linear morphea. (Photograph by Dr Nina Madnani.)

Linear psoriasis is an uncommon presentation of psoriasis characterized by erythematous linear plaque with silvery scales. Various treatments like topical corticosteroids, topical calcipotriol and even biologics have been used for the treatment of linear psoriasis with varied results.

An 8-year-old child with asymptomatic depigmented, atrophic patches involving the mons pubis extending down the anterior aspect of the left thigh (Figure 16.15).

Linear morphea is the commonest type of morphea seen in school children. Early lesions may be indurated, while older lesions may be sclerotic/atrophic. It may extend deeper to involve the subcutaneous fat, underlying muscle and bone. Treatment modalities include phototherapy, topical super potent corticosteroid, topical calcineurin inhibitors and topical calcipotriene. Severe cases may require systemic therapy with corticosteroids or methotrexate.

Nutritional dermatosis

A well-defined erythematous plaque with areas of crusting, scaling and fissuring is seen on the periorificial area and buttocks in an 11-month-old child (Figure 16.16a and b).

Acrodermatitis enteropathica is a rare, autosomal recessive disorder caused due to a defect in the zinc transport protein leading to a defect in

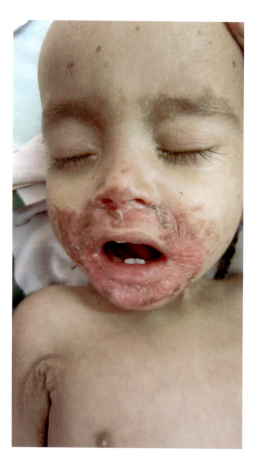
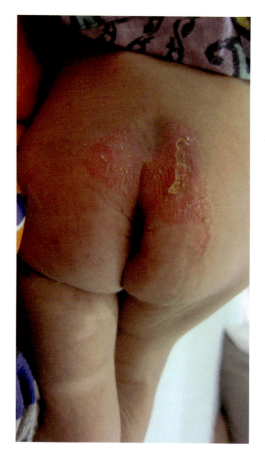

FIGURE 16.16 **(a and b)** Acrodermatitis enteropathica. (Photograph by Dr Bela Shah.)

zinc absorption. The symptoms usually start at the time of weaning. Cutaneous lesions can be vesiculobullous, eczematous or papulosquamous seen on the perioral, perianal and distal extremities. Other features include lethargy, alopecia, diarrhea, photophobia, angular cheilitis, irritability, growth retardation and secondary infections. A lifelong treatment with oral zinc sulfate (1–3 mg/kg/day) resolves the symptoms.

Recommended reading

1. Simpson RC, et al. Best Pract Res Clin Obstet Gynaecol (2014). PMID: 2513445.
2. Fischer G, et al. Pediat Dermatol (2000). PMID: 10720979.
3. Powell J. J Obstet Gynaecol (2006). PMID: 17071420.
4. Orszulak D, et al. Int J Environ Res Public Health (2021). PMID: 34281089.
5. Fivozinsky KB, et al. J Reprod Med (1998). PMID: 9777614.

17

MENOPAUSE AND VULVOVAGINAL DISEASE

Nina Madnani

Contents

Menopause, a period in a woman's life when estrogen levels are depleted, is often fraught with various problems related to her genitourinary system. Genitourinary syndrome of menopause (GSM), previously known as atrophic vaginitis, is a condition that severely compromises the woman's quality of life and needs to be recognized early and managed adequately. Lichen sclerosus and lichen planus, both chronic inflammatory diseases are seen during menopause (see Chapter 6, section Vulvar lichen planus and section Lichen sclerosus), when untreated, predispose to the development of differentiated vulvar intraepithelial neoplasia (dVIN) (see Chapter 7, section Vulvar intraepithelial neoplasia).

Genitourinary syndrome of menopause

Introduction

Estrogen levels are important to maintain the vagina in a moist and supple state and at an optimal pH between 3.5 and 4.5. Post-menopause, these levels get reduced and depleted, and the mucosa becomes pale, thin, and dry. The pubic hair reduces over the mid-section, and turns white. The labia minora shrink, mimicking a picture of lichen sclerosus. With the pH moving towards the alkaline range, candidial infections are almost non-existent (except in diabetics, immunosuppressed, and post-antibiotic use). These post-menopausal changes were previously labeled as atrophic vaginitis and vulvovaginal atrophy. The new nomenclature is genitourinary syndrome of menopause (GSM).

Epidemiology

Women are unaware that certain symptoms they face post-menopause, such as itching dyspareunia etc, may be due to menopause and could be improved with therapy. Hence, it is not disclosed in a normal consult. A study from Delhi, India, reported a prevalence of 67% among 200 women screened for the symptoms of GSM. This matched an international report which published an incidence of 70%.

Pathophysiology

The urogenital system has estrogen receptors which respond to circulating estrogens, helping to maintain normal functioning. As estrogen levels and the number of its receptors deplete, structural and functional changes occur. The pH becomes alkaline. The mucosa gets dry and easily injured, and the tissues become more prone to trichomoniasis and bacterial vaginosis (BV). Various problems related to the vagina and the lower urogenital system ensue.

Presenting complaints

The women may complain of dryness, itching, irritation, pain, soreness, post-coital bleeding, or a smelly discharge. Urinary incontinence, frequency or dysuria, and dyspareunia severely impairs the woman's quality of life (QoL). Vulvar itch and rashes are consequences of urinary incontinence. Menopausal women may also complain of low sexual desire, recurrent urinary tract infections, and the feeling that something is coming down through their vagina.

Clinical examination

Dryness of the mucosa, vaginal and peri-urethral pallor, flattening of the vaginal rugae, and shrinkage of the labia minora are the common findings (Figure 17.1). A thin yellowish watery discharge is seen on speculum examination. Reduction in the

DOI: 10.1201/9781003284116-17

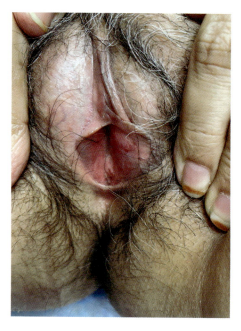

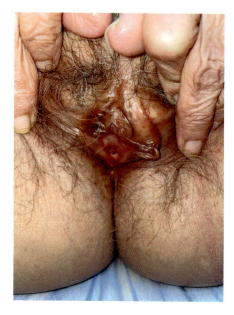

FIGURE 17.1 During menopause, the vulva appears pale and the labia minora fused. (Photograph by Dr Nina Madnani.)

FIGURE 17.2 Vulva shows canites, pallor with dilated veins, and peri-urethral fullness. (Photograph by Dr Nina Madnani.)

subcutaneous fat results in loss of volume and sagging of the labia majora. Due to inadequate lubrication, erosions and fissures occur at the introitus, especially post-intercourse. The vulva may show erythema or excoriations secondary to contact dermatitis (incontinence-associated dermatitis) due to urinary or fecal incontinence, or a vaginal discharge. Urethral polyps, mucosa eversion, cystocele, rectocele, and cervicoceles may be concomitant findings. The vestibule may be read due to mucosal atrophy. There is evidence of labia minora fusion and canites (Figure 17.2).

Laboratory examination
Smears from the vagina will show reduced numbers of superficial cells, with an increased number of parabasal cells. The pH will be more than 4.5. Occasionally, evidence of trichomoniasis or BV may be seen.

- A pap smear will support the diagnosis.
- Endometrial ultrasound shows a thinned endometrium.
- Estrogen levels if tested are low.

Differential diagnosis
The vaginal discharge needs to be distinguished from that of other vulvovaginal infections.

The labia minora fusion may mimic lichen planus or lichen sclerosus.

Course and prognosis
Women tend to suffer in silence and their QoL gets seriously impaired due to the development of a cystocele or rectocele. Sexual satisfaction is significantly reduced. A rise in the vaginal pH predisposes the woman to trichomoniasis and BV.

Treatment
Many modalities are available to assist women with GSM. These include moisturizers, lubricants, non-hormonal and hormonal medication, and lasers and radiofrequency devices. Hormone replacement therapy (HRT) and topical estrogens are useful in alleviating this distressing condition. Ospimephine, a selective estrogen receptor modulator is approved for the treatment of dyspareunia in women with GSM. Fractional lasers and radiofrequency tightening devices have been reported to improve many of the symptoms, but more studies with larger cohorts are required before which this procedure can be recommended as a standard of care. Pelvic floor rehabilitation is extremely useful as a supportive therapy. Recommendations of lubricants which may be water-based, oil-based, or silicone-based are necessary, especially in those with lichen sclerosus and lichen planus.

Pearls

A menopausal woman should be questioned in detail about the various symptoms of GSM, as many are unaware that these are reversible.

Recommended reading

1. Gupta N, et al. J Midlife Health (2018). PMID: 30294184.
2. Calleja-Agius J, et al. Climacteric (2015). PMID: 26366796.
3. Patni R. J Midlife Health (2019). PMID: 31579156.
4. Juhász MLW, et al. Dermatol Surg (2021). PMID: 33165070.

Incontinence-associated dermatitis

Introduction

Both bladder and bowel incontinence are common in menopause due to the laxity of the muscle tone as an outcome of low estrogen level. The incontinence may be episodic or continuous, large volumes keeping the diapers, or bed linen completely soaked.

Epidemiology

The exact incidence is difficult to calculate as many women would be embarrassed to talk about their incontinence. Both urine and fecal incontinence are prevalent worldwide.

When the skin is exposed to intermittent/continuous urine and stool incontinence, the skin barrier is breached, leading to inflammation, erosion, and ulceration.

Presenting complaints

The patient may complain about burning pain or ulcers in the genital and buttock area.

Clinical examination

Early dermatitis may be very mild where there is barely any erythema. As dermatitis progresses, the convex areas of the genitals and buttock show erythema and edema, with areas of tenderness that may further get eroded and ulcerated (Figure 17.3). Bed sores may be an additional outcome in patients who are bedridden or immobile.

Lab work up

A swab for bacteriology and antibacterial sensitivity is required for ulcers and erosions.

A biopsy is rarely performed.

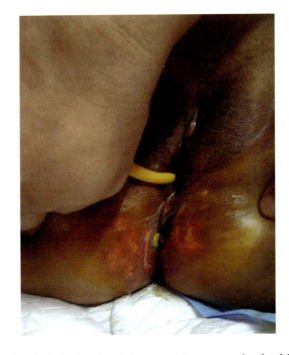

FIGURE 17.3 Multiple erosions in a bedridden patient with incontinence. (Photograph by Dr Nina Madnani.)

Management

All patients with incontinence dermatitis must be advised of local skin care. The area must be cleansed after each episode with water or a soap-free cleanser, dried thoroughly and a zinc oxide barrier cream applied. Moribund patients need active assistance from a caregiver. Cold compresses prior to application of the barrier cream can allay the burning. In more advanced cases, before an erosion or ulceration sets in, a topical antifungal–steroid combination may be applied twice a day under the barrier cream for a period of 7–10 days. When the area has become eroded, special absorbent dressings are helpful, and the patient needs to be encouraged to change the sleeping position every 2 hours to avoid the formation of bed sores.

Pearl

Diaper dermatitis in a menopausal woman is a clue to bladder or bowel incontinence.

Recommended reading

1. Sharma P, et al. Indian J Crit Care Med (2021). PMID: 33707893.
2. Beeckman D. J Tissue Viability (2017). PMID: 26949126.

18

VULVAR INJURIES INCLUDING SEXUAL ABUSE

Smitha Prabhu S

Contents

Introduction

Vulvar injury is not infrequent and can be sexual or non-sexual in nature. Often, it is associated with anogenital injury due to the close proximity of these regions. Vaginal injury is more common than vulvar injury. Genital trauma in girls accounts for 0.2–8% of all pediatric trauma. Mechanisms of vulvar injuries are given in Table 18.1.

Classification of genital injuries based on location:

- *External injuries* – Labia majora and minora, periurethral area, posterior fourchette and perineum
- *Internal injuries* – Fossa navicularis, hymen, vagina and cervix
- *Anal injuries* – Anus and rectum

TABLE 18.1: Mechanisms of Vulvar Injuries

Type of Injury	Causes
Blunt trauma	Straddle injuries, athletic injuries
Penetrating trauma	High-pressure jet ski accidents, pelvic fracture and bone penetration, sexual trauma, insertion of foreign objects
Cuts, wounds, ulcers	Intentional harm
Burns	Cigarette burns, marking nut injury, scalds

Non-sexual vulvar injuries

Common non-sexual causes for vulvovaginal injuries are given in Table 18.2.

Straddle injury: In these types of injuries, the vulva or perineum is forcibly hit on an object, and the injury is caused by force generated by the female's body leading to compression of soft tissue against the bony perineal outlet. These can be blunt or penetrating.

Patients present with pain, bruising, edema and/or bleeding of varying severity. Lacerations of labia majora are usually seen anterior or lateral to the hymen. There may be associated dysuria if the injury involves urethral meatus.

TABLE 18.2: Common Non-Sexual Causes for Vulvovaginal Injuries

- Straddle injuries
- Playground injuries in children – landing on a metal bar or rod, bicycle rod injuries
- Falls – on bedpost, on bathtub fixtures, during athletics
- Pedestrian injury in road traffic accidents
- Physical abuse not mounting to sexual abuse
- Insertion of a foreign body into the vagina
- Burns – accidental or induced
- Marking nut injury
- Female genital mutilation
- Intrapartum injuries

DOI: 10.1201/9781003284116-18

In the majority of patients, the injuries involve mons, labia majora, clitoris and hood, labia minora and are anterolateral to hymen. Injury to hymen, posterior fourchette, vaginal bleeding, perineal lacerations, hematuria and bleeding at urethral meatus suggests penetrating or intentional trauma. Hematomas, ecchymoses and lacerations are seen corresponding to the trauma sustained. Hymenal injury bleeding is minimal and subsides soon, whereas vaginal laceration will bleed profusely and for a longer period of time.

Road traffic and other accidents: The injuries vary depending upon force and mechanism of injury and vary from contusions, hematoma, lacerations, abrasions to penetrating injury, even involving internal organs.

Physical abuse: The causes of the injury vary from burns, irritant dermatitis, bite, contusion, bruise or even self-mutilation (Figure 18.1).

Marking nut injury: *Semicarpus anacardium,* the marking nut, contains irritant fluid that can cause irritant contact dermatitis. It is deliberately used in certain patriarchal communities to punish women who are deemed as sexually promiscuous by smearing the fluid to the genital area.

Intrapartum genital trauma: This includes lacerations, episiotomy wound infection and dehiscence, hematoma, uterine rupture and uterine inversion. Severe trauma is very rare, though minor ones are relatively common.

Female genital mutilation: This is a cultural practice prevalent in certain regions of Africa, Middle East and Asia. In India, this practice exists in small pockets of certain communities in Kerala and Gujarat and is termed 'khatna' or 'khafz'. The process involves partial or complete removal of external female genitalia to satisfy cultural beliefs and norms. It is classified depending on the structures removed (Figure 18.2; Table 18.3).

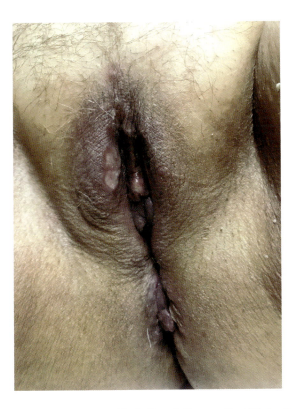

FIGURE 18.1 Well-defined linear factitial ulcer of left labia majora. (Photograph by Dr Nina Madnani.)

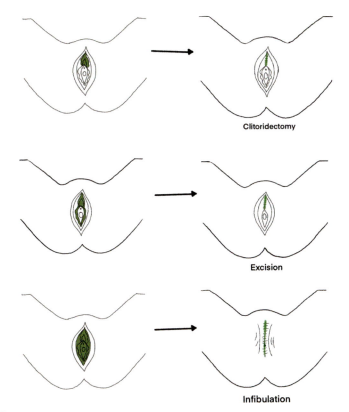

Clitoridectomy

Excision

Infibulation

FIGURE 18.2 Various stages of female genital mutilation (FGM). (Photograph by Aashka Mehta.)

TABLE 18.3: Types of Female Genital Mutilation

Type 1	partial or total removal of glans of the clitoris with or without prepuce and clitoral hood
Type 2	partial or total removal of glans of the clitoris with labia minora with or without labia majora
Type 3	infibulation, wherein the vaginal opening is narrowed by creating a covering seal formed of labia minora or majora, with or without removing the clitoris
Type 4	includes all other processes of non-medical mutilation of female genitalia and may include pricking, piercing, incision, cauterization

Sexual injuries

Sexual injuries can be genital as well as non-genital, with a prevalence of up to 5–87% and 30–76%, respectively. Consensual (in up to 32% women) as well as forced sex can lead to trauma. Consensual injuries are generally less severe. Non-consensual injuries vary considerably depending upon the age of the victim, previous sexual experience, parity, time gap between incident and examination and the method of examination used.

Types of genital injuries: tears, ecchymosis, abrasions, erythema (redness) and swellings [acronym **TEARS**].

Consensual sex: Widespread hypervascularity of the genital area, especially within 6 hours of intercourse is the most consistent finding. Common injuries seen are hymenal and fourchette tears, increased vascularity and telangiectasia, petechiae, erythema, abrasions, and edema.

Internal genital injury may occur in up to 10% of women, but are minor and focal, and usually higher up than seen with rape.

Rape: The prevalence of injuries range from 5 to 87% depending upon the method of visualization used (naked eye examination versus colposcopic).

External injury: Entry injury is most common, wherein the vagina is penetrated by the penis or other parts/objects. Common sites involved are posterior fourchette (70%), labia minora (53%), hymen and fossa navicularis. Periurethral area, perineum and anorectal injuries too can occur in severe cases.

Hymenal rupture and ecchymosis are seen in virgins.

Anal injuries occur in forced anal penetration and are manifested as anal pain, bleeding per rectum and fissuring.

Internal injury: About one-fourth of rape victims sustain injury to the vagina or cervix, in the form of ecchymosis or rarely lacerations, especially in older women.

If there is lower abdominal or pelvic pain and discomfort, deep pelvic contusions should be ruled out by imaging techniques.

Important differentiating factors between consensual, non-consensual sexual and non-sexual injuries are given in Table 18.4.

Examination in a case of genital injury

A thorough examination of vulva, perineum and vagina is mandatory, and patient may even be sedated if the pain is severe.

Position of the patient: Classical lithotomy position, 'frog leg' or 'butterfly' position, or knee-chest position.

Examine labia, clitoris, urethra, vestibule, hymen and fourchette, anorectal area in detail.

Look for tears, lacerations, erythema, edema, ecchymosis, tenderness and hematoma formation. Examination of the vaginal outlet and hymen should be attempted by gentle downward and outward traction of the lower aspect of labia minora. Any hymenal tear between 3 0' clock and 9 0' clock position in children is highly indicative of penetrating vaginal injury, most likely sexual abuse. A thorough inspection, evaluation and photography of the following anatomical areas are recommended in suspected sexual abuse injury: labia majora and minora, periurethral area, posterior

TABLE 18.4: Differentiating Points between Sexual and Non-Sexual Injuries

Non-Sexual Injuries	Consensual Sexual Injuries	Non-Consensual Sexual Injuries
The area involved depends on the type of injury/accident – penetrating, contusions, blunt trauma, intentional harm	Posterior fourchette, labia minora and vagina are commonly involved	Posterior fourchette, hymen, fossa navicularis and labia minora are commonly involved
Lacerations anterior or lateral to hymen.	Milder tear of posterior fourchette and posterior part of hymen	Posterior fourchette and posterior hymen (between 3 O' clock and 9 O' clock in lithotomy position) invariably involved
Associated pelvic bone fracture, contusions and bruises depending upon the pattern of trauma	Internal genital injury minor or focal, higher up in the vagina	Internal injury is more severe and lower down in the vagina
Hypervascularity not seen	Widespread hypervascularity of the genital area, which lasts for up to 6 hours	Hypervascularity without injury not seen
Teeth mark and suck marks are absent	Love bites which are less severe in nature	Severe bite marks, contusions on the external genitalia, breasts,, thighs, lower abdomen
Vaginal bleeding is more common	Minimal bleeding	Transient bleeding from posterior fourchette, hymen.
No association with sexually transmitted infections, though other secondary infections may occur	Sexually transmitted infections may occur	Frequently associated with sexually transmitted infections at a later date
Post-traumatic stress disorder may be seen based on the severity of trauma	No post-traumatic stress or psychological complications	Post-traumatic stress disorder and psychological complications are very common
May need surgical correction and long-term treatment	No treatment is required other than an ice pack and analgesics. Rarely, treatment of sexually transmitted diseases (STDs)	May need surgical correction, long-term treatment, treatment of STDs

fourchette and fossa navicularis, hymen, vagina, cervix, perineum and anorectal region.

If there is profuse bleeding, gentle irrigation with normal saline can be done.

A speculum examination for visualizing posterior fornix and lateral vaginal walls must be done as these are usually lacerated by forcible or forceful vaginal intercourse. If the injury is missed, which later heals naturally, it can lead to a fistula between the vagina and bladder or bowel. Perineal tears vary in severity from first to fourth degree (only skin involved in first, perineal body involved in addition in second, muscles and capsule of rectal sphincter involved in third, rectal mucosa affected in fourth).

If severe genital trauma has occurred, urethral and urinary bladder injury should be ruled out by catheterization, which will reveal hematuria in case of injury.

Per rectal examination should be done to assess bleeding, tenderness, tone and integrity. Pelvic and perineal bones should be palpated for any tenderness which may suggest fracture.

Further urological studies like cystogram and ultrasonogram may be needed to elucidate the extent of injury. If required trans-labial ultrasound can differentiate between inflammatory edema and hematoma. Ultrasound of the pelvic area can delineate internal injuries missed by clinical examination.

Management

Investigations in a case of vulvar injury should include test for sexually transmissible organisms including HIV, Syphilis, Hepatitis B, Hepatitis C. Vaginal/cervical smears for gonococci, chlamydia (Nucleic Acid Amplification Test – NAAT) from the site of penetration.

NAAT from urine or vaginal specimen for Trichomonas vaginalis should be done. Wet mount test, measurement of vaginal pH and KOH test for evidence of bacterial vaginosis and candidiasis should be done. Urine routine examination and urine culture and sensitivity must be done.

Treatment: For minimal contusion, bruising or swelling:

- Warm water soaks
- Ice packs to the injured tissue
- Oral analgesics and anti-inflammatory agents
- Rest to the affected area
- Topical antibiotics and emollients

Straddle injuries usually heal without any long-term sequelae.

Empirical treatment for STIs like chlamydia, gonorrhea, trichomonas, HIV should be given when a sexual injury is suspected.

Penetrating injuries are more extensive and often require surgical repair as peritoneal, urethral and rectal injury too can occur in addition.

For severe injuries, surgical correction may be required. Female genital mutilation can be reversed to some extent, though the genitalia never assume their natural shape and function.

Pearls

Most injuries that cause vaginal bleeding are accidental, and most sexual assaults do not result in major visible genital injuries.

Blunt injuries lead to labial bruising or lacerations anterolateral to the hymen, whereas sexual abuse can injure the hymen, posterior fourchette or perineal tears.

Recommended reading

1. Laufer MR, Makai G. (2021). Evaluation and management of female lower genital tract trauma. Accessed on Nov 2022: https://www.uptodate.com/contents/evaluation-and-management-of-female-lower-genital-tract-trauma.
2. Sommers MS. Trauma Violence Abuse. 2007. PMID: 17596344.
3. Fan SM, et al. Pediatr Surg Int. 2020. PMID: 32851470.
4. Female Genital Mutilation. WHO. Available at: Female genital mutilation (who.int) Accessed on 28.05.2021.
5. Garg M, Jain R. Female genital mutilation: (A Socio-Legal Perspective In Indian Context). Int J Law Legal Jur Stud; 4(3). ISSN: 2348-8212.
6. Orellana-Campos C. Rev Bras Ginecol Obstet. 2020. PMID: 32227326.
7. Saxena AK, et al. Indian J Pediatr. 2014. PMID: 23824694.

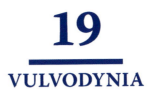

19

VULVODYNIA

Nina Madnani

Contents

Introduction

Vulvodynia has been such an enigma that over the years several definitions have been put forward. In 2003, at the International Society for the Study of Vulvovaginal Disease (ISSVD) World Congress, vulvodynia was defined as "vulvar discomfort, most often described as burning pain, occurring in the absence of relevant visible findings or a specific, clinically identifiable neurological disorder". Later in 2015, various societies met and defined vulvodynia as "vulvar pain lasting at least 3 months, without a clear identifiable cause, which may have potential associated factors". Hence, essentially, vulvodynia is a diagnosis of exclusion.

Etiology

This condition is complex and is prevalent worldwide with an incidence of 8–10%, but in some studies, the incidence was reported above 20%. Although more common in menopausal women, it has been reported in younger women and adolescents too. Premenopausal women and those on estrogen replacement therapy seem to be affected.

Marital status, age, and ethnicity seem to modulate the incidence. Data from Asia seems to be sparse with a study of vulvodynia in Nepal reporting an incidence of 0.95%. A study from Taiwan included vulvodynia as one of the causes of dyspareunia. It has been compared to diabetic neuropathy in its similarity, with a hypothesis that all women with diabetes should be questioned about vulvar pain and vice versa.

Pathophysiology

The exact pathophysiology is still evolving, but inflammation, pelvic floor dysfunction, microbiomes, psychological, central and peripheral neurological disorders have been hypothesized. Also, increased mast cell activity, genetic polymorphism, and as a component of complex pain syndromes are the other theories considered in the pathogenesis.

Presenting complaints

The commonest complaints are dyspareunia, pain either at rest (unprovoked) or during an activity (provoked), over the entire vulva (generalized) or a small area (localized), all the time (continuous) or for a short time (episodic). Burning, stinging, stabbing or shooting pain, and rawness are the other adjectives patients use to describe their discomfort. They complain of low self-worth and frustration due to their inability to have a satisfactory sexual life. Non-sexually active women often complain of pain on tampon insertion, cycling, sitting, or when wearing tight trousers.

DOI: 10.1201/9781003284116-19

A good history is essential while evaluating a patient with suspected vulvodynia. Past surgeries, per vaginal (PV) deliveries with/without episiotomy, depression or psychiatric complaints, other myalgias, and bladder or bowel problems are important questions.

Clinical examination

The vestibule may be erythematous and minute fissures may be seen at the fourchette. The rectum, anal orifice, and bladder are palpated to rule out pathology. It is important to carefully examine the vulva for evidence of a disease which could be contributing to the pain, especially evidence of injury. Look out for episiotomy scars. A speculum or PV examination is often impossible, although topical lidocaine gel applied 10 min prior to the examination may facilitate this procedure. A PV examination is good for determining the tone of the pelvic musculature. Also, the patient is asked to cough and examined for evidence of urinary incontinence or bladder/vaginal prolapse.

The "cotton swab" test is a simple test to evaluate a patient of vulvodynia. A cotton swab is gently pressed against various areas of the vulva in a clockwork fashion in order to elicit the area of pain. This is done to elicit "provoked" vulvodynia (Figure 19.1).

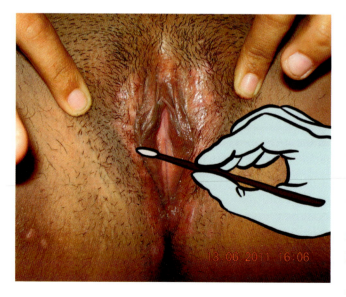

FIGURE 19.1 A "cotton swab" test to elicit "provoked" vulvodynia. (Photograph by Aashka Mehta.)

Laboratory examination

A few investigations like a wet mount, pH stick evaluation, and cultures are useful for excluding other diseases like candidiasis, trichomoniasis, herpes, and cytolytic vaginosis, which may cause pain.

Differential diagnosis

Before a patient can be labeled as vulvodynia, other conditions like post-herpetic/pudendal neuralgia, irritant contact dermatitis, hidradenitis suppurativa, Crohn's disease, lichen planus, vulvar malignancies, and post-trauma need to be ruled out. Candidiasis should be ruled out in patients with provoked vulvodynia.

Post-herpetic pain, pudendal neuralgia, and post-trauma/surgical are a form of neuropathic pain, and a careful history can differentiate each of them, although all would have symptoms of burning, lancing pain, and hypersensitivity to light touch.

Management

Management of vulvodynia needs to be holistic and should include a gynecologist, dermatologist, physical therapist, psychiatrist, counsellor, microbiologist, and plastic surgeon. Therapy is not protocol based and should be individualized for each patient.

Three aspects need to be addressed:

- Drugs to relieve the pain
- Psychotherapy
- Physical therapy

The patient should be counselled about the longevity of the treatment and compliance adherence for a successful outcome.

Drugs to relieve pain include medication which relieve skin pain, pelvic muscle pain, and neuropathic and emotional pain.

Topicals like Xylocaine, lidocaine, and prilocaine mixture are useful when applied 10 min prior to intercourse. Compounded amitriptyline 2% with baclofen 2% cream applied twice a day is useful.

Systemic medications include:

- **TCAs (tricyclic anti-depressants)**
  - Amitriptyline, nortriptyline, and desipramine. Start at 10–25 mg and titrate up by 10–25 mg every 7 days to the maximum dose.
- **Anticonvulsants**
  - *Gabapentin*: 100–3600 mg/d in 3 divided doses. Start at 100 mg and titrate up by 100 mg/d every 5–7 days if well-tolerated.
  - *Pregabalin*: Start at 150 mg and titrate up to 300 mg after 1 week if well-tolerated.
- **Serotonin or norepinephrine reuptake inhibitors**
  - *Duloxetine*: Start at 20 mg and titrate up by 20 mg/d every 7 days to the maximum dose. 150–300 mg/d in 2–3 divided doses.

Physical therapy plays an essential role in pain relief and includes pelvic relaxation exercises, biofeedback, ultrasound therapy, use of dilators, trigger-point release etc.

Cognitive behavior therapy to turn off the pain loop either with group or single sessions.

Nerve blocks and botulinum toxin injections are resorted to when the previous treatments are unsuccessful. Localized vestibulectomy is a last resort to remove the trigger point.

Pearls

If you have found a cause for the pain, then it is not vulvodynia.

Systemic medications are to be started in low doses and gradually stepped up.

Recommended reading

1. Ridley CM. International Society for the Study of Vulvovaginal Disease (ISSVD). Report of committee on vulvodynia. J Reprod Med (1993);38:14.
2. Kalra B, et al. Indian J Endocrinol Metab (2013). PMID: 24083157.
3. Moyal-Barracco M, et al. J Reprod Med (2004). PMID: 15568398.
4. Torres-Cueco R, et al. Int J Environ Res Public Health (2021). PMID: 34205495.

20

FREQUENTLY ASKED QUESTIONS BY PATIENTS ON COMMON VULVAR CONDITIONS

Nina Madnani and Nisha Chaturvedi

Contents

Lichen sclerosus

1. What is lichen sclerosus (LS) (Figures 20.1 and 20.2)?
   a. LS is an autoimmune condition where the body reacts to its own cells.
2. Why do I have LS?
   a. We don't know the exact cause, but genetics, trauma and chronic irritation with urine have been blamed.

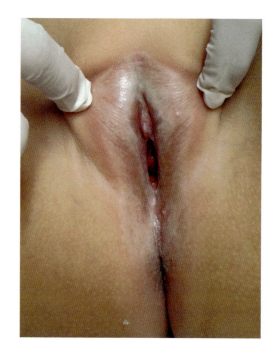

FIGURE 20.2 Lichen Sclerosus in an child. (Photograph by Dr Nina Madnani.)

3. Can my child get LS?
   a. This condition is not contagious. But it can occur in prepubertal children.
4. Why do I need blood tests for this condition?
   a. LS has been associated with diseases like thyroid, diabetes, pernicious anemia, and hence we need to rule them out.
5. Is there a treatment for LS?
   a. Yes, treatment is available and is very effective in managing this condition.

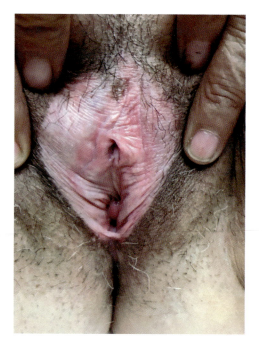

FIGURE 20.1 Lichen Sclerosus in an adult. (Photograph by Dr Nina Madnani.)

DOI: 10.1201/9781003284116-20

6. How long do I need treatment?
   a. As this is a chronic condition similar to other chronic diseases like diabetes, hypertension and hypothyroidism, it requires long-term treatment and lifelong follow-ups. The treatment frequency may be modified as the disease improves.
7. What happens if I don't treat the condition?
   a. If untreated, studies have shown that a small percentage of women can develop vulvar cancers. Also, since this condition causes scarring, it may lead to painful intercourse and problems in urination.
8. What is the treatment I need?
   a. You will be prescribed applications, usually containing steroids. Tablets may be co-prescribed to reduce the itching.
9. Are there any side effects of this treatment?
   a. If done under proper medical supervision, there are no side effects.
10. Can my treatment prevent me from developing vulvar cancers?
   a. Studies have shown that when patients have been consistent with their treatment and follow-ups, the incidence of vulvar cancers is reduced to zero.

Lichen planus

1. What is lichen planus (LP) (Figures 20.3 and 20.4)?
   a. LP is an autoimmune condition wherein one's own cells attack the cells of the skin and mucous membrane.
2. Does it only affect the genitals?
   a. No, it can also affect the mouth, nails, scalp and skin.
3. Is this condition treatable?
   a. LP can be controlled effectively with the help of creams and oral medications prescribed by your physician after evaluating the extent of involvement.
4. What type of treatment is prescribed?
   a. It could be topical creams which may or may not containing steroids. In severe cases, oral medications which suppress the autoimmune process may be prescribed.

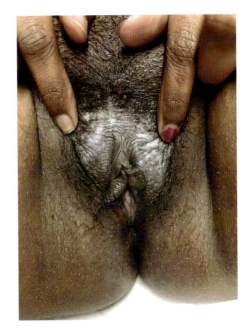

FIGURE 20.3 Thick, greyish patches of lichen planus. (Photograph by Dr Nina Madnani.)

5. What happens if I don't treat this condition?
   a. Since LP is a chronic inflammatory and scarring process if left untreated, it can lead to the total obliteration of the vulva leaving behind just a tiny residual vaginal opening. In a small percentage of patients, it may develop into vulvar cancer.

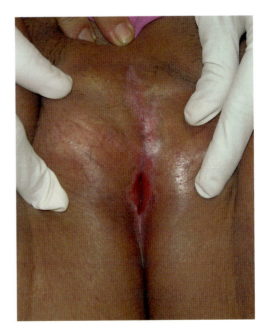

FIGURE 20.4 Complete scarring secondary to lichen planus. (Photograph by Dr Nina Madnani.)

Eczema (contact dermatitis/lichen simplex chronicus)

1. What is eczema (Figures 20.5 and 20.6)?
   a. Eczema is a condition that can be described as an itch that rashes.
2. What causes eczema?
   a. Genetics plays a major role in its causality. There is a defect in the barrier function of the skin. Eczema can be triggered by factors like harsh detergents, friction, warmth, humidity, tight clothing and stress.
3. Can I transfer my eczema to anyone in close contact?
   a. Eczema is not infectious or contagious and cannot be transferred to anyone else by close contact.
4. Can it spread to other parts of the body?
   a. Eczema can occur in various parts of the body. It may occur independently of the vulva.
5. Can eczema be treated?
   a. Yes, eczema can be treated. Your treatment will include barrier repair and anti-inflammatory creams which may contain

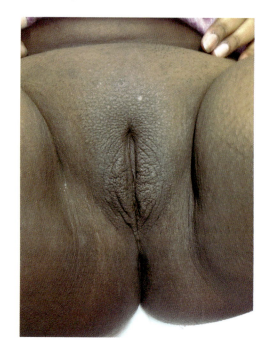

FIGURE 20.6 Contact dermatitis to sanitary napkin. (Photograph by Dr Nina Madnani.)

steroids or non-steroidal agents. In severe cases, oral medications may be added.
6. How do I cleanse the area which has eczema?
   a. Plain water or a mild soap-free cleanser can be used twice a day to keep the area clean. Make sure to dab dry the area completely. Avoid using douches, wet wipes and strong detergents as cleansers.

Herpes genitalis

1. What causes herpes genitalis (HG) (Figures 20.7 and 20.8)?
   a. HG is a sexually transmitted viral infection caused by the herpes simplex virus.
2. How did I get it?
   a. This condition is usually sexually transmitted from your partner who may not have evidence of infection at that particular time. Very rarely, if you have an infection around the mouth, you could transfer the virus via your fingers.
3. Can it be transferred to another person?
   a. Yes, it is a contagious condition and is transmitted by skin-to-skin contact but not by common articles like towels, napkins or toilet seats.

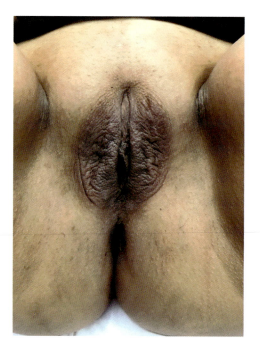

FIGURE 20.5 Thick, pigmented, wrinkled skin of lichen simplex chronicus. (Photograph by Dr Nina Madnani.)

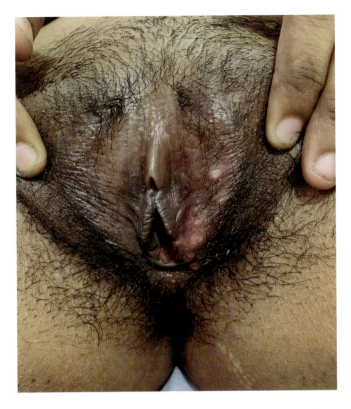

FIGURE 20.7 Ulcers of Herpes simplex. (Photograph by Dr Nisha Chaturvedi.)

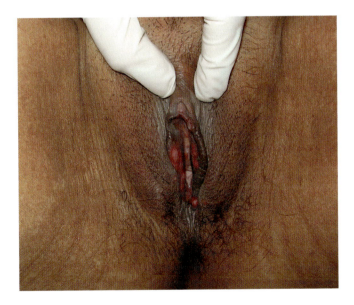

FIGURE 20.8 Extensive ulcers of Herpes simplex. (Photograph by Dr Nina Madnani.)

4. What treatment will I be given?
   a. Antivirals like acyclovir, famciclovir or valacyclovir are prescribed for 5–10 days. Pain can be managed by taking anti-inflammatory medications like paracetamol or ibuprofen. Topical antiviral or antibacterial creams may also be added to the prescription.

5. Can I be cured of HG?
   a. HG cannot be cured as the virus remains in the body and resurfaces from time to time.

6. Can I have sexual intercourse once I am diagnosed with this infection?
   a. It is recommended not to have sexual intimacy when you have the active infection. Your significant other should be encouraged to use condoms.

7. How do I know I have HG again?
   a. A repeated attack may give a warning sensation of pricking or burning followed by blisters which then heal in 5–7 days.

Genital warts (human papillomavirus infections)

1. What are genital warts (Figures 20.9 and 20.10)?
   a. Genital warts are an infection caused by human papillomavirus (HPV). There are innumerable HPV types, of which few strains can cause vulvar, cervical, vaginal and anal cancer.

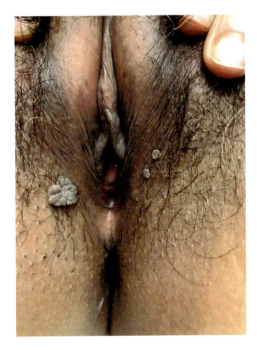

FIGURE 20.9 Fleshy growths of vulvar warts. (Photograph by Dr Nina Madnani.)

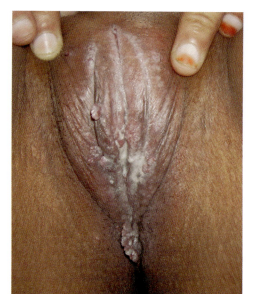

FIGURE 20.10   Vulvar warts with vaginal discharge. (Photograph by Dr Nisha Chaturvedi.)

2. How did I get genital warts?
   a. Genital warts are generally sexually transmitted. Occasionally, they can be transmitted to the genital area from the infected hands of a caregiver/mother/self. Beauty procedures like waxing the vulvar area can often disseminate the warts.
3. Can these warts be treated?
   a. Genital warts can be treated by physical destruction or by stimulating the bodies' immune response to fight the infection.
4. Can I transfer this to my family members/partner?
   a. Yes, HPV infections are contagious and can pass on to susceptible individuals by skin-to-skin contact or through shared linen.

5. Are these warts dangerous?
   a. Certain HPV types, if contracted, may lead to cancers (vulvar, cervical, vaginal, anal).
6. Is sexual intimacy allowed while I have this infection?
   a. Sexual intimacy is not recommended with active infection as it can disseminate the virus deeper into the vagina.
7. Can I or my family members take preventive steps against genital warts?
   a. HPV vaccines (Cervarix, Gardasil/Gardasil 9) protect against certain HPV types and are recommended by the WHO for girls and boys from ages 9 to 26 years. Women above this age can be administered the vaccine at the discretion of the treating physician.
8. Can I develop warts again once I am treated?
   a. Yes, since there are many strains of HPV virus, you can be reinfected from a different strain.
9. Can I plan pregnancy when I have the infection?
   a. It is recommended to get the warts completely treated before you get pregnant, as during the pregnancy, the warts get larger and more extensive due to the increased blood supply to the genitals. Also, during childbirth, the infection can pass on to the newborn during its passage through the birth canal.

FLOWCHARTS

Nina Madnani, Kaleem Khan, and Nisha Chaturvedi

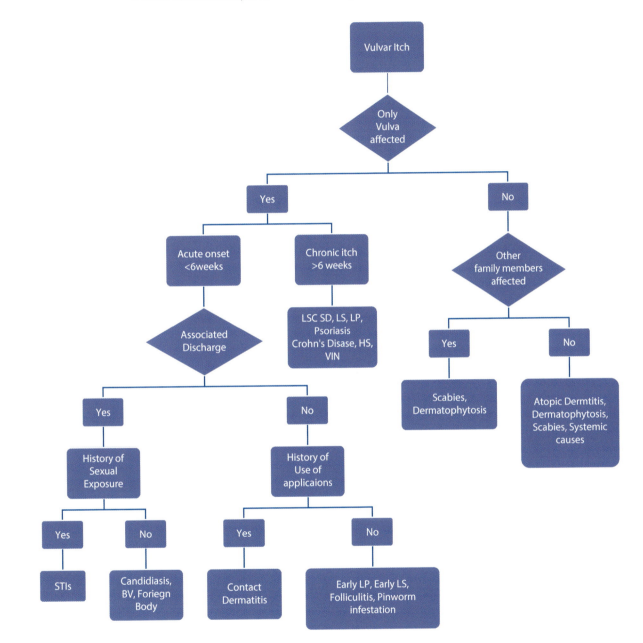

FLOWCHART 20.1 History taking in vulvar itch.

Note: History taking provides key insights into possible causes of vulvar itch. For further information on the above-mentioned diseases, please refer to their individual chapters.

Legends: LP: Lichen Planus, **LS**: Lichen Sclerosus, **HS**: Hidradenitis Suppurativa, **LSC**: Lichen Simplex Chronicus, **SD**: Seborrheic Dermatitis, **VIN**: Vulvar Intraepithelial Neoplasia, **BV**: Bacterial Vaginosis, **STI**: Sexually Transmitted Infections – including Herpes Genitalis, Verruca Vulgaris, Gonorrhea, Chlamydia.

DOI: 10.1201/9781003284116-21

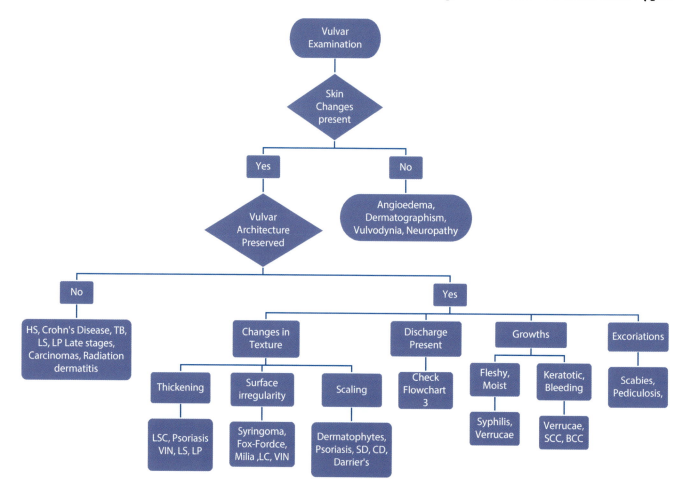

FLOWCHART 20.2   Clinical examination in vulvar itch.

Note: Often, an extragenital site may give a clue to the cause of the vulvar itch. A perianal examination is equally important in patients with vulvar itch. For further information on the above-mentioned diseases, please refer to their individual chapters.

Legends: LP: Lichen Planus, **LS**: Lichen Sclerosus, **HS**: Hidradenitis Suppurativa, **LSC**: Lichen Simplex Chronicus, **TB**: Tuberculosis, **VIN**: Vulvar Intraepithelial Neoplasia, **LC**: Lymphangioma Circumscriptum, **SD**: Seborrheic Dermatitis, **CD**: Contact Dermatitis, **SCC**: Squamous Cell Carcinoma, **BCC**: Basal Cell Carcinoma.

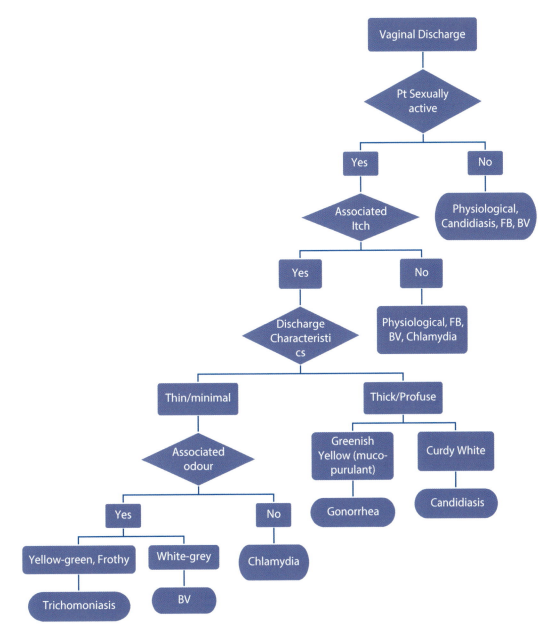

FLOWCHART 20.3 Vaginal discharge.

Note: Discharge characteristics can change with mixed infections. pH evaluation of discharge is necessary. A pH less than 4.5 is suggestive of a candidial infection. A pH of more than 4.5 is suggestive of BV and trichomoniasis. For further information on the above-mentioned diseases, please refer to their individual chapters.

Legends: BV: Bacterial Vaginosis, **FB:** Foreign Body.

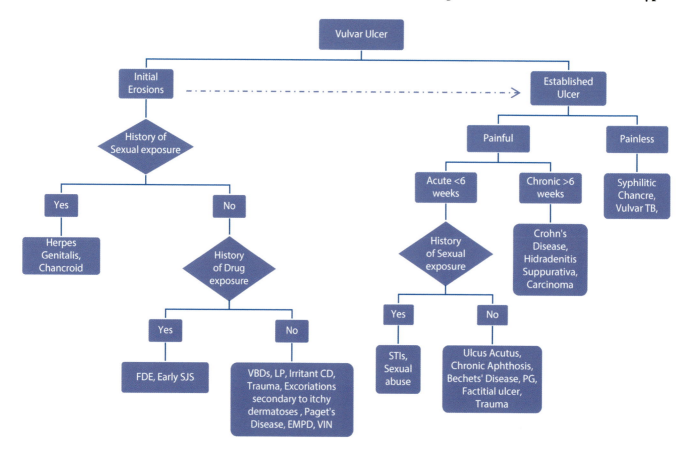

FLOWCHART 20.4   Vulvar ulcer.

Note: Initial erosions can progress to ulcerations due to trauma, secondary infection including HIV and in immunocompromised states. In immunocompromised states, the presentation may be florid. For further information on the above-mentioned diseases, please refer to their individual chapters.

Legends: FDE: Fixed Drug Eruption, **SJS:** Steven–Johnson Syndrome, **CD:** Contact Dermatitis, **HS:** Hidradenitis Suppurativa, **EMPD:** Extra Mammary Paget's Disease, **VIN:** Vulvar Intraepithelial Neoplasia, **PG:** Pyoderma Gangrenosum, **TB:** Tuberculosis, **STIs:** Sexually Transmitted Infections – including Chancroid, Lymphogranuloma Venereum, Granuloma Inguinale, Amoebic Ulcer, **VBDs:** Vesiculo-Bullous Disorders – including Pemphigus Vulgaris, Bullous Pemphigoid, Cicatricial Pemphigoid, Linear IgA Disease.

INDEX

Note: Locators in *italics* represent figures and **bold** indicate tables in the text.